For my

in (

sincerely yours

Ronald v Meerwaarde

Editors **Philipp Lobenhoffer**
Ronald J van Heerwaarden
Alex E Staubli
Roland P Jakob

Co-editors **Mellany Galla**
Jens D Agneskirchner

Osteotomies around the Knee

Indications—Planning—Surgical techniques using plate fixators

Editors **Philipp Lobenhoffer**
Ronald J van Heerwaarden
Alex E Staubli
Roland P Jakob

Co-editors **Mellany Galla**
Jens D Agneskirchner

Osteotomies around the Knee

Indications—Planning—Surgical techniques using plate fixators

530 figures and illustrations

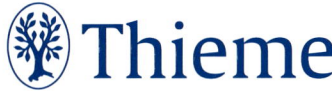

Library of Congress Cataloging-in-Publication Data is available from the publisher.

ISBN 978-3-13-147531-2

Table of contents

Foreword

The fundamental principles of osseous deformity correction were defined by Friedrich Pauwels in 1964 and Paul Maquet in 1976. Since the biomechanical basis of our clinical work was established, many techniques have been developed for osteotomies around the knee. Mark Coventry published his technique for closed-wedge high-tibial osteotomy in 1965, which became the gold standard for many years. The success of an osteotomy around the knee depends on the biomechanics of the lower extremity, the load distribution in the knee, Wolff's law of continuous transformation of bone under stress, and also on the mechanical property of the implants used for osteotomy fixation. The surgeon must be aware of all these factors if he wants to achieve good long-term results.

Even today the process of patient selection and evaluation, of preoperative planning, and of surgical correction of a deformity around the knee is demanding. The definition of the site of correction, of the angle of correction, the choice of the osteotomy procedure, and the fixation device is complex, and various pitfalls may compromise the result. Osteotomies around the knee have had a significant complication rate in the past and many surgeons abandoned these procedures although the favorable long-term results were well known. The main problems were the intraoperative choice of the correction angle and the risk of a postoperative loss of correction. After many years of closed-wedge osteotomy of the proximal tibia, open-wedge valgization osteotomy has become popular.

I appreciate the work of Prof Philipp Lobenhoffer, a very well-known knee surgeon, and the other editors and co-editors, who assembled this excellent book on osteotomies around the knee using specific plate fixators for internal fixation. The broad experimental basis and vast clinical experience on the TomoFix tibia implant including that of the Luzern development group of Dr Alex Staubli are presented in a systematic way. This book starts with an original chapter on the history of osteotomy by Prof Roland P Jakob et al. Furthermore, it includes chapters on the physiology and pathophysiology of the human leg axis, the effect of osteotomy on cartilage pressure, patient examination, preoperative assessment and planning, the principles of internal plate fixators, and their application in tibial and femoral osteotomies. The role of osteotomies for frontal plane correction, for sagittal plane correction, and for treatment of knee instability is discussed. Double osteotomies and rotation corrections are discussed with special expertise by Dr Ronald J van Heerwaarden. Prof Robert A Teitge has described his expert knowledge on osteotomies for failed osteotomies, and chapters on selected complications with open-wedge HTO and knee joint replacement after osteotomy complete the book. A chapter on future developments has been added, and improved implants are also presented. The layout is clear and didactic, allowing the reader to follow the authors' meaning very easily.

I consider this book an important tool for future clinical practice, since I feel strongly that osteotomies will remain an important procedure in the spectrum of joint-preserving knee surgery.

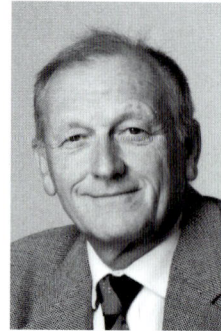

Prof Dr Werner Müller, Riehen
Professor emeritus University of Basel

Editors' foreword

Worldwide one out of four human beings had already developed or will develop osteoarthritis in the future. In 2020, osteoarthritis will rank number four of reasons for permanent invalidity worldwide. Presently over 500,000 patients in the USA and over 120,000 patients in Germany per year receive a total knee replacement due to osteoarthritis. About one third of the patients scheduled for total joint replacement of the knee are potential candidates for an osteotomy.

Osteotomy around the knee is an established procedure, which was widely used before the development of knee prostheses. Many studies have proven significant improvements of joint function and pain level for 10–20 years. Osteotomy allows the patient to safely load his leg, even in sports activities and strenuous labor, without risking failure of an artificial joint implant. The development of total knee replacement, the short-term success of this operation, and the attractive conditions the industry offered to many surgeons led to an inappropriate overuse of total joint replacement worldwide in the last decade. However, endoprosthesis registers established in many countries (Sweden, Norway, Great Britain, Australia, and New Zealand) clearly show that 20% of all patients with total knee prostheses are not satisfied with the result, mainly because of residual pain and stiffness. This holds true especially in the younger age group (under 60 years). It became apparent that the risk of severe complications, especially infection, may count up to 3% if acute postoperative and secondary hematogenous infections are considered.

This experience and the development of new techniques for axis correction around the knee have led to a revival of knee osteotomy procedures. 90% of all osteotomies around the knee are valgization osteotomies of the proximal tibia (high-tibial osteotomy = HTO). Whereas in the past closed-wedge osteotomy from the lateral side with fibula osteotomy was the gold standard in many countries; 15 years ago a method of open-wedge osteotomy from the medial side with fixation by a spacer plate was introduced. This procedure looked very attractive to many surgeons because of the small incision and the simple surgical steps. However, the implant was biomechanically rather unsafe and its wide-spread use resulted in a significant number of failures, often associated with implant loosening and breakage. In 2000, Staubli and De Simoni developed an alternative technique and implant which was based on the LCP system (TomoFix). With the aid of the Knee Expert Group (KNEG) and the AO Technical Commitee, the surgical technique and the implant were gradually improved, and similar plates were developed for other osteotomy locations around the knee. More than 14 scientific papers were published by Lobenhoffer, van Heerwaarden, and Staubli, many courses have been given in Germany, Netherlands, Switzerland, England, USA, and Japan. The book "Kniegelenknahe Osteotomien" was produced in German by Thieme Verlag in 2006, which included the main developments around the TomoFix concept and is the basis for this AO book. Over the last years, the TomoFix technique received wide-spread acceptance in the German speaking part of Europe. Osteotomy is still gaining in popularity and an increasing number of patients request preservation of their knee in monocompartimental osteoarthritis. Interest has also been raised in entire Europe and there is a huge potential in other European countries which have a long tradition in osteotomies. Valgization HTO has also been widely performed in Japan. There is a traditional concern about total knee replacement, because it often limits maximum knee flexion, which is necessary for traditional Japanese sitting. A first TomoFix course in Tokyo with 35 participants in April 2008 was very successful. The problem of oversized implants has been solved by KNEG with the development of a small version of the TomoFix, which has recently been launched. The potential patient group in Japan is enormous due to the high incidence of varus/internal rotation tibia deformation in the population. This would hold true in other Asian countries such as Korea,

India, or China, where bow legs are also very common and this type of surgery would offer huge advantages compared to joint replacement regarding complications and aftercare.

HTO is presently not commonly performed in the USA, but patients there will certainly be attracted by the idea of joint-preserving surgery as well, if the information on the benefit of these new techniques is spread. Due to the high interest in physical activity and sports in this country, the potential for osteotomy procedures will be huge.

The development of specific locked bolt implants for osteotomies around the knee has increased the safety of these procedures significantly, and enables the surgeon to perform even multi-plane corrections acutely without the risk of secondary loss of correction. The implants have an extremely high biomechanical strength, allowing for a functional rehabilitation and rapid weight bearing. Open-wedge osteotomy of the tibia can be performed without bone grafting or bone substitution in most cases.

This book reflects the experience from the first 10 years of application of internal plate fixators in osteotomies around the knee, based on over 2,000 cases treated personally by the editors. Deformity correction is a complex process involving patient examination, radiographic deformity analysis, preoperative planning, surgical correction, and internal fixation. All aspects are addressed closely and we hope that the book offers a comprehensive review on this subject. We recommend that the surgeon interested in these techniques after studying the book visits a course, workshop, or practical training session before starting this type of procedure. The AO network offers many opportunities to gain deeper insight in the fascinating subject of deformity correction around the knee.

Prof Dr Philipp Lobenhoffer
on behalf of the editors and co-editors: Dr Ronald J van Heerwaarden, Dr Alex E Staubli, Prof Dr Roland P Jakob, Prof Robert Teitge, Dr Mellany Galla, Dr Jens D Agneskirchner

Acknowledgements

The editors would like to acknowledge the help we received in the past years from our co-workers in the orthopedic departments at the Henriettenstift, Hannover, the Limb deformity reconstruction unit Sint Maartenskliniek Nijmegen and Woerden, the Kantonsspital Luzern and Fribourg. The biomechanical experiments described in this book have all been performed at the Laboratory for Biomechanics and Biomaterials, Orthopedic University Department, Hannover Medical School under the guidance of Dr Ing C Hurschler. Members of the KNEG in recent years as André Gächter and Peter Holzach from Switzerland, Takeshi Sawaguchi and Rohei Takeuchi from Japan, and Brent Norris and Robert Teitge from the USA have been of great help in the development of innovative osteotomy techniques and the TomoFix concept. Mathys medical group and Synthes International (M Portmann and M Rettenmund) have provided us with prototype implants and many new tools that enabled ever improving surgical technique.

For this book excellent illustrations have been made by Jecca Reichmuth from AO Publishing. Terrific pictures have been provided by Rolf Zimmerman and Hans Radenborg. Our personal secretaries have been of great help in preparing the manuscripts. Last but not least, we are greatly indebted to Dr Mellany Galla, co-editor, and Cristina Lusti and her team from AO Publishing for final manuscript preparation.

Contributors

Editors

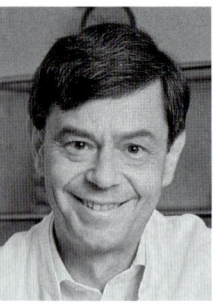

Philipp P Lobenhoffer, Prof Dr
Klinik für Unfall- und
Wiederherstellungschirurgie
DK Henriettenstiftung Hannover
Marienstrasse 72–90
30171 Hannover
Germany

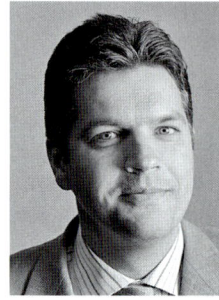

Ronald J van Heerwaarden, MD, PhD
Orthopedic Surgeon
Limb Deformity Reconstruction Unit
Sint Maartenskliniek Nijmegen
Hengstdal 3
6500 GM Nijmegen

Medical Director
Sint Maartenskliniek Woerden
Polanerbaan 2
3447 GN Woerden
Netherlands

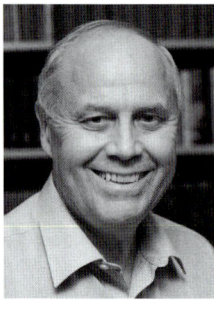

Alex E Staubli, Dr med
FMH Orthopädische Chirurgie
Sonnmatt Luzern
Kurhotel Residenz Privatklinik
6000 Luzern 15
Switzerland

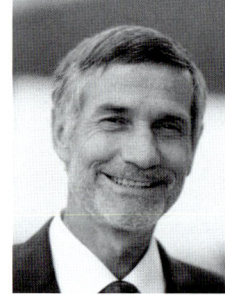

Roland P Jakob, Prof Dr
Freiburger Spital
Standort Tafers
Maggenberg 1
1712 Tafers
Switzerland

Co-editors

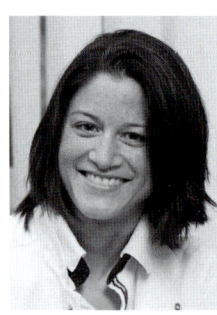

Mellany Galla, Dr med
Klinik für Unfall- und
Wiederherstellungschirurgie
DK Henriettenstiftung Hannover
Marienstrasse 72–90
30171 Hannover
Germany

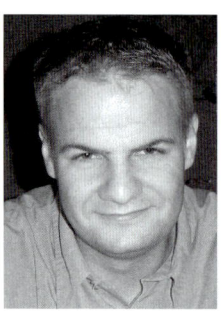

Jens D Agneskirchner, Dr med
Klinik für Unfall- und
Wiederherstellungschirurgie
DK Henriettenstiftung Hannover
Marienstrasse 72–90
30171 Hannover
Germany

Authors

Jens D Agneskirchner, Dr med
Klinik für Unfall- und
Wiederherstellungschirurgie
DK Henriettenstiftung Hannover
Marienstrasse 72–90
30171 Hannover
Germany

Koen C Defoort, MD
Orthopedic Department
Sint Maartenskliniek Nijmegen
Hengstdal 3
6500 GM Nijmegen
Netherlands

Denise Freiling, Dr med
Klinik für Unfall- und
Wiederherstellungschirurgie
DK Henriettenstiftung Hannover
Marienstrasse 72–90
30171 Hannover
Germany

Mellany Galla, Dr med
Klinik für Unfall- und
Wiederherstellungschirurgie
DK Henriettenstiftung Hannover
Marienstrasse 72–90
30171 Hannover
Germany

Siegfried Hofmann, Dr med
Universitäts-Dozent
Allgemeines und Orthopädisches
Landeskrankenhaus Stolzalpe
8852 Stolzalpe
Austria

Christof Hurschler, PhD
Biomedizinische Technik, Biomechanik
Abteilung Orthopädie
Medizinische Hochschule Hannover
Carl-Neuberg-Strasse 1
30625 Hannover
Germany

Matthias Jacobi, MD
Departement of Orthopedic Surgery
Kantonsspital Fribourg
1708 Fribourg
Switzerland

Roland P Jakob, Prof Dr
Freiburger Spital
Standort Tafers
Maggenberg 1
1712 Tafers
Switzerland

Paul Koning, MD
Orthopedic Department
Sint Maartenskliniek Nijmegen
Hengstdal 3
6500 GM Nijmegen
Netherlands

Philipp P Lobenhoffer, Prof Dr
Klinik für Unfall- und
Wiederherstellungschirurgie
DK Henriettenstiftung Hannover
Marienstrasse 72–90
30171 Hannover
Germany

Urs W Müller, Dr
Co-Chefarzt Orthopädie
Kantonsspital Luzern
Spitalstrasse
6000 Luzern 16
Switzerland

Werner Müller, Prof Dr
Professor emeritus for Orthopedic Surgery,
University of Basel
4125 Riehen
Switzerland

Lutz-Peter Nolte, Prof Dr Ing
ME Müller Forschungszentrum
für Orthopädische Chirurgie
Institut für chirurgische Technologien
und Biomechanik
Stauffacherstrasse 78
3014 Bern
Switzerland

Dietrich Pape, Dr med
Centre du l'Appareil Locomoteur de
Médicine du Sport et de Prévention
Centre Hospitalier de Luxembourg
Clinique d'Eich
78, Rue d'Eich
1460 Luxembourg
Luxembourg

Robert A Teitge, Prof Dr
Department of Orthopaedic Surgery
Wayne State University, Detroit, MI, USA
3272 E Twelve Mile Road
Warren, MI, 48092
USA

Ibo B van der Haven, MD
Orthopedic Department
Sint Maartenskliniek Nijmegen
Hengstdal 3
6500 GM Nijmegen
Netherlands

Ronald J van Heerwaarden, MD, PhD
Orthopedic Surgeon
Limb Deformity Reconstruction Unit
Sint Maartenskliniek Nijmegen
Hengstdal 3
6500 GM Nijmegen

Medical Director
Sint Maartenskliniek Woerden
Polanerbaan 2
3447 GN Woerden
Netherlands

Gijs G van Hellemondt, MD
Orthopedic Department
Sint Maartenskliniek Nijmegen
Hengstdal 3
6500 GM Nijmegen
Netherlands

Alex E Staubli, Dr med
FMH Orthopädische Chirurgie
Sonnmatt Luzern
Kurhotel Residenz Privatklinik
6000 Luzern 15
Switzerland

Frank Wagenaar, MD
Orthopedic Department
Sint Maartenskliniek Nijmegen
Hengstdal 3
6500 GM Nijmegen
Netherlands

Peter Wahl, MD
Departement of Orthopedic Surgery
Kantonsspital Fribourg
1708 Fribourg
Switzerland

Gongli Wang, Dr
M. E. Müller Forschungszentrum
für Orthopädische Chirurgie
Institut für chirurgische Technologien
und Biomechanik
Stauffacherstrasse 78
3014 Bern
Switzerland

Christiane D Wrann, Dr
Klinik für Unfall- und
Wiederherstellungschirurgie
DK Henriettenstiftung Hannover
Marienstrasse 72–90
30171 Hannover
Germany

Ate B Wymenga, MD, PhD
Orthopedic Department
Sint Maartenskliniek Nijmegen
Hengstdal 3
6500 GM Nijmegen
Netherlands

Guoyan Zheng, Dr phil, PhD
M. E. Müller Forschungszentrum
für Orthopädische Chirurgie
Institut für chirurgische Technologien
und Biomechanik
Stauffacherstrasse 78
3014 Bern
Switzerland

Authors Roland P Jakob, Matthias Jacobi, Philipp Lobenhoffer

The history of osteotomy

1 Introduction

Osteotomies are now an important and accepted treatment of different pathologies of the knee joint. The development of osteotomy from the 19th to the 21st century was only possible due to the introduction of anesthesia [1, 2], blood spearing surgical techniques [3] and asepsis [4, 5], as well as the detection of radiography [6–8]. Indications for osteotomy have changed fundamentally: Whereas osteotomy is now mainly used to treat unicompartimental osteoarthritis, in the past the main indications were severe genu valgum, posttraumatic deformities, rickets, and other bowing deformities [9, 10].

2 Osteotomy in the 16th century

It was only in the 16th century that the armourer's art first made the development of surgical equipment possible. "Osteoclasia" was a common treatment for malalignment at that time. It consisted of breaking the bone in a controlled manner to correct deformity. Originally this was done manually, but as precision was not high enough, machines were developed to control and guide the force. A machine made by Bosch, which was an ordinary bookbinder press, became the prototype for following instruments. It was first used to treat a malunited femoral fracture. As these instruments became more sophisticated, they were not only used for bony anklyosis but also for genu valgum and varum (Fig 1).

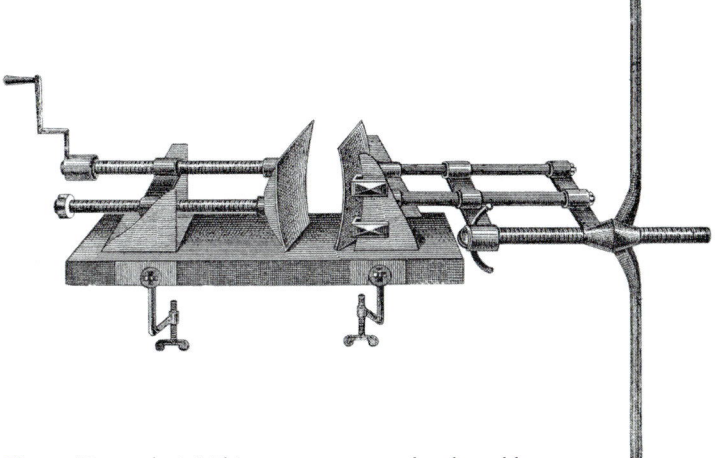

Fig 1 "Osteoclasia". This apparatus was developed by Lorenz and was the best of its time [11].

3   Osteotomy before the 20th century

In literature, the first modern osteotomy is commonly contributed to the American **John Rhea Barton** (1794–1871) from Pennsylvania [12].

On November 22, 1826, Barton performed a subtrochanteric osteotomy on a 21-year-old sailor with flexion/adduction ankylosis—an osteotomy therefore to loosen up a flexion deformity of the hip and meant to create a pseudarthrosis which became also the first arthroplasty [13]. The operation was done with a keyhole saw without anesthesia and asepsis, and took only seven minutes (Fig 3). Bone healing was avoided through daily mobilization and led to the intended pseudarthrosis which was successful for 6 years. Thereafter the pseudarthrosis ankylosed again. In 1835 Barton performed a supracondylar wedge osteotomy of the femur for bony ankylosis of the knee curved at a right angle. The osteotomy healed with only minor complications such as "minor infection and extrusion of some small sequestra".

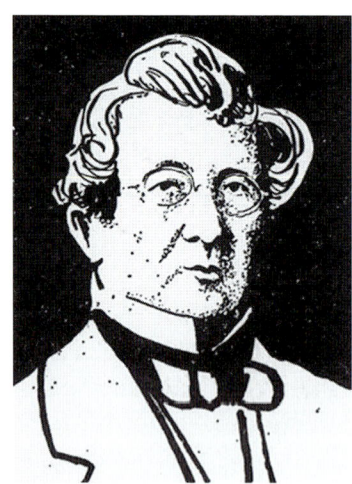

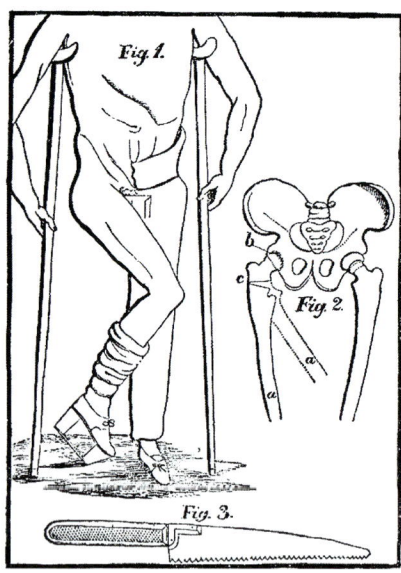

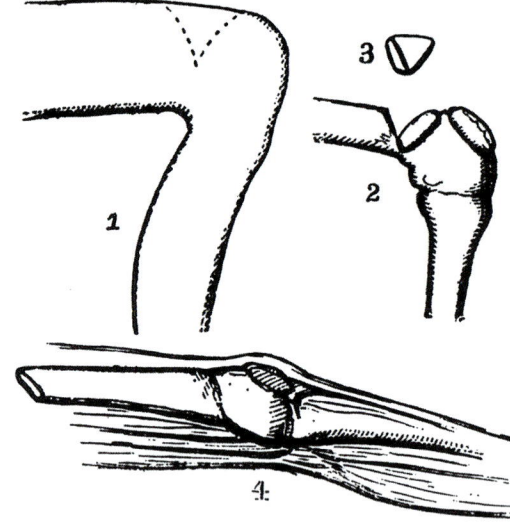

Barton: Osteotomy. 1. Gives the position of the flap just above the knee; 2. Shows the operation on the femur; 3. The piece of bone removed; 4. The manner in which the gap in the bone was closed by the overlapping of the surfaces consequent to the extension of the leg. These uniting restored the integrity of the limb.

Fig 2   John Rhea Barton (1794–1871) from Pennsylvania [12].

Fig 3a–b
a   Barton's first osteotomy for hip ankylosis [12].
b   Wedge osteotomy for knee ankylosis by Barton [12].

August Friedrich Wasserfuhr, a German military surgeon, performed a corrective osteotomy of a 90° malunited femoral fracture on a 5-year-old boy in 1828 [14].

John Karney Rodgers from New York was the first to perform a wedge osteotomy in 1830 [14].

Joseph Anton von Mayer from Würzburg, Professor of Morbid Anatomy, was the first German to perform an osteotomy. Mayer named the operation "resectio tibiae cuneiformis" and avoided the term osteotomy because with "resectio" it was easier to convince patients to agree to this type of surgery. From 1839–1854 he performed 20 osteotomies in rickets-induced deformities. All osteotomies healed with no or only minor complications. He used a variety of osteotomy instruments such as different kinds of saws, sizzles, and osteotomes. Most of his cases were performed using open surgery, but he also performed three subcutaneous surgeries [9, 10].

In the same city worked the famous instrument maker **Joseph G Heine** (1770–1838). For the first time the skills of an instrument maker were combined with the surgeon's science. Heine took his nephew **Bernhard Heine** (1800–1846) into apprenticeship, and he would later develop the "Osteotome", an instrument designed to perform an osteotomy. This made him famous throughout Europe when Heine, now a Professor in Würzburg, presented this medical tool to his colleagues in 1830. It was a bone saw which revolutionized surgical treatment (Fig 4), and was a great success among medical experts. Heine travelled to other parts of Germany, France, and even Russia to present it to other surgeons. By 1836 a doctoral thesis on the "Osteotome and its application" had been published in München, Germany [14, 15].

Bernhard Rudolf Konrad von Langenbeck (1810–1887) professor in Göttingen, Kiel, and Berlin, Germany, was the first to describe a subcutaneous osteotomy technique. He specialized in military surgery. In 1848, he experimentally osteotomized a humerus during the war between Prussia and Denmark in Schleswig-Holstein. In 1854 he described two cases of rickets with varus deformity and a case of fracture malunion in which he performed a subcutaneous osteotomy under chloroform anesthesia. He made a stab wound, then a short skin incision straight to the bone on the inner aspect of the tibia. A drill hole was made passing this incision in transverse direction through the tibia. A fret saw was introduced into this hole, and the tibia was subtotally cut. After that, the tibia could be broken and placed in a straight position either immediately or later—the method of subcutaneous osteotomy was born. All cases suffered from osteomyelitis in the follow-up but subsequently healed [16].

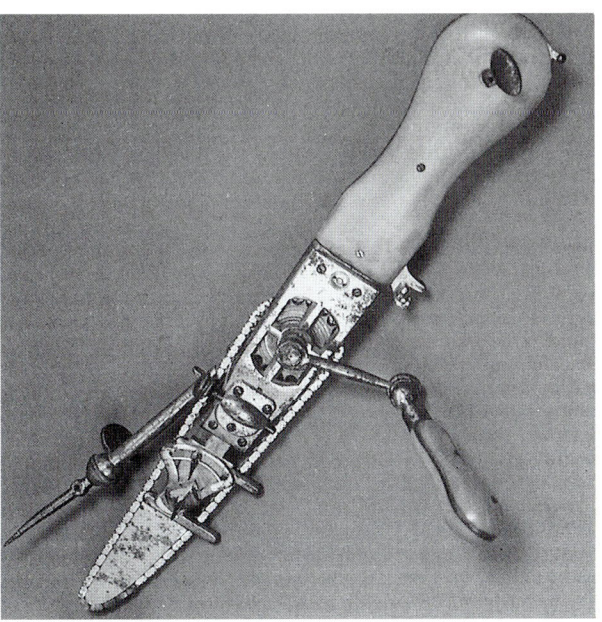

Fig 4 Bernhard Heine's osteotome.

Theodor Billroth (1829–1894) Professor in Zürich, Switzerland and Wien, Austria is known as the originator of modern abdominal surgery [17]. In March 1868 Billroth performed his first osteotomy using the subcutaneous technique of Langenbeck with a chisel in a patient with a malunited tibial fracture. In his publication of the case he advised the use of a chisel (Fig 5). In his opinion this instrument was more useful than both the Heine osteotome (see Fig 4) and the fret saw used by Langenbeck [16].

Sir William Macewen (1848–1924), Professor in Glasgow, performed the first antiseptic osteotomy in Great Britain on April 11, 1875. In 1884, he presented his series of 1,800 cases without major complications except for three deaths not related to surgery [19]. Of these cases, 810 were done in the "proper" supracondylar closed-wedge technique of Macewen (Fig 6) [3, 18, 19]. In 1880 Macewen published a book on osteotomy [19]. This book was probably the first one exclusively on osteotomies. He used for most of his osteotomies either the open- or closed-wedge technique (Fig 7).

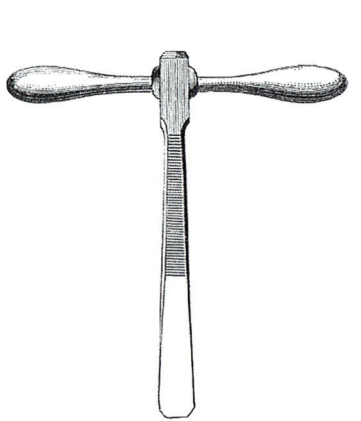

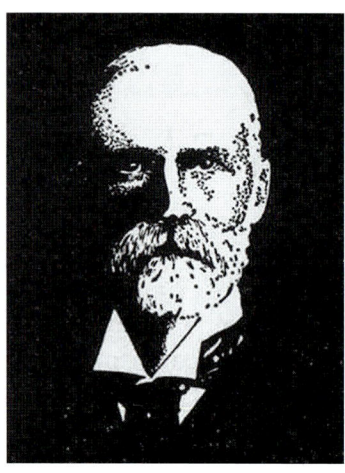

Fig 5   Chisel as used by Billroth for his osteotomies [11].

Fig 6   Sir William Macewen, 1848–1924 [19].

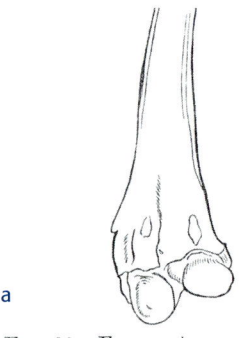

a

FIG. 36.—FEMUR AFFECTED WITH GENU VALGUM — SHOWING DE-FORMITY TO BE RECTIFIED.

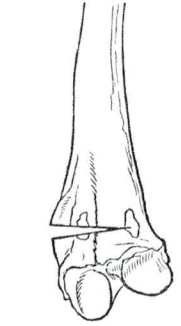

b

FIG. 37.—FIRST STAGE OF OPERATION ON INNER SIDE.

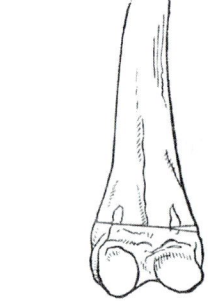

c

FIG. 38.—RESULT AFTER OPERATION ON INNER SIDE. PERIOSTEUM PRESERVED.

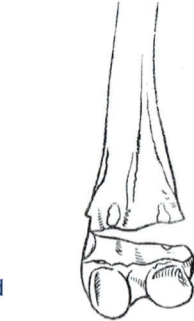

d

FIG. 39.—RESULT AFTER OPERATION ON OUTER SIDE. PERIOSTEUM CUT ACROSS.

Fig 7a–d   Description of varization osteotomy on distal femur from Macewen [19].

Location of osteotomy		Kind of osteotomy	Author and year
Femur	Both condyles	Linear	Annandale 1875
	One condyle	Linear	Ogston 1876
			Reeves 1878
		Cuneiform	Macewen 1878
			Chiene 1877
	Above the condyles	Cuneiform	Macewen 1878
	Diaphysis	Linear	Reeves 1878
			Neudörfer 1874
Tibia	Metaphysis	Linear	Billroth 1874
		Cuneiform	Mayer 1854
Tibia and fibula	Metaphysis	Cuneiform	Schede 1877
Femur and tibia	Metaphysis	Linear	Barwell 1879

Table 1   Different options for osteotomy described by Hoffa [11].

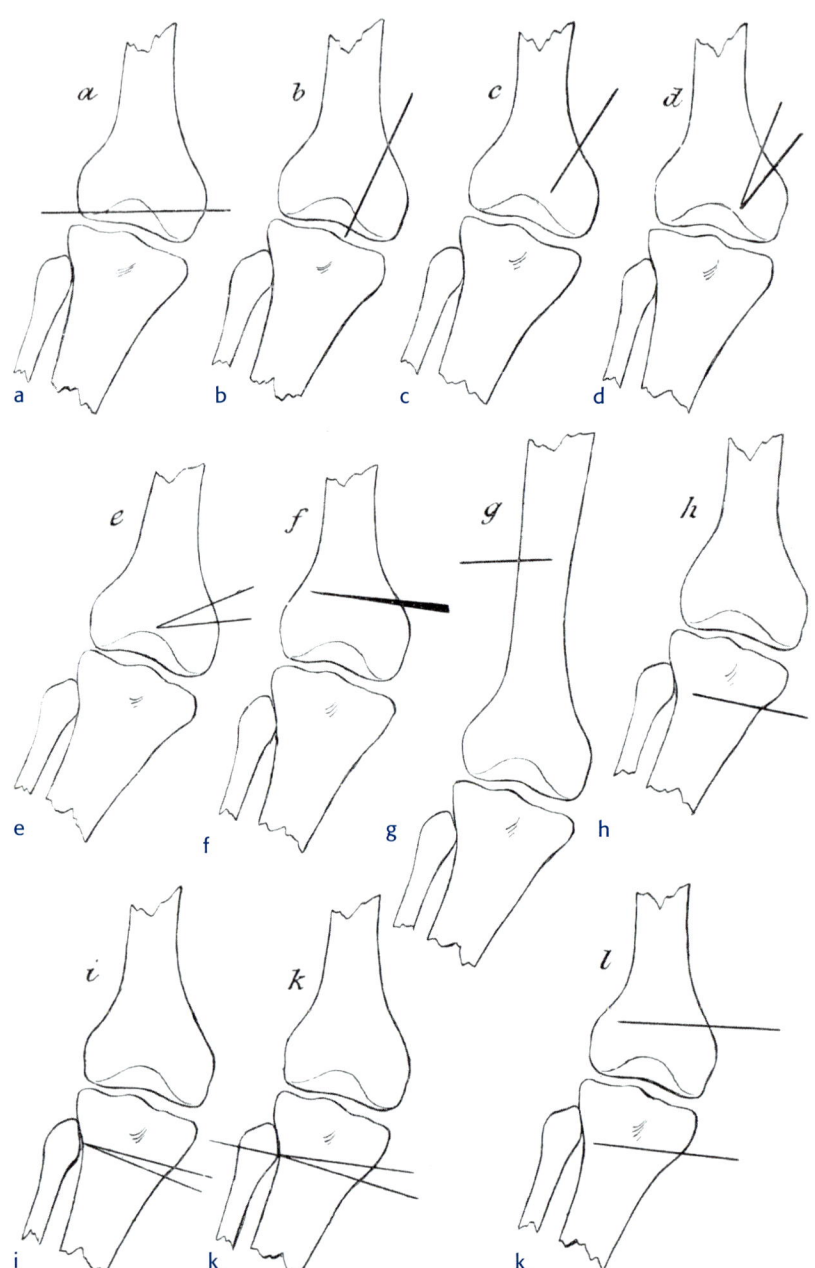

Fig 8a–k   Osteotomy options described in Hoffa's book [11].

4 Osteotomy since the 20th century

Although osteotomies were performed regularly in the first half of the 20th century, the real breakthrough came only with the publications of Jackson, Waugh, Gariépy, Coventry, and others in the late 1950s and 60s [20–23] (Fig 9). Osteotomy became a standard treatment option for unicompartimental osteoarthritis of the knee. Whereas Jackson operated distal to the tibial tuberosity [20, 21], the classic osteotomy of Coventry was a closed-wedge valgization type including a fibula osteotomy, and was performed proximal to the tibial tuberosity [23]. This was the most widely used technique for a long time.

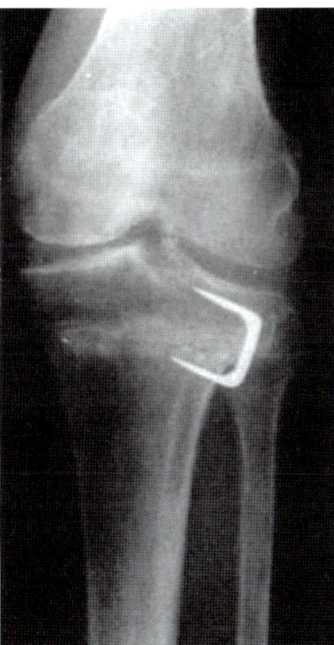

Fig 9   Staple fixation as used by Coventry and others. This fixation needed additional casting and therefore a functional rehabilitation protocol was not possible [23].

Open-wedge osteotomy was first described by Lexer 1931 and Brett 1935 in cases of genu recurvatum [24, 25]. Brett performed the first osteotomy immediately below the joint surface.

Osteotomy of the tibia combined with division of the fibula has been practiced in Liverpool since 1928 by Wardle [26]. The operation was repopularized by Jackson and Waugh [20, 21]. Their original osteotomy was performed just below the tibial tubercle. Wardle reported on the osteotomy at the junction of the upper and middle third of the tibia [27]. The operative site was next moved proximally to the tibial tubercle. In Germany, Steindler [28] recommended 1940 osteotomy as a treatment of osteoarthritis.

In France the first official description of open-wedge correction in the frontal plane dates from 1961 by Debeyre [29, 30]. Publication of a larger series did not appear until 1987 (Hernigou), although the technique has been regularly performed since 1951 [31]. Maquet's technique of barrel vault osteotomy was reported in 1976 [32]. In this period postoperative stabilization was routinely done with cast fixation alone, and sometimes augmented with staples (Fig 9). Stable fixation of osteotomy around the knee was not standard until the 1970s [33].

When the AO was founded in 1958, the main goal was to improve fracture treatment, and the AO principles could also be applied to osteotomies. In the first edition of the "Manual of Osteosynthesis" from 1969, an osteotomy technique with angular plate fixation was already advocated [34] (Fig 10).

In the 1980s and 90s, osteotomy around the knee lost importance due to the success of knee arthroplasty. However, the development of new plates, particularly plates with angular stability, during the last ten years has led to a revival of osteotomy around the knee, especially for younger patients. The TomoFix plate system which is based on an internal fixator principle with angular stability of the screws, allows open-wedge osteotomy without bone grafting because of its excellent stability [35] (Fig 11).

With these new products the open-wedge osteotomy became the favored technique, being easier to perform, and is nowadays probably the most commonly used technique with the advantage that it is more precise, quicker, has no risk of peroneal nerve injury, and preserves the proximal tibia better when considering a future total knee arthroplasty.

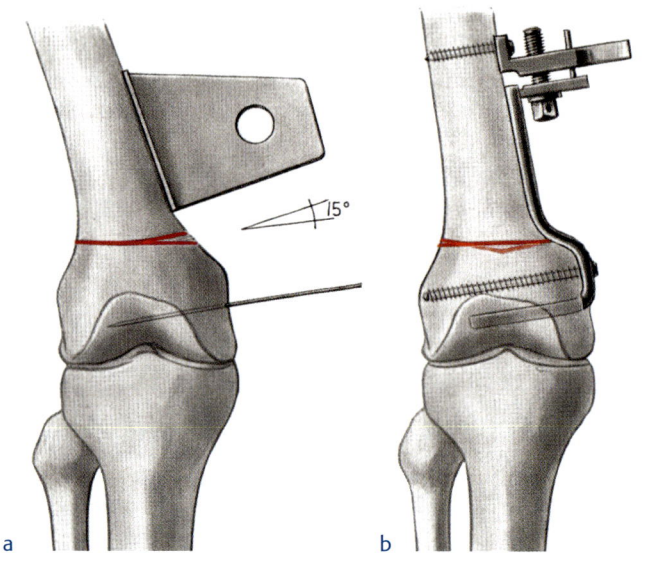
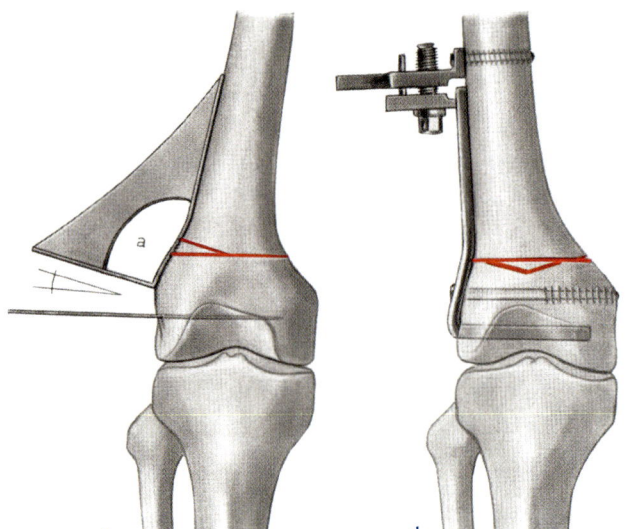

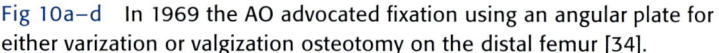

Fig 10a–d   In 1969 the AO advocated fixation using an angular plate for either varization or valgization osteotomy on the distal femur [34].

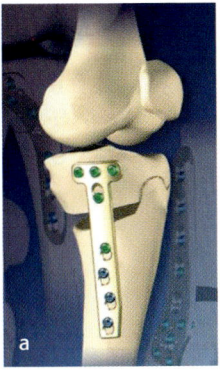 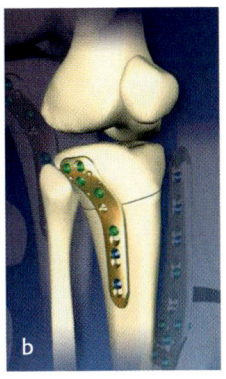 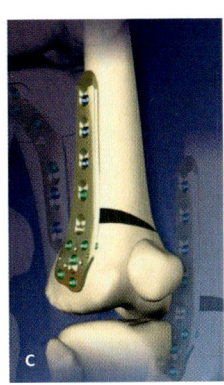 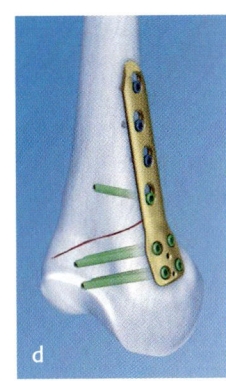

Fig 11a–d   The TomoFix system allows rigid fixation, and in cases of open-wedge osteotomy, the osteotomy gap can be left open (source: Synthes Inc).

5   Conclusions

The history of osteotomy teaches us that the past should not simply be forgotten, and that in many aspects the knowledge and techniques of our predecessors are still of great worth.

"Those who cannot remember the past, are condemned to repeat it." Quoted from *Reason in Common Sense*, the first volume of his philosophical work *"The Life of Reason"* by George Santayana, 1905.

6   Bibliography

[1]   **Long CW** (1849) An account of the first use of sulfuric ether by inhalation as an anaesthetic in surgical operations. *South Med Surg J*; 5:705–713.

[2]   **Rae S, Wildsmith J** (1997) So just who was James "Young" Simpson? *Br J Anaesth*; 79(3):271–273.

[3]   **von Esmarch F** (1873) [On Artificial Bloodlessmess during operations.] *Volkmanns Sammlung klinischer Vorträge, Chirurgie*; 58(1):373–84. German.

[4]   **Lister J** (1867) On a New Method of Treating Compound Fractures, Abscesses, Etc., with Observations on the Conditions of Suppuration. *The Lancet 1*; 326–329.

[5]   **Lister J** (1867) On a New Method of Treating Compound Fractures, Abscesses, Etc., with Observations on the Conditions of Suppuration. *The Lancet 2*; 353–356.

[6]   **Röntgen W** (1895) [On a new kind of rays.] *Sitzungsberichte der Physik.-med. Gesellschaft zu Würzburg*; 132–141. German.

[7]   **Röntgen W** (1896) [On a new kind of rays.] *Sitzungsberichte der Physik.-med. Gesellschaft zu Würzburg*; 11–16. German.

[8]   **Röntgen W** (1897) [Further observations on characteristics of x-rays.] *Sitzungsberichte der Königlich Preussischen Akademie der Wissenschaften zu Berlin*; 576–592. German.

[9] **Mayer A** (1851) [The osteotomy as a new orthopaedic operation method.] *Verhandlungen der physikalisch-medizinischen Gesellschaft in Würzburg*. German.

[10] **Mayer A** (1856) [Reports from German clinics and hospitals— Historical and statistical notes about the osteotomies performed by Dr A Mayer in Würzburg.] *German clinic*. German.

[11] **Hoffa A** (1902) *[Orthopaedic surgery.]* 4th ed. Stuttgart: Verlag von Ferdinand Enke. German.

[12] **Barton J** (1835) Views and treatment of an important fracture of the wrist. *Medical Examiner*; (1):365.

[13] **Barton J** (1827) On the treatment of anchylosis by the formation of artificial joints. *North Am Medical Surg J*; (3):279, 400.

[14] **Kunz M** (1993) [The beginning of the osteotomy and the development in the orthopedic.] *Mannheim, Clinic of Orthopedics*. German.

[15] **Noodth C** (1836) [The osteotome and its application.] München.

[16] **Langenbeck B** (1854) [The subcutaneous osteotomy.] *German Clinic*; 6:327. German.

[17] **Billroth T** (1870) [About the use of the chisel as a sculptor in osteotomies.] *Wien Med Wochenschr*;18. German.

[18] **James C** (1974) Sir William Macewen. *Proc Roy Soc Med*; 67(4):237–242.

[19] **Macewen W** (1880) *Osteotomy with an inquiry into the aetiology and pathology of knock-knee, bow-leg, and other osseous deformities of the lower limbs*. London: Churchill.

[20] **Jackson JP** (1958) Osteotomy for Osteoarthritis of the Knee. Proceedings of the Sheffield Regional Orthopaedic Club. *J Bone Joint Surg*; 40(4):826.

[21] **Jackson JP, Waugh W** (1961) Tibial Osteotomy for Osteoarthritis of the Knee. *J Bone and Joint Surg*; 43(4):746–751.

[22] **Gariépy R** (1964) Genu varum treated by high tibial osteotomy. In Proceedings of the Joint Meeting of Orthopaedic Associations. *J Bone Joint Surg*; 46(4):783–784.

[23] **Coventry MB** (1965) Osteotomy of the upper portion of the tibia for degenerative arthritis of the knee. A preliminary report. *J Bone Joint Surg*; 47:984–990.

[24] **Lexer E** (1931) *Revascularization osteotomy*. 2nd ed. Barth JA.

[25] **Brett AL** (1935) Operative correction of genu recurvatum. *J Bone Joint Surg Am*; 17:984–989.

[26] **Wardle EN** (1964) Osteotomy of the Tibia and Fibula in the Treatment of Chronic Osteoarthritis of the Knee. *Postgrad Med J*; 40:536–542.

[27] **Wardle EN** (1962) Osteotomy of the tibia and fibula. *Surg Gynecol Obstet*; 115:61–64.

[28] **Steindler A** (1940) *Orthopedic Operations: Indications, Technique, and End Results*. Springfield, Illinois:Charles C Thomas.

[29] **Debeyre J, Patte D** (1962) [Value of corrective osteotomies in the treatment of certain knee diseases with axial deviation.] *Rev Rhum Mal Osteoartic*; 29:722–729. French.

[30] **Debeyre J, Patte D** (1961) [The place of corrective osteotomies in the treatment of gonarthrosis.] *Acta Orthop Belg*; 27:374–383. French.

[31] **Hernigou P, Medevielle D, Debeyre J, et al** (1987) Proximal tibial osteotomy for osteoarthritis with varus deformity. A ten to thirteen-year follow-up study. *J Bone Joint Surg Am*; 69(3):332–354.

[32] **Maquet P** (1976) Valgus osteotomy for osteoarthritis of the knee. *Clin Orthop Relat Res*; 120:143–148.

[33] **Sprenger TR, Weber BG, Howard FM** (1979) Compression osteotomy of the tibia. *Clin Orthop Relat Res*; 140:103–108.

[34] **Müller M, Allgöwer M, Willenegger H** (1969) *[Manual of Osteosynthesis—AO Technique]* Berlin, Heidelberg, New York: Springer-Verlag.

[35] **Staubli AE, Simoni CD, Babst R, et al** (2003) TomoFix: a new LCP-concept for open wedge osteotomy of the medial proximal tibia - early results in 92 cases. *Injury*; 34 Suppl 2:55–62.

Indications and planning

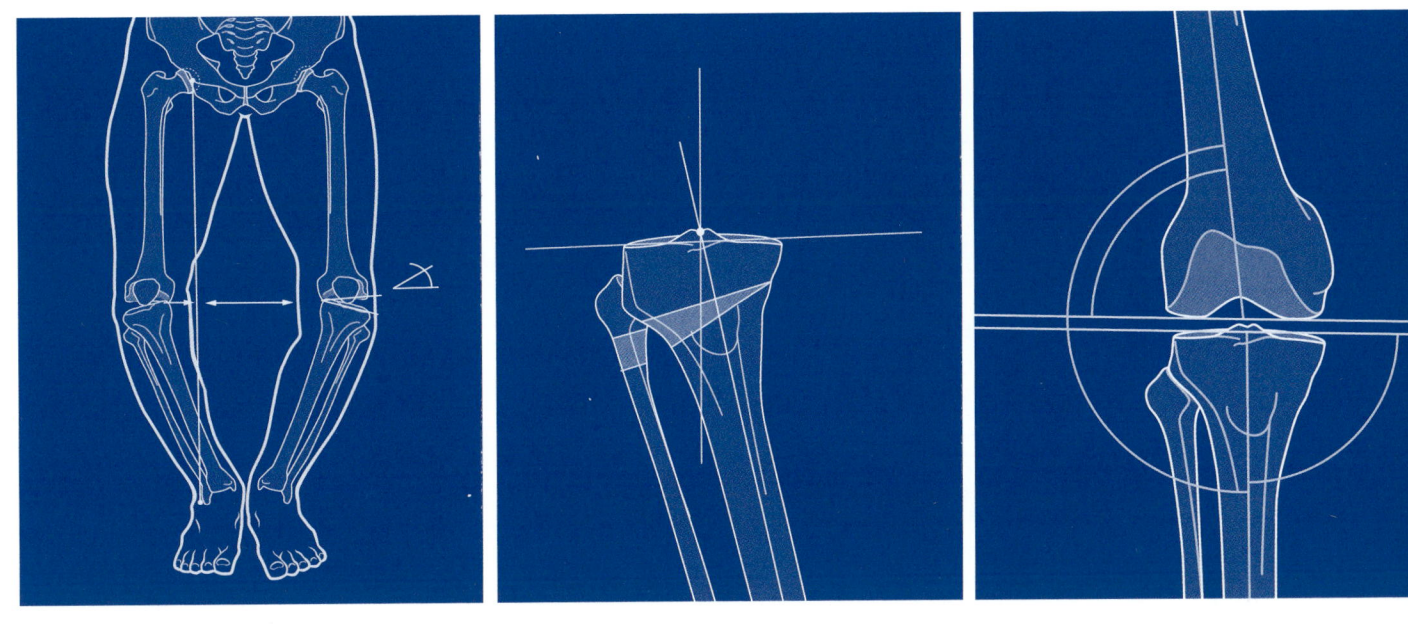

Authors **Mellany Galla, Philipp Lobenhoffer**

1 Physiological axes of the lower limb

1 Introduction

The knee joint is the largest and most complex joint in the human body and has the longest lever arms. The joint transmits muscle forces into motion of the human body. The large lever arms of the knee joint produce substantial loading moments.

Axial load causes high mechanical stress in the knee joint. The mechanical load during walking on even ground amounts to 3.4 times body weight and as much as 4.3 times body weight when climbing stairs [1, 2].

2 Physiological axes of the leg

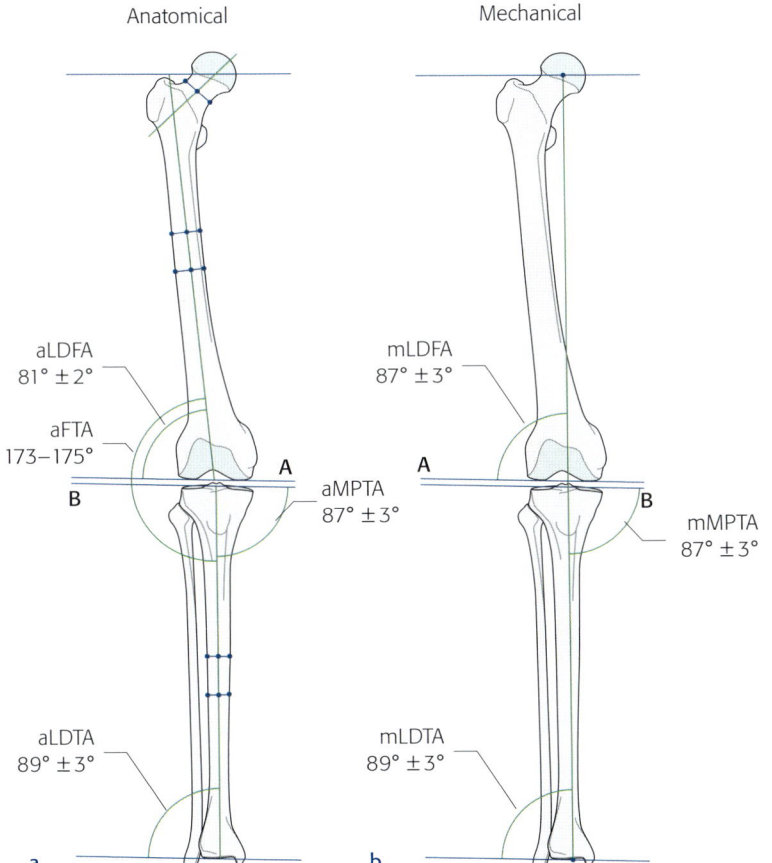

Anatomical

Mechanical

aLDFA
81° ±2°

mLDFA
87° ±3°

aFTA
173–175°

A

A

aMPTA
87° ±3°

B

B

mMPTA
87° ±3°

aLDTA
89° ±3°

mLDTA
89° ±3°

a

b

It is necessary to differentiate between anatomical and mechanical axes when considering the axes of the lower extremity.

The anatomical axes of the femur and tibia correspond to the diaphyseal midline of these long bones. The diaphyseal axis of the femur is not on a straight line with the anatomical axis of the tibia because of the orientation of the femoral neck. The anatomical axes of the femoral and tibial diaphyses form a laterally opened angle of 173–175° (aFTA) (Fig 1-1a).

Fig 1-1a–b Diagram of the leg axes and joint angles in the frontal plane.
a   Anatomical axes and joint angles with standard values. Anatomical femorotibial angle (aFTA) = 173–175°, anatomical lateral distal femoral angle (aLDFA) = 81° ±2°, anatomical medial proximal tibial angle (aMPTA) = 87° ±3°, anatomical lateral distal tibial angle (aLDTA) = 89° ±3°.
b   Mechanical axes and joint angles with standard values. Mechanical lateral distal femoral angle (mLDFA) = 87° ±3°, mechanical medial proximal tibial angle (mMPTA) = 87° ± 3°, mechanical lateral distal tibial angle (mLDTA) = 89° ±3°.

A = Tangent to the femoral condyles (knee base line).
B = Tangent to the tibial plateau.

The mechanical axis of the femur runs from the center of the femoral head to the center of the knee joint and forms an angle of 6° ± 1° with the anatomical axis of the femoral diaphysis (aMFA) (Fig 1-2). The mechanical and the anatomical axes of the tibia are almost identical. Both lines run parallel, whereby the anatomical tibial axis lies a few millimeters medial to the mechanical tibial axis. The mechanical axis of the leg (Mikulicz line) is the connecting line between the center of the femoral head and the center of the ankle joint (Fig 1-3). This line physiologically runs on average 4 (±2) mm medial to the center of the knee joint [3]. If the mechanical axis runs lateral or medial to this point, this indicates either a valgus or a varus deformity (see below). Due to the greater distance between the centers of the hip joints than between the centers of the knee joints and ankle joints, the weight-bearing axis of the leg runs slightly oblique from craniolateral to mediocaudal at an approximate angle of 3° to the perpendicular axis of the body (Fig 1-3).

- The mechanical axis of the leg (Mikulicz line) runs from the center of the femoral head to the center of the ankle joint. Under physiological conditions this line runs on average 4 (±2) mm medial to the center of the knee joint.

  The anatomical and mechanical femoral axes form an angle of 6° (±1°) (aMFA).

Under physiological conditions the knee base line (tangent to the femoral condyles) and the tangent to the tibial plateau run almost parallel to each other (joint line convergence angle = JLCA, 0–1° medial convergence) (see Fig 1-1, Fig 1-6). Since the mechanical and anatomical axes of the tibia run parallel, the medial proximal angle between the tangent to the tibial plateau and the anatomical and mechanical axes is 87° ± 3° in both cases; the standard value for the lateral distal tibial angle at the line of the ankle joint is 89° ± 3° (see Fig 1-1a–b).

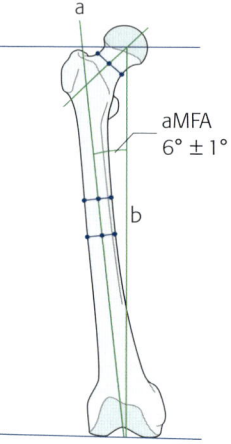

Fig 1-2   Angle between the mechanical (a) and the anatomical (b) femoral axis. The anatomical mechanical femoral angle (aMFA) is 6° ± 1° physiologically.

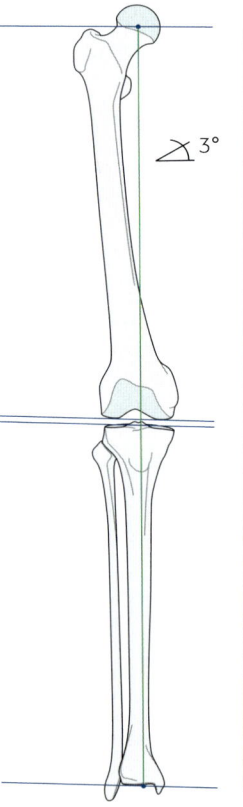

Fig 1-3   The mechanical axis of the leg (green line) runs slightly oblique from craniolateral to mediocaudal at an approximate angle of 3° to the perpendicular axis of the body (black line).

The lateral distal angle between the mechanical femoral axis and the base line of the knee is also 87° ± 3°. Due to aMFA, the knee base line forms an angle of approximately 81° ± 2° with the anatomical axis of the femur (see **Fig 1-1a–b, Table 1-1**).

Joint angle	Abbreviation	Standard value
Anatomical femorotibial angle	aFTA	173–175°
Anatomical mechanical femoral angle	aMFA	6° ± 1°
Anatomical lateral distal femoral angle	aLDFA	81° ± 2°
Mechanical lateral distal femoral angle	mLDFA	87° ± 3°
Anatomical medial proximal tibial angle	aMPTA	87° ± 3°
Mechanical medial proximal tibial angle	mMPTA	87° ± 3°
Anatomical lateral distal tibial angle	aLDTA	89° ± 3°
Mechanical lateral distal tibial angle	mLDTA	89° ± 3°

Table 1-1   Physiological joint angles of the lower extremity.

3 Orientation of the joint surfaces

The anatomy of the femoral and tibial diaphyses and the joint condyles is ideally matched to the functions of the knee joint. Both the femoral and the tibial diaphyses have a concave posterior curvature (Fig 1-4a–b). The tibial plateau is slightly shifted in a posterior direction in relation to the axis of the femoral diaphysis in the sagittal plane (Fig 1-4b). Moreover, the tibial joint surface is tilted by about 10° caudally in the sagittal plane at the posterior aspect of the tibia (tibial slope) (Fig 1-4c). The anatomy with the axial curvature as described above, and the specific anatomy of the femoral and tibial joint are prerequisites for the extensive range of movement and above all, for flexion of the knee joint without bone impingement or trapping of posterior soft tissues or muscular masses.

- The tibial plateau is slightly shifted in a posterior direction in relation to the axis of the femoral diaphysis and is tilted caudally by 10° in relation to the horizontal line in the sagittal plane (tibial slope).

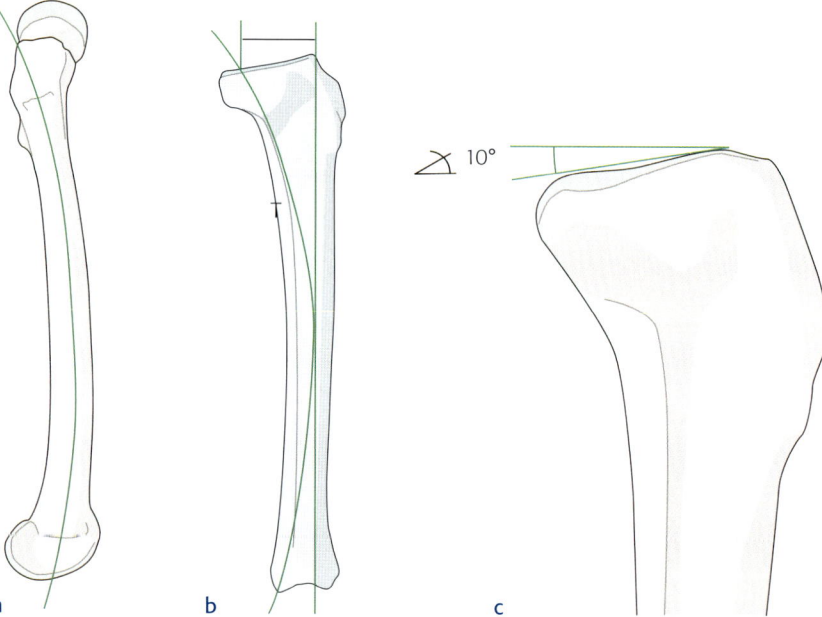

10°

Fig 1-4a–c

a   Physiological posterior-concave curvature of the femoral diaphysis in the sagittal plane.

b   Physiological posterior-concave curvature of the tibial diaphysis in the sagittal plane with physiological posterior shift of the tibial plateau in relation to the axis of the femoral diaphysis (T).

c   Schematic diagram of the tibial slope. The tibial joint surface tilts approximately 10° caudally in the posterior aspect of the tibial head in the sagittal plane in relation to the horizontal line.

4   Etiology of leg deformities

Deformities of the lower limb are defined as a deviation of the physiological axes. The joint angles and axes described above can be pathologically altered in the frontal, sagittal or transverse plane and cause malalignment of the entire lower extremity. If several parameters are affected simultaneously, a complex leg deformity results. Alterations of the physiological longitudinal torque of the femoral and/or tibial diaphyses result in so-called torsional deformities of the leg. Torsional malalignment of the lower leg and its analysis and treatment by correction osteotomy will be described in detail in chapter 15 "Rotational osteotomies of the femur and the tibia".

The causes of leg deformities are manifold [4]. Deformities may be of congenital or constitutional etiology. They may develop during childhood, eg, due to a growth disorder with premature partial closure of the epiphyseal plate or due to metabolic disorders (eg, rachitis) and osteopathies (eg, renal osteopathy).

Deviations of the leg axis are often observed as part of systemic myopathic and neurogenic disorders. In adults, posttraumatic deformities are mostly the result of a fracture healed in malalignment. Destruction of the joint surface due to bone necrosis, bone tumor, or rheumatoid arthritis can lead to secondary deviation of the mechanical axes of the lower limb. The most frequent cause of secondary varus and/or valgus malalignment is secondary cartilaginous damage following meniscectomy (Table 1-2).

- The deviation of the physiological axis constitutes a deformity of the lower limb. The joint angles and axes may be pathologically altered in the frontal, sagittal and/or transverse plane. The most frequent pathologies and therefore those of greatest clinical relevance are varus-valgus deformities in the frontal plane.

Etiology of axial deformities
Congenital deformities
Constitutional deformities
Growth disorders with premature partial closure of the epiphyseal plate
Metabolic diseases (eg, rachitis)
Osteopathies (eg, renal osteopathy)
Systemic myopathic disorders
Systemic neurogenic disorders
Posttraumatic deformities due to incorrectly healed fracture
Secondary deviation due to destruction of the joint surface as a result of bone necrosis, bone tumor, or rheumatoid arthritis
Varus or valgus deformity due to secondary cartilaginous damage after meniscectomy

Table 1-2   Etiology of axial deformities of the lower extremity.

5 Systematic analysis of axial deformities

The most frequent leg deformities occur in the frontal plane (varus-valgus deviations). Malalignment in the frontal plane is analyzed by application of the "malalignment test" [3]. Malalignment is the manifestation of the deviation of a mechanical axis (MAD = mechanical axis deviation). A significant deviation in the frontal plane is diagnosed when the weight bearing axis of the lower extremity lies more than 15 mm medial of the center of the knee joint (varus deviation) or more than 10 mm lateral of the center (valgus deviation) [3]. To differentiate between a femoral and a tibial cause of malalignment, the mechanical lateral distal femoral angle (mLDFA, standard value 87° ±3°) and the mechanical medial proximal tibial angle (mMPTA, standard value 87° ±3°) (Fig 1-5) must be considered. If the mLDFA value is smaller than the standard value, the cause of the valgus deformity is a femoral

one. If the mechanical medial proximal tibial angle (mMPTA) is increased, the valgus malalignment is due to a tibial deviation. Conversely, an increased femoral angle (mLDFA) indicates a femoral cause of varus malalignment, whereas an mMPTA < 87° ±3° indicates a tibial cause. The joint line convergence angle (JLCA) is subsequently analyzed. Under physiological conditions the knee base line (tangent to the femoral condyles) and the tangent to the tibial plateau run almost parallel to each other (0–1° medial convergence). A medially increased joint line convergence angle may result from medial ligamentocapsular laxity, ligamentous instability, or loss of cartilage in the lateral articular compartment. Conversely, loss of cartilage, destruction of the joint surface on the medial side or laxity of the lateral ligamentocapsular structures leads to a laterally widened joint [3].

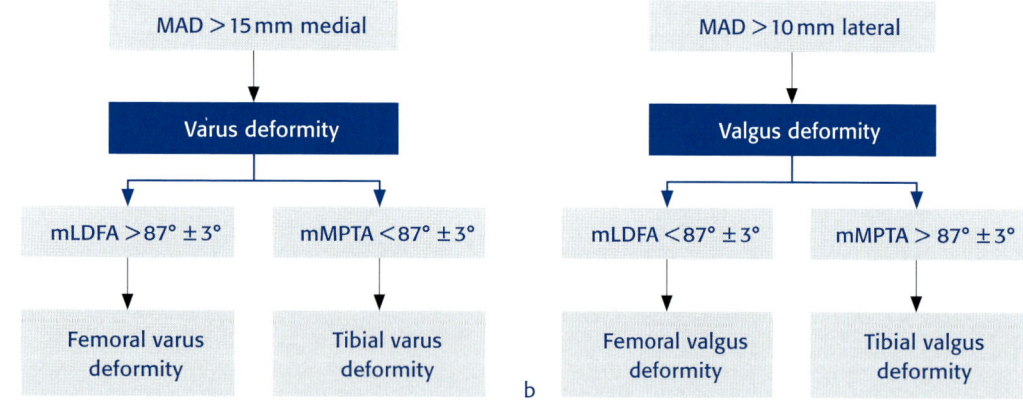

a

b

Fig 1-5a–b Systematic analysis of deformity based on the "malalignment test" [3].
MAD = mechanical axis deviation, significant for a displacement of >15 mm medially (varus deformity) (a) and by >10 mm laterally (valgus deformity) (b) from the center of the knee joint.

mLDFA = mechanical lateral distal femoral angle, standard value 87° ±3°.
mMPTA = mechanical medial proximal tibial angle, standard value 87° ±3°.

Genu varum
Anatomical femorotibial angle >173–175°
Mikulicz line runs medial to the 4 mm point, significant in MAD >15 mm medial to the center of the knee joint
Increased intercondylar distance

Table 1-3   Characteristics of genu varum.

Genu valgum
Anatomical femorotibial angle <173–175°
Mikulicz line runs lateral to the 4 mm point, significant in MAD >10 mm lateral to the center of the knee joint
Increased intermalleolar distance

Table 1-4   Characteristics of genu valgum.

5.1   Genu varum

In genu varum the lateral angle between the anatomical femoral axis and the axis of the tibial diaphysis (aFTA) is greater than 173–175°. The weight-bearing line from the center of the femoral head to the midpoint of the upper ankle joint runs more than 4 (±2) mm medial to the center of the knee joint, ie, in the case of a significant varus malalignment, the deviation of the mechanical axis (MAD) from the center of the knee joint will be more than 15 mm medially [3]. The distance between the femoral condyles (intercondylar distance) is increased (Fig 1-6a–b, Table 1-3).

5.2   Genu valgum

In valgus malalignment of the lower extremity the anatomical femorotibial angle (aFTA) is less than 173–175° and the Mikulicz line lies laterally to the 4 mm point. The deviation of the mechanical axis from the center of the knee joint is larger than 10 mm laterally if there is a significant valgus deviation [3]. The distance between the medial malleoli is increased (Fig 1-6a, Fig 1-6c, Table 1-4).

The systematic analysis of leg deformities in the sagittal and transversal plane is described in chapter 11 "Osteotomy and ligament instability: tibial slope corrections and combined procedures around the knee joint" and chapter 15 "Rotational osteotomies of the femur and the tibia".

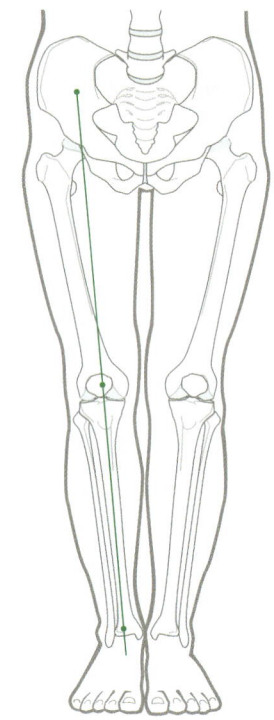

a

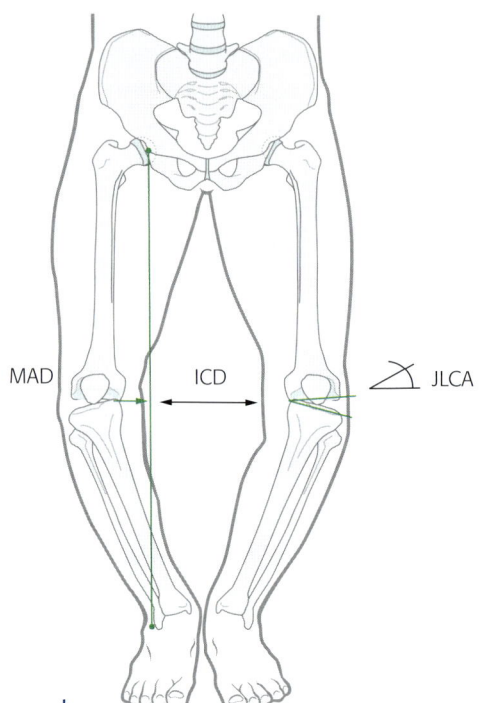

b

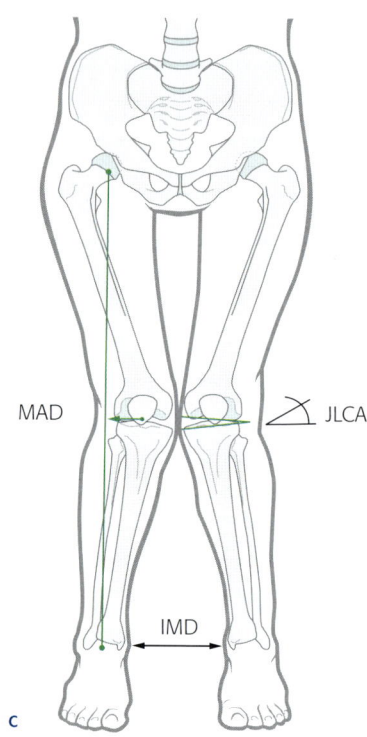

c

Fig 1-6a–c   Lower limb deformities in the frontal plane.

a   Physiological axes of the lower extremity. The mechanical axis runs 4 (±2) mm medial to the center of the knee joint.

b   Genu varum with an increased anatomical femorotibial angle (aFTA >173–175°). The Mikulicz line runs medial to the 4 mm point (MAD >15 mm medially, green line) and the intercondylar distance (ICD) is increased. The joint forms an open angle laterally (JLCA).

c   Genu valgum with decreased anatomical femorotibial angle (aFTA <173–175°). The weight-bearing axis runs lateral to the 4 mm point and the distance between the medial malleoli (intermalleolar distance = IMD) is increased. The angle between the tibial plateau and the tangent to the femoral condyles (JLCA) is opened medially.

6   Consequences of lower limb deformities

In the presence of tibial or femoral deviations in the frontal plane, forces can no longer be transferred uniformly at the knee joint. Instead, nonphysiological load distribution with mechanical stress occurs in the medial or lateral compartment. The mechanical overload of a joint compartment correlates with cartilage damage [5] and promotes the development of degenerative joint disease or accelerates its progress [6, 7]. Deformities of the lower extremity are regarded as so-called prearthritic deformities [4].

- In the presence of tibial or femoral deviations, the transfer of mechanical stress in the joint is no longer uniform because load is distributed nonphysiologically more to the medial or lateral compartment. Deviations of lower extremity axes are regarded as so-called prearthritic deformities.

Osteotomies around the knee that alter the weight-bearing axis of the lower extremity have a substantial effect on the load balance and the distribution of pressure at the knee joint [8]. Both proximal tibial head osteotomies and supracondylar femoral osteotomies can be performed in additive technique (open-wedge) or subtractive technique (closed-wedge), and are regarded as established procedures for the restoration of the physiological axes and the treatment of varus and valgus osteoarthritis, provided that the deformity is situated adjacent to the knee joint. If the deformity is not located around the joint but in the diaphysis of the long bones, the correction should be performed at the site of the diaphyseal deviation [3].

- Femoral and tibial osteotomies around the knee facilitate the restoration of the physiological axes of the lower limb and are regarded as an established procedure in the treatment of varus and valgus osteoarthritis.

7 Bibliography

[1] **Morrison J** (1968) Bioengineering analysis of force actions transmitted by the knee joint. *Bio-Med Eng;* 3:164–170.

[2] **Morrison J** (1969) Function of the knee in various activities. *Bio-Med Eng;* 4:573–580.

[3] **Paley D, Pfeil J** (2000) [Principles of deformity corrections around the knee.] *Orthopäde;* 29(1):18–38. German.

[4] **Schmitt E, Heisel J, Jani L, et al** (2002) [Axial deformities around the knee joint.] Leitlinien der Orthopädie. Deutsche Gesellschaft für Orthopädie und orthopädische Chirurgie. Köln: Ärzte-Verlag. German.

[5] **Cicuttini F, Wluka A, Hankin J, et al** (2004) Longitudinal study of the relationship between knee angle and tibiofemoral cartilage volume in subjects with knee osteoarthritis. *Rheumatology;* 43(3):321–324.

[6] **Cerejo R, Dunlop DD, Cahue S, et al** (2002) The influence of alignment on risk of knee osteoarthritis progression according to baseline stage of disease. *Arthritis Rheum;* 46(10):2632–2636.

[7] **McKellop H A, Sigholm G, Redfern FC** (1991) The effect of simulated fracture-angulations of the tibia on cartilage pressures in the knee joint. *J Bone Joint Surg Am;* 73(9):1382–1391.

[8] **Maquet PG** (1984) *Biomechanics of the knee: with applications of the pathogenesis and the surgical treatment of osteoarthritis.* 2nd ed. Berlin Heidelberg New York: Springer-Verlag.

2   Clinical and radiological evaluation

1   Clinical examination

Patient history and clinical examination are the baseline of any preoperative work up for osteotomies around the knee. History of trauma or previous surgery, and professional activity and sports, are of special interest. The expected patient activity level is to be considered. Contraindications such as nicotine abuse, which often leads to delayed consolidation of the osteotomy, overweight, rheumatoid arthritis, and patient age over 60–70 years, where knee arthroplasty leads to better results [1, 2], must be ruled out. Nevertheless, consideration of biological age should take priority over chronological age.

Clinical examination includes evaluation of soft tissue and skin as well as vascular and neurological status of the lower extremity. Systemic or local infection should be ruled out.

The range of motion of the knee should be inspected. At least 120° of flexion and not more than 20° extension deficit are mandatory. Anteroposterior and mediolateral ligamenteous stability should be examined and the leg length must be inspected. The alignment of the lower extremity is evaluated under full weight bearing and in the supine position. If the medial compartment is involved, movement under varus stress is painful, whereas valgus stress should reduce pain.

The authors classify three different groups of patients which can be treated by osteotomy around the knee:
- Patients with unicompartmental arthritis
- Patients with malalignment of the leg and ligamenteous instability of the knee
- Patients with complex deformities

1.1   Unicompartmental osteoarthritis

The most common group of patients presents with unicompartmental medial or lateral femorotibial osteoarthritis. These patients complain about pain in the affected joint compartment during weight bearing. If pain is not located exclusively either over the medial compartment or the lateral joint space, the indication for osteotomy should be reconsidered. Femoropatellar pain with significant degenerative changes of the cartilage is considered as a relative contraindication for osteotomy. Special attention should be addressed to the subjective pain level, for example with the visual analog scale (VAS). In the authors' experience, patients suffering higher pain levels often have less relief and benefit from osteotomy.

1.2   Knee instability

Another group of patients that can be treated by osteotomy around the knee are patients with varus malalignment of the leg and ligamenteous instability of the knee. Signs of cartilage damage in the medial joint are often present in these patients. In contrast to patients with osteoarthritis, where pain is the leading symptom, instability and giving way of the knee is prominent. Combined procedures with correction osteotomy and ligament reconstruction or two-plane osteotomy (valgization-flexion or valgization-extension osteotomy) are established treatment methods for these patients (see chapter 11 "Osteotomy and ligament instability: tibial slope corrections and combined procedures around the knee joint").

1.3 Complex deformities

Mishealed fractures, metabolic and neurological diseases, and congenital disorders can lead to complex deformities of the lower extremity. In patients with complex leg deformities accurate examination is mandatory to localize the level and the character of the deformity. Deviation of the axis is present in more than one plane and/or one level. For example, a varus/ valgus malalignment in the frontal plane might be associated with a flexion/extension deformity in the sagittal plane. Special attention must be given to torsion of the femur and tibia. The clinical and radiological examination of patients with torsional malalignment is described in chapter 15 "Rotational osteotomies of the femur and the tibia".

2 Radiological diagnostics

2.1 Radiographic views

For preoperative assessment of the anatomy and the leg axis radiography of the knee joint in three planes (AP view, lateral view, patella tangential view) (Fig 2-1a–c) and a weight-bearing x-ray of the entire lower limb (Fig 2-1g) are necessary. The weight-bearing x-ray of the leg is essential to assess the correct indication and for the planning of any osteotomy around the knee. The examination is performed in AP projection with a horizontally focused x-ray beam with the patient weight bearing on both legs. Malrotation must be avoided by aligning the patella to the front in the center of the femoral condyles [3].

Weight-bearing x-rays with the knee in a flexion of 45° (so-called "Rosenberg view") (Fig 2-1d) may give information about the degree of changes and the joint collapse, respectively the joint-space narrowing of the affected compartment [4], but are not absolutely necessary.

Varus and valgus stress views of the knee (Fig 2-1e–f) might be helpful to visualize stability of medial and lateral collateral ligaments. Especially in case of lateral laxity in a varus osteo- arthritic knee, overcorrection can be avoided by identifying ligamenteous insufficiency during preoperative planning (see chapter 4 "Basic principles of osteotomies around the knee").

2.2 Magnetic resonance imaging

Magnetic resonance imaging (MRI) is an established imaging technique for assessment of meniscal and ligamenteous lesions and cartilage damage (Fig 2-2). It may give information about the degree of changes in the affected compartment, but it is not mandatory, since the authors always perform a diagnostic arthroscopy of the knee under the same anesthesia prior to the osteotomy to evaluate and document the state of the cartilage.

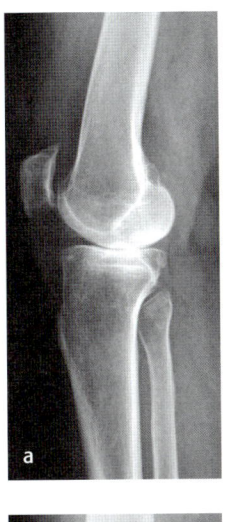
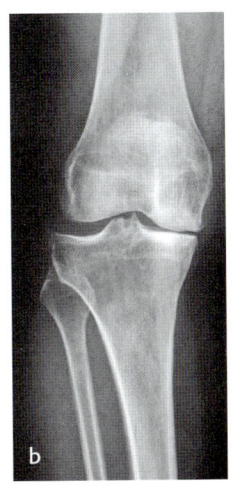
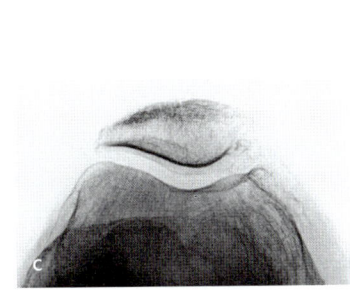
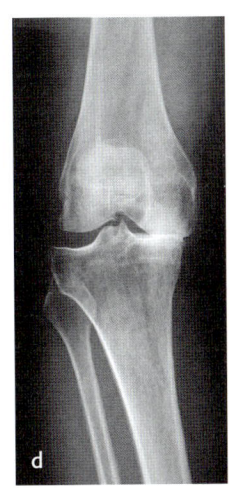
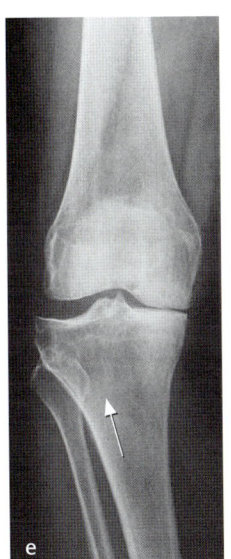
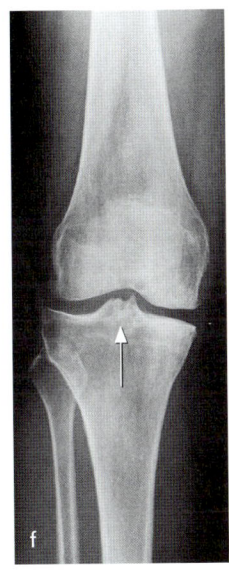
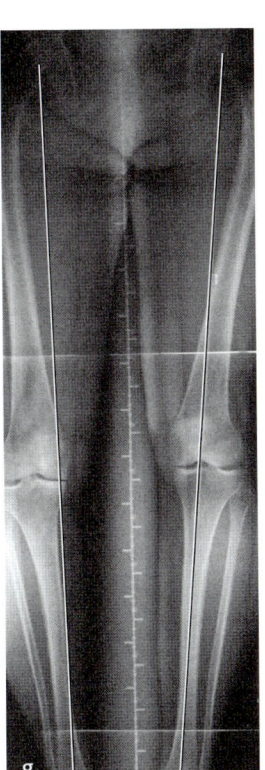

Fig 2-1a–g   Case example. 58-year-old active female with medial osteoarthritis and varus deformity.

a–c Radiographic views show medial osteoarthritis with an intact femoropatellar and lateral femorotibial compartment.

d   The "Rosenberg view" in 45° flexion shows the joint space narrowing under weight bearing.

e–f The varus (e, arrow) stress view and the valgus (f, arrow) stress wwan overcorrection by osteotomy if not considered during preoperative planning.

g   A weight-bearing view of the leg shows that the right mechanical axis runs through the medial compartment.

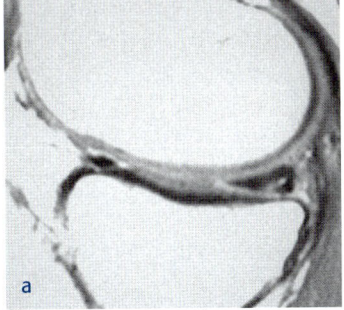
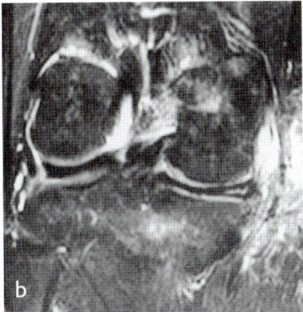

Fig 2-2a–b   MRIs showing a lesion of the posterior horn of the medial meniscus.

2.3 Scintigraphy

Scintigraphy (Fig 2-3) is usually not needed in osteotomy procedures. However, it facilitates identification of overload of the joint before morphological changes are apparent in radiographic views. Hypercaptation beyond the compartment that is to be unloaded might pose a contraindication for shifting of the weight-bearing axis by osteotomy.

2.4 Computer tomography

Computer tomography (CT scan) (Fig 2-4) is rarely indicated in the planning of an osteotomy around the knee. However, in cases with posttraumatic defects or bone lesions, the CT scan facilitates more precise visualization of the deformity. In patients with torsional malalignment of the lower extremity, CT scan is the gold standard for preoperative examination (see chapter 15 "Rotational osteotomies of the femur and the tibia").

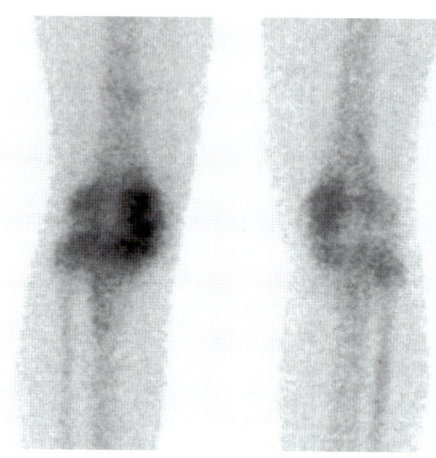

Fig 2-3 Scintigraphy visualizing metabolic hypercaptation in the medial compartment as a sign of overload.

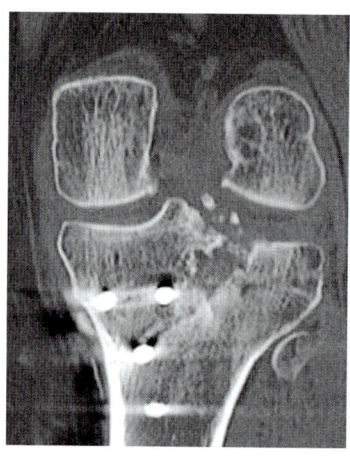

Fig 2-4 CT scan of a 29-year-old patient after open reduction and internal fixation (ORIF) of a tibial head fracture. The CT scan shows the defect of the lateral joint space and the intraarticular fragments.

3 Bibliography

[1] **Job-Deslandre C, Languepin A, Benvenuto M, et al** (1991) [Tibial valgization osteotomy in gonarthrosis with or without chondrocalcinosis. Results after 5 years.] *Rev Rhum Mal Osteoartic;* 58(7):491–496. French.

[2] **Coventry MB** (1987) Proximal tibial varus osteotomy for osteoarthritis of the lateral compartment of the knee. *J Bone Joint Surg Am;* 69(1):32–38.

[3] **Jakob RP, Jacobi M** (2004) [Closing wedge osteotomy of the tibial head in treatment of single compartment arthrosis.] *Orthopäde;* 33(2):143–152. German

[4] **Rosenberg TD, Paulos LE, Parker RD, et al** (1988) The forty-five-degree posteroanterior flexion weight-bearing radiograph of the knee. *J Bone Joint Surg Am;* 70(10):1479–1483.

3   Indications for high-tibial osteotomy, unicondylar knee arthroplasty, and total knee prosthesis

1   Introduction

Monocompartmental osteoarthritis is a common pathology occurring among all age groups. The surgeon is confronted with numerous treatment options and high patient expectations especially in the younger patient group. Medical factors as well as cultural differences have to be taken into account. If the institution treats a large number of knee patients, the entire spectrum of operative procedures should be available. In the author's department, we perform almost the same quantity of osteotomies and unicondylar knee replacements in contrast to a double number of total knee prostheses yearly (Fig 3-1).

This chapter summarizes the present knowledge on indications for high-tibial osteotomy (HTO), unicondylar knee arthroplasty (UKA), and total knee arthroplasty (TKA).

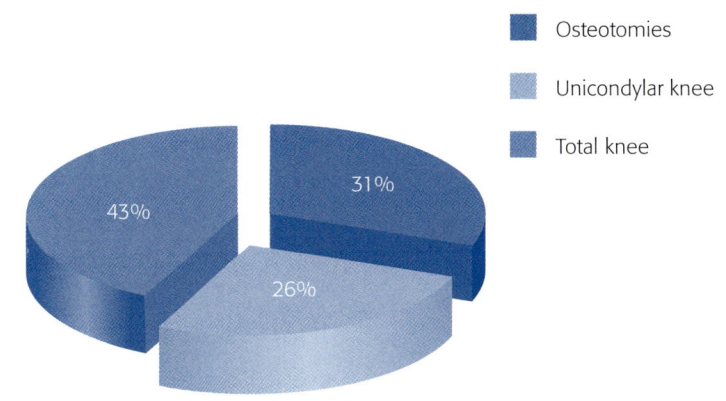

■ Osteotomies

■ Unicondylar knee

■ Total knee

Fig 3-1   Procedures done in the author's institution for monocompartmental osteoarthritis in 2007.

2   Patient selection guidelines

The main patient-derived factors for decision making are:
■ Stage of osteoarthritis
■ Ligamentous status
■ Type of deformity and reducability
■ Age
■ Range of motion
■ Obesity
■ General medical status

2.1   Stage of osteoarthritis

An osteotomy is a biological procedure which aims to shift peak load areas from the medial compartment to central and lateral areas. The best results are obtained in limited chondral defects on the medial side and the outcome will be compromised the more the osteoarthritis has progressed. The patient should be informed that limited pain relief must be expected if there is already 4th degree osteoarthritis on the medial side with relative medial instability [1]. HTO is not indicated in pagoda-type tibiae, meaning severe bone loss on the medial side and a sloped lateral compartment (Fig 3-2). It is very difficult to choose the correction angle in this situation, and failures by under- or overcorrection are common. Unicompartmental knee replacement is advisable in this situation. Obviously HTO is not indicated after substantial lateral meniscectomy and in severe lateral osteoarthritis. MRI scans should not be relied upon in decision-making, since the sensitivity and specifity for chondral defects are low. Arthroscopy tends to overestimate chondral pathology on the lateral side. Softening of the tibial chondral surface is a normal finding in adults and no contraindication against HTO. Superficial fraying of the femoral cartilage is not relevant and can be ignored. Important findings are defect zones in the load-bearing areas and ruptures or deficiencies of the lateral meniscus. We rely more on stress x-rays in questionable cases and consider significant closure of the lateral joint side under valgus stress as an exclusion criteria for HTO and also for a UKA (Fig 3-3).

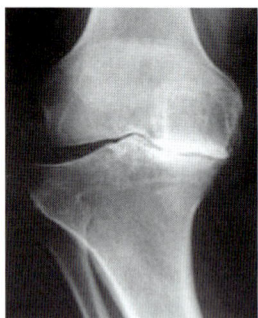

Fig 3-2   Severe osteoarthritis and tibial deformity (Pagoda type) are contraindications for an osteotomy.

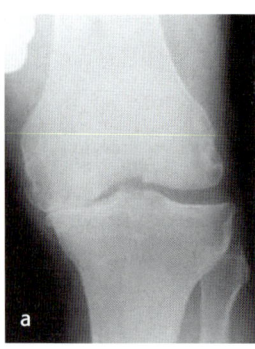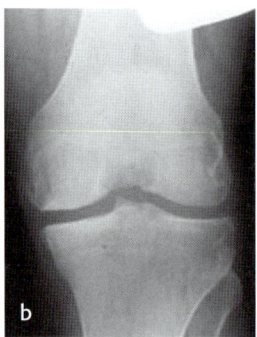

Fig 3-3a–b   Stress x-rays are important for the indications of HTO and UKA.
a   This x-ray was made under varus stress with the beam parallel to the joint plane and demonstrates full-thickness defect of the cartilage on the medial side.
b   This x-ray was made under valgus stress and demonstrates a functionally intact lateral compartment. HTO as well as UKA require such an intact lateral compartment.

2.2   Patellofemoral joint

Many patients with medial joint pain have degenerative changes in the patellofemoral joint as well. If the clinical symptoms are clearly those of medial osteoarthritis, these changes can be ignored in the decision-making process and should not guide the surgeon towards a TKA. Certainly the patient has to be informed that stair climbing or downhill walking may be compromised after the procedure but the leading symptoms of joint-line pain will be cured, as in patients without patellofemoral joint pathology. In open-wedge HTO it is advisable to use the modified biplanar technique with the anterior osteotomy plane sloped downwards (see chapter 15 "Rotational osteotomies of the tibia and femur", Fig 15-4). This modification avoids patella infera and rules out pressure increases in the patellofemoral joint [2, 3]. Current literature indicates that at least mobile bearing UKAs can be safely implanted in patients with patellofemoral degeneration without increasing the middle- and long-term revision rate [4–6].

2.3   Ligamentous status

HTO has a wide indication range in patients with instable knees and is a fundamental part of the therapeutic repertoire. The common combination of persistent instability, meniscectomy, and medial osteoarthritis in patients with varus morphotype can be treated ideally by an open-wedge valgus/extension osteotomy of the tibia. The combination of posterior/posterolateral instability and varus morphotype requires a flexion/valgization osteotomy (see chapter 11 "Osteotomy and ligament instability: tibial slope corrections and combined procedures around the knee joint"). The only contraindication for HTO would be a significant deficiency of the medial collateral ligament (MCL) with risk of secondary ligamentous valgus, a situation the author has encountered very rarely. In contrast, in many cases of preexisting MCL injuries the ligament can be retensioned by open-wedge osteotomy if the distal part is not detached during the procedure (see chapter 16 "Total knee arthroplasty after osteotomy around the knee", Fig 16-8).

On the other hand, the correct function of a UKA is strongly dependent on an intact anterior cruciate ligament (ACL). The revision rate is unacceptably high if a UKA is implanted in an ACL deficient knee [5]. In this respect, it is important to understand the morphological differences between medial osteoarthritis in ACL-intact and ACL-deficient knees. If the ACL is intact, the relative position of the tibia on the femur is constant and the osteoarthritis is obligatory anterior on the tibia and distal on the femur which corresponds to the areas with highest physiological load. Since the posterior part of the femur and the tibia will still have a chondral surface, the deformity is restricted to the extended and slightly flexed position of the knee and will reduce completely in flexion. The MCL will be slack in extension due to the wear, and tight in flexion because the intact chondral surfaces retension the ligament.

In ACL deficiency, the tibia will shift to an anterior position relative to the femur. The contact point shifts posterior on the tibial plateau and the osteoarthritis will develop posteromedially, often resulting in a dished-form defect of the posteromedial tibia (cupula). At this stage the anterior subluxation of the tibia is fixed and cannot be reduced anymore, meaning that the clinical instability may appear less obvious, although the ACL is completely deficient.

Knowing these mechanisms, the surgeon may rule out cases for UKA simply by carefully assessing the plain lateral x-rays (Fig 3-4), whereas the indication for a HTO may still be given even in chronic ACL deficiency.

If there is concern about the stage of osteoarthritis especially in the lateral compartment, we recommend performing stress x-rays with manual or instrumented varus and valgus stress. If the lateral joint space closes under stress, neither HTO nor UKA are indicated any more, and a total knee replacement is necessary. If the narrowed medial joint space does not open to

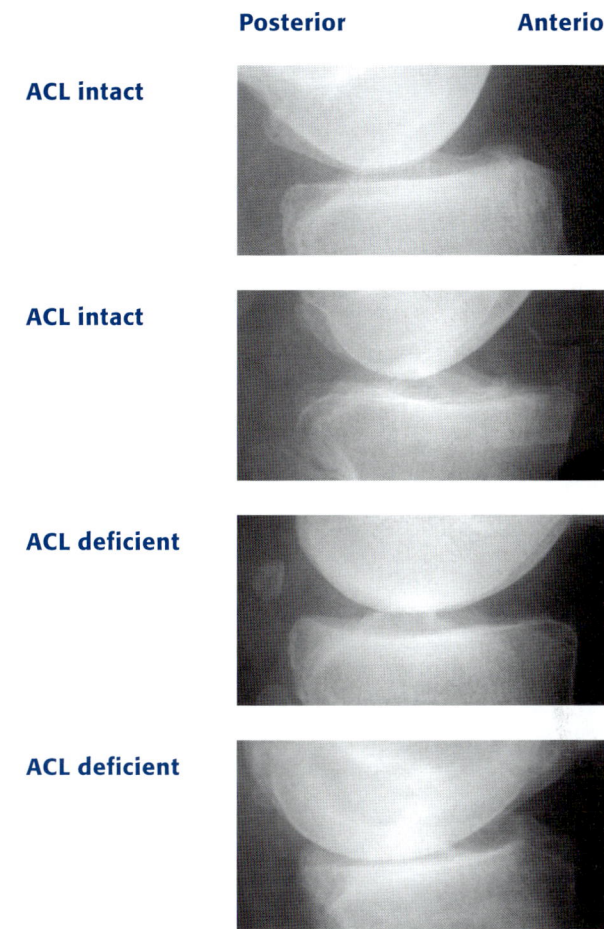

Posterior   **Anterior**

ACL intact

ACL intact

ACL deficient

ACL deficient

Fig 3-4   The localization of the osteoarthritis is important for the indication of HTO and UKA. Careful study of lateral x-rays reveals that with intact ACL the tibial wear is anterior and only with deficient ACL extends to the back of the tibia [5]. At the end of the process the tibia is fixed in the anterior position and a dished-type defect exists on the posteromedial tibia, in which the femur rests (cupula) (from [5]).

the regular width in 20° knee flexion, a contracture of the MCL is present which rules out the typical situation of anteromedial osteoarthritis (see Fig 3-3) and a UKA should not be implanted. For the same reason, a UKA is also not indicated if the osteoarthritis involves the entire medial tibia on a lateral x-ray. In these cases the degeneration has either progressed to general osteoarthritis or is correlated with chronic ACL deficiency and will not respond sufficiently to monocompartmental arthroplasty.

2.4 Type of deformity

Varus malalignment of the leg and overload of the medial side may be caused by three factors:

(1) Meniscectomy and wear on the medial joint side can cause narrowing of the medial joint space with resulting varus deformation.

(2) An osseous deformity mostly of the proximal tibia (metaphyseal varus) will lead to varus morphotype (Fig 3-5).

(3) Theoretically, a lateral ligament deficiency could also induce a deformity, but in practical terms this is extremely unusual and will not be discussed here.

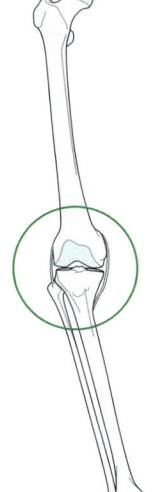
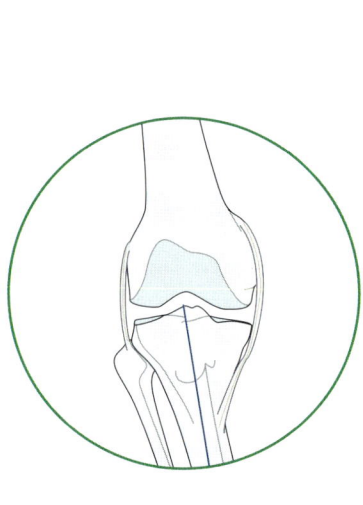
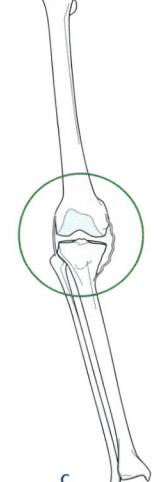
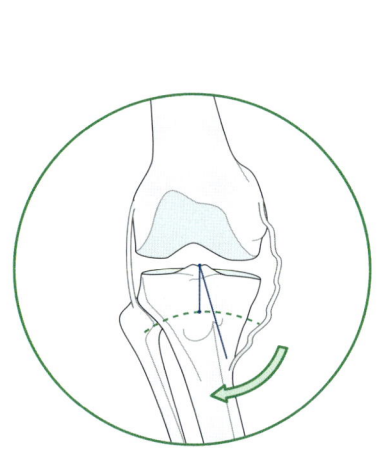

Fig 3-5a–c The different causes for a varus malalignment of the leg.

a A pathological mechanical axis deviation (MAD) should be analyzed for the main factor—wear or bony deformity.

b Intraarticular wear, eventually combined with loss of the medial meniscus may cause collapse of the medial joint space. No extraarticular deformity exists and the entire pathology is intraarticular. This is the ideal scenario for a UKA, as long as the ACL is functionally intact.

c Preexisting metaphyseal varus induces overload and degeneration of the medial joint space. Wear is a secondary phenomenon in this situation. This is the ideal scenario for a HTO, as long as the degeneration has not progressed too far. Implantation of a UKA will not correct the extraarticular deformity and a residual varus will exist which induces significant load on the implant.

Regarding the indications, it is important to understand that an osteotomy is a procedure which best corrects an inherent bony deformity when performed in the region where the bone is angled (level of deformity). In this case the osteotomy will restore the anatomy and especially correct all joint angles to normal (see chapter 1 "Physiological axes of the lower limb"). A slight overcorrection, as is typically aimed for in valgization HTO, creates only a minimal obliquity of the joint line. However, if there is no bony deformity, the osteotomy may correct the mechanical leg axis but will induce a new deformity and a significant obliquity of the joint line (Fig 3-6). It has been proven that in this situation, despite mechanical axis correction, the pain relief is short lived and inconstant, and the revision rate of such osteotomies is high (Table 3-1).

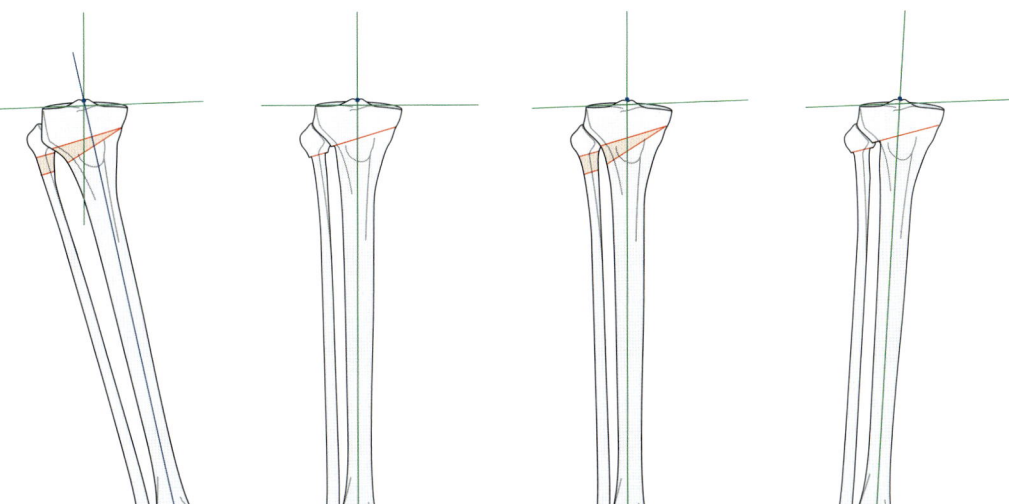

a   b   c   d

Fig 3-6a–d The importance of metaphyseal varus for the result of HTO.
a–b In a case with significant tibial bone varus angle (TBVA) an osteotomy corrects the deformity. The joint line is normalized and knee and ankle joint lines are horizontal.
c–d In a case with a normal tibia morphotype a HTO will create a new deformity. The knee joint line is oblique and knee and ankle joint lines are incongruent. This scenario results in only an inconstant pain relief and a short survival time of an osteotomy.

Tibial bone metapysis axis (°)	Clinical result of high-tibial osteotomy (%)
< 0	36
0–2	56
2–5	71
> 5	83

Table 3-1 Results of high-tibial osteotomy in relation to tibial metaphyseal axis [1].

By contrast, a unicondylar arthroplasty is a surface replacement designed to work in a knee with normal ligament function. This implant can only substitute intraarticular wear and has no influence on any present extraarticular deformity. This means that in cases with an osseous deformity like the common tibia varus, a significant residual varus will persist after the UKA procedure and—unlike the current policy in TKA—the mechanical axis will remain shifted to the medial side. This may compromise the long-term result due to overload of the implant. In addition, implantation of a monocompartmental knee prosthesis in a tibia with metaphyseal varus deformity causes problems because of the medially sloped joint line. Implanting the UKA in line with the healthy cartilage on the lateral side will place the tibial implant obliquely and induce shear stress on the polyethylene. Implanting the tibial tray 90° to the mechanical axis (as in TKA) will cause a discongruency between the medial and lateral tibia plateau in the frontal plane. This may be a problem in fixed-bearing tibial components, whereas mobile bearings seem to tolerate this scenario quite well.

In conclusion, differentiation between the origin of a varus deformity of the leg is important for the indication of HTO versus UKA. Detection of a metaphyseal varus of the tibia is crucial and should guide the surgeon's decision more towards an osteotomy. Identification of intraarticular wear as the main reason of the deformity usually indicates that implantation of an UKA is the correct treatment. In clinical practice, it may be difficult to analyze the anatomy of the proximal tibia because the joint line is no longer apparent on the medial side due to the development of osteoarthritis. The construction of the mechanical medial proximal tibial angle (mMPTA) in the frontal plane will not be precise in this situation. It is advisable to either project the joint line of the healthy joint compartment over to the medial compartment in order to define the former medial joint line [7] or to use the tibial bone varus angle (TBVA) (see chapter 5 "Detailed planning algorithm for high-tibial osteotomy").

This angle depends on the radiological residual of the proximal tibia epiphysis, and indicates the axis of the epiphyseal segment of the tibia. If there is a significant varus between this real joint line and the axis of the tibia shaft, an osteotomy should be considered.

2.5   Obesity

The discussion on the importance of body weight on the development of osteoarthritis and on the outcome of orthopedic procedures is never ending. Generally speaking, the obese patient loads his knee joint more, however, on a lower activity level. There is no clear correlation between body weight and results either for HTO or for unicondylar or total knee prosthesis, except for extreme obesity [1]. In the new generation of plate fixators the mechanical stability and load-bearing tolerance is sufficient enough to abandon patient weight as a risk factor for fixation. In more than 1,000 HTOs performed in the author's institution in the last 8 years, no implant failure or specific surgical complication was observed in direct correlation to weight. Regarding unicondylar knee prosthesis in obese patients the present systems can be implanted via a limited anteromedial arthrotomy, which is also feasible in these patients, without invasive soft-tissue dissection. We feel that no patient should be excluded from these procedures only due to overweight. In contrast, the implantation of a total knee prosthesis often requires an extended approach in these patients and is a significant surgical stress with increased risk.

2.6   Age

If a HTO is performed in a patient with metaphyseal varus deformity of the tibia, a preexisting deformity is corrected. Since this is a prophylactic indication, no lower age limit for this procedure (besides open physes) exists. In young patients without osteoarthritis we would correct to a normal weight-bearing situation, meaning that the mechanical axis runs through the medial spine of the tibial eminence postoperatively (MAD zero) (see chapter 1 "Physiological axes of the lower limb"). Regarding the upper age limit of HTO, the results of HTO tend to be inferior in higher-age groups. Literature and clinical practice in Europe and America indicate that the age limit for an osteotomy in males is 65 years and in females even may be as low as 55 years [1]. The impaired results may be explained by the general progression of osteoarthritis, leading to a disease of the entire knee in many individuals and restricting tolerance of the joint to increased loads on the lateral side. However, in Asia, due to ethical and cultural factors, osteotomies are commonly performed in higher age groups, and these are often successful. Certainly, these age values are arbitrary and strongly depend on the individual patient.

2.7   Activity

HTO is the procedure which allows for the highest postoperative activity level of a patient with monocompartmental osteoarthritis. However, the patient must be informed that he may not be completely pain free during strenuous activity. A correctly implanted UKA allows for a moderate activity level which becomes relevant especially in the middle-aged patient group. There is no outcome data available for patients under 55 years. The outcome studies in patients between 55 and 65 are controversial. Whereas favorable 10-year survival rates comparable to elder patient groups have been published [8, 9] the Finnish arthroplasty register shows a 1.5-fold higher revision rate in patients under 65 years [10] and this finding is supported by recent data from the Australian register. It is certainly wise to counsel patients with a UKA that high-impact sports like running should be avoided, and to consider that presently only sparse outcome data for younger patients (50–65 years) with a hemiarthroplasty is available. The indication in younger patients should be restricted and a too widespread use of these implants in the younger age group will certainly cause a significant revision rate. On the other hand, the UKA is the ideal implant for older patients since the risks of surgery are minimal ("UKA is the meniscectomy of the old patient"). As long as the typical anteromedial osteoarthritis is

treated, there is no upper age limit for this procedure and the risks of a total knee implantation can be avoided. Especially with the use of mobile bearing implants, up to one third of all patients scheduled for a total knee arthroplasty may be potential candidates for a unicondylar arthroplasty.

2.8   Range of motion

Full extension is an important prerequisite for a good result after HTO. Many patients with medial osteoarthritis develop a flexion contracture. With the techniques described in this book, we are able to correct 10° of flexion contracture during the open-wedge high-tibial osteotomy. If more than 10° of extension deficit is present, the indication for HTO should be questioned. A flexion deficit is usually not in the foreground in this patient group and the range-of-motion for flexion will not decrease in consequence of a tibial osteotomy.

Implantation of a unicompartmental prosthesis does not correct range of motion of the knee. In patients with a flexion contracture over 10° and a maximum flexion below 100° an UKA is not indicated. However, in contrast to a total knee replacement the UKA usually allows preservation of the range of motion of the patient and is the best high-flex knee presently available.

2.9   Lateral osteoarthritis

Decision making for patients with isolated lateral osteoarthritis and valgus deformity is similar. If there is an osseous deformity (usually in the femur) and if the patient is suitable for a reconstructive procedure, an osteotomy is advisable (see chapter 13 "Supracondylar varization osteotomy of the femur with plate fixation"). If the deformity is caused by pure wear of the lateral compartment, for example after lateral meniscectomy, and if no bony deformity is detected, a lateral unicondylar arthroplasty should be considered [11]. Good results have been reported with fixed-bearing implants as well as recently with a mobile bearing implant with a biconcave meniscus inlay.

In conclusion, the above mentioned factors allow defining guidelines for the indication for HTO in contrast to UKA [10–13].

The ideal patient for a HTO:
- Is younger than 65 years (male) respectively 55 years (female)
- Has congenital metaphyseal varus deformity of the tibia (TBVA > 5°)
- Has an intact lateral compartment
- Has almost normal range of motion (10° extension deficit may be corrected by the surgery)
- Is a non-smoker
- Has a certain pain tolerance
- May have ACL or PCL deficiency (can be addressed by the surgery)
- Should preferably have a BMI under 30

The ideal candidate for a UKA:
- Is older than 55 years
- Has no osseous deformity and mere intraarticular wear
- Has intact ligaments (ie, ACL, MCL)
- Has a deformity which reduces completely in 20° of flexion under valgus stress
- Has an intact lateral compartment
- Has an almost normal range of motion
- Has no inflammatory disease
- Should preferably have a BMI under 30

The ideal candidate for a TKA:
- Is older than 75 years
- Has generalized and manifest osteoarthritis of the knee
- Has significant and continuous pain during activities of daily life
- May have extension or flexion deficits
- May have axis deviation and bone deficiencies
- Has limited expectations regarding activity and range of motion

4   Bibliography

[1] **Bonnin M, Chambat P** (2004) [Current status of valgus angle, tibial head closing wedge osteotomy in medial gonarthrosis.] *Orthopäde*; 33(2):135–142. German.

[2] **Gaasbeek RD, Sonneveld H, van Heerwaarden RJ, et al** (2004) Distal tuberosity osteotomy in open wedge high tibial osteotomy can prevent patella infera: a new technique. *Knee*; 11(6):457–461.

[3] **Stoffel K, Willers C, Korshid O, et al** (2007) Patellofemoral contact pressure following high tibial osteotomy: a cadaveric study. *Knee Surg Sports Traumatol Arthrosc*; 15(9):1094–1100.

[4] **Beard DJ, Pandit H, Gill HS, et al** (2007) The influence of the presence and severity of pre-existing patellofemoral degenerative changes on the outcome of the Oxford medial unicompartmental knee replacement. *J Bone Joint Surg Br*; 89(12):1597–1601.

[5] **Goodfellow J, O'Connor J, Dodd C, et al** (2006) *Unicompartmental arthroplasty with the Oxford knee.* New York: Oxford University Press.

[6] **Murray DW, Goodfellow JW, O´Connor JJ** (1998) The Oxford medial unicompartmental arthroplast: a ten-year survival study. *J Bone Joint Surg B*; 80(6):983–989.

[7] **Jenny JY, Boéri C, Ballonzoli L, et al** (2005) [Difficulties and reproducibility of radiological measurement of the proximal tibial axis according to Lévigne.] *Rev Chir Orthop Réparatrice Appar Mot*; 91(7):658–663. French.

[8] **Pennington DW, Swienckowski JJ, Lutes WB, et al** (2003) Unicompartmental knee arthroplasty in patients sixty years of age or younger. *J Bone Joint Surg Am*; 85(10):1968–1973.

[9] **Cartier P, Khefacha A, Sanouiller JL, et al** (2007) Unicondylar knee arthroplasty in middle-aged patients: a minimum 5-year follow-up. *Orthopedics*; 30(8 Suppl):62–65.

[10] **Koskinen E, Paavolainen P, Eskelinen A, et al** (2007) Unicondylar knee replacement for primary osteoarthritis: a prospective follow-up study of 1,819 patients from the Finnish Arthroplasty Register. Acta Orthop; 78(1):128–135.

[11] **Servien E, Aitsiseli T, Neyret Ph, et al** (2007) How to select candidates for lateral unicomppartmental prosthesis. *Techn Knee Surg*; 6(1):51–59.

[12] **Robertsson O, Borgquist L, Knutson K, et al** (1999) Use of unicompartmental instead of tricompartmental prostheses for unicompartmental arthrosis in the knee is a cost-effective alternative. 15,437 primary tricompartmental prostheses were compared with 10,624 primary medial or lateral unicompartmental prostheses. *Acta Orthop Scand*; 70(2):170–175.

[13] **Stukenborg-Colsman C, Wirth CJ, Lazovic D, et al** (2001) High tibial osteotomy versus unicompartmental joint replacement in unicompartmental knee joint osteoarthritis: 7-10-year follow-up prospective randomised study. *Knee*; 8(3):187–194.

4   Basic principles of osteotomies around the knee

1   Introduction

After detailed examination of the patient, correct planning is the key to a successful osteotomy. A variety of approaches can be used to achieve a good result. The choice of surgical technique might be influenced by personal preference and experience of the surgeon.

Computer-aided surgery, especially computer-guided navigation, is of increasing interest for osteotomy procedures. It may become a common tool in performing osteotomies around the knee in the future [1] (see chapter 19 "Computer-assisted navigation in proximal tibial osteotomy"). This would of course change the entire planning process. Nevertheless, computer-aided surgery is not standard in all clinics and nowadays, the majority of osteotomies are still planned and performed using conventional techniques.

Understanding normal anatomy of the lower extremity and its physiological angles and axes is essential for planning. The anatomical and mechanical axes and angles are described in detail in chapter 1 "Physiological axes of the lower limb".

The weight-bearing line (Mikulicz line, mechanical axis) of the leg is the connecting line between the center of the femoral head and the center of the ankle joint (see chapter 1 "Physiological axes of the lower limb", Fig 1-3). The point where it crosses the joint line of the knee is of special interest. The distance from this line to the middle of the knee identifies and quantifies mechanical axis deviation (see chapter 1

"Physiological axes of the lower limb", Fig 1-6). Under physiological conditions the crossing point should be located at the center or slightly medial in the knee joint. A deviation can be defined in different ways:

- It can be measured in millimeters from the center of the knee [2–4].
- Fujisawa [6] scales of each compartment separately, from the center of the knee as 0%, to the medial or lateral border as 100% (Fig 4-1). The devation is defined in percentage.
- Another possibility is to scale the entire width of the tibial plateau from the medial border (0%) to the lateral border (100%) (see chapter 9 "High-tibial open-wedge valgization osteotomy with plate fixator", Fig 9-15).

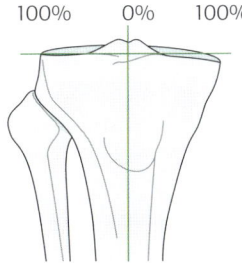

Fig 4-1   Fujisawa scale [6]. The center of the knee is defined as 0% and the medial and lateral border of the joint as 100%.

2   Localization of deformity

The nature of the deformity should be understood before planning is done. The malalignment test described in chapter 1 "Physiological axes of the lower limb", subchapter 5 "Systematic analysis of axial deformities" helps to localize the level of the deformity (see chapter 1 "Physiological axes of the lower limb", Fig 1-5). Axial deformities can exist due to isolated deformity of either femur or tibia, or due to combined deviations of the long bones. It is important to identify patients with complex deformities, as they need more detailed analysis and planning (see chapter 14 "Double osteotomies of the femur and the tibia") [2–4]. However, the majority of patients who are candidates for a correction osteotomy present with minor deformities localized around the knee joint. Even with a mechanical axis deviation within the physiological range, an unloading osteotomy might be indicated in order to prevent further development of osteoarthritis.

3   Planning step A

Prerequisites for the planning process are:
- A good quality weight-bearing x-ray of the entire lower extremity
- Definition of the type and localization of the deformity
- Knowledge of any associated ligamenteous instability

3.1   Level of the osteotomy

Determination of the level and kind of correction is the first step in planning an osteotomy procedure. Several planning methods with different advantages and disadvantages exist. The choice might be guided by the technique the surgeon is most comfortable with. However, the following principles must be considered in all methods:

- The osteotomy should be performed at the apex of the deformity. This will result in an optimal correction. Performing an osteotomy at a different level will not restore the physiological axes but create a new deformity.
- The metaphysis of a long bone is the region of best healing capacity. Bone healing is significantly decreased at the diaphyseal bone. The anatomy of the distal femur needs for osteotomy at the metadiaphyseal junction, whereas tibial osteotomy can easily be performed in the metaphysis. Therefore, healing time favors tibial osteotomy. Especially open-wedge osteotomy of the distal femur can result in delayed union or nonunion. The most favorable location of hinge points for different types of osteotomies around the knee are displayed in Table 4-1.
- Open-wedge osteotomies are generally easier and more precise to perform than closed-wedge osteotomies. Furthermore, the opening procedure allows for intraoperative "fine-tuning" by adjusting the opening with a spreader. In most cases bone grafting is unnecessary when angular stable implants are used [7, 8].
- A closed-wedge osteotomy at the lateral proximal tibia has been the classic procedure for treatment of varus osteoarthritis. Long-term results are good to excellent [9–13]. Nevertheless, the necessity of an osteotomy of the proximal fibula might damage the peroneal nerve. The incidence of postoperative lesions ranges from 2–16% [14–16].

- Sagittal instability can be influenced favorably by alteration of the tibial slope (see below and in chapter 11 "Osteotomy and ligament instabilitiy: tibial slope corrections and combined procedures around the knee joint").
- Restoring or preserving the horizontal joint line (midjoint line) is mandatory for achieving a good result [17].

3.2   Correction of the sagittal plane

If anterior knee instability (ie, ACL insufficiency) is present, the tibial slope should be decreased, whereas in posterior cruciate ligament (PCL) insufficiency the slope should be increased [18–20]. If the slope exceeds 8–10° in case of chronic anterior knee instability, it is advisable to decrease the slope to 5° in order to minimize the anterior force vector, provided the sagittal correction does not cause hyperextension of the knee joint.

Chronic PCL instability will improve at a tibial slope of about 12° since the increased slope creates an anterior force vector. The effect of tibial slope correction is described in detail in chapter 11 "Osteotomy and ligament instabilitiy: tibial slope corrections and combined procedures around the knee joint".

3.3   Correction of the transversal plane

Transversal plane or rotation deformities of the lower limb should be corrected at the level where the deformity is present. As patellar tracking may be changed significantly after corrections around the knee, it is important to analyze patellofemoral alignment. Evaluation, planning, and correction are described in detail in chapter 15 "Rotational osteotomies of the femur and the tibia".

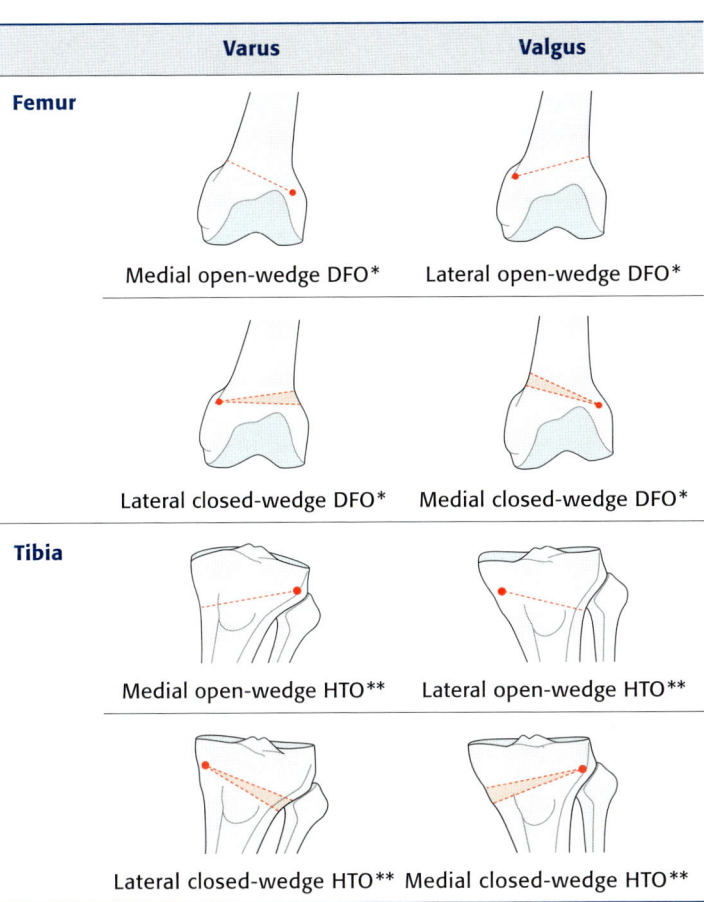

Table 4-1   Location of hinge points for planning of varus (left) and valgus (right) corrections of the distal femur (above) and proximal tibia (below) in a left knee.
*DFO = distal femur osteotomy
**HTO = high-tibial osteotomy

3.4 Amount of correction

Under physiologic conditions, the mechanical axis passes through the center of the knee or slightly medial of it (see chapter 1 "Physiological axes of the lower limb"). However, in a well-aligned knee, load distribution is not well-balanced but physiologically 60% in the medial and 40% in the lateral compartment [21]. Therefore it is not sufficient to restore a physiological alignment in cases of medial osteoarthritis. Instead, overcorrection by shifting the weight-bearing line slightly to the lateral compartment is recommended. The authors define the corrected axis between 10% and 35% laterally on the Fujisawa-scale [6] (Fig 4-2), whereby higher corrections are chosen for cases with more severe osteoarthritis. The aim of the mechanical axis is at 10–15% of the scale in the lateral compartment for patients who have lost one third of their medial compartment cartilage, 20–25% if two thirds of medial cartilage is lost, and at 30–35% if the medial cartilage is completely lost [18].

In patients with valgus deformity together with lateral compartment osteoarthritis, the corrected mechanical axis can be planned at 0–20% medially on the scale depending on cartilage loss. Overcorrection to the opposite compartment does not seem to be as important as in case of varus osteoarthritis, as the load distribution in the knee is not symmetric (Fig 4-2) [21].

Residual cartilage	Planned axis
Two third	10–15%
One third	20–25%
None	30–35%

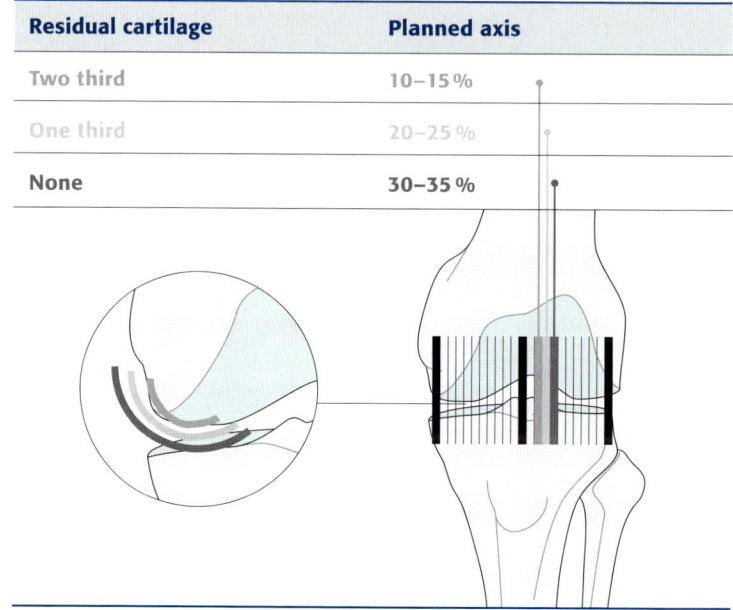

Fig 4-2 Fujisawa scale. Determination of the correction depending on residual cartilage thickness in the involved compartment, eg, if only one third of the cartilage thickness is left in the medial compartment, the mechanical axis should be corrected to 20–25% on the Fujisawa scale in the lateral compartment.

4   Planning step B (Miniaci method)

Once the localization and kind of osteotomy is defined the preoperative drawing can be done. This can be done either on the weight-bearing x-ray of the leg or at a digital work station. Several methods of planning an osteotomy are described in the literature [5, 22–24]. Based on a study by Fujisawa et al [6] and the planning method described by Miniaci [23], the authors have developed a technique to define the correction angle. The planning procedure includes three steps [23, 25–27] and is demonstrated in this chapter for a varus osteoarthritis knee.

Step 1

The first step is only necessary in cases of lateral knee instability in a valgization osteotomy: To avoid overcorrection, instability or laxity of the lateral collateral ligament must be taken into account. A virtual "push view" image is drawn (Fig 4-3a–c). Valgus and varus stress x-rays are required. First, the bony contour of the tibia is traced on a transparent paper. Then the height of the joint spaces of the stressed compartments, as seen in the stress views, is added to the drawing. The tibia is now superimposed on the weight-bearing x-ray of the leg in the corrected position, whereby the distracted medial and lateral joint space are included. The corrected x-ray is the scaffold for further planning. This method helps to avoid overcorrection due to lateral instability.

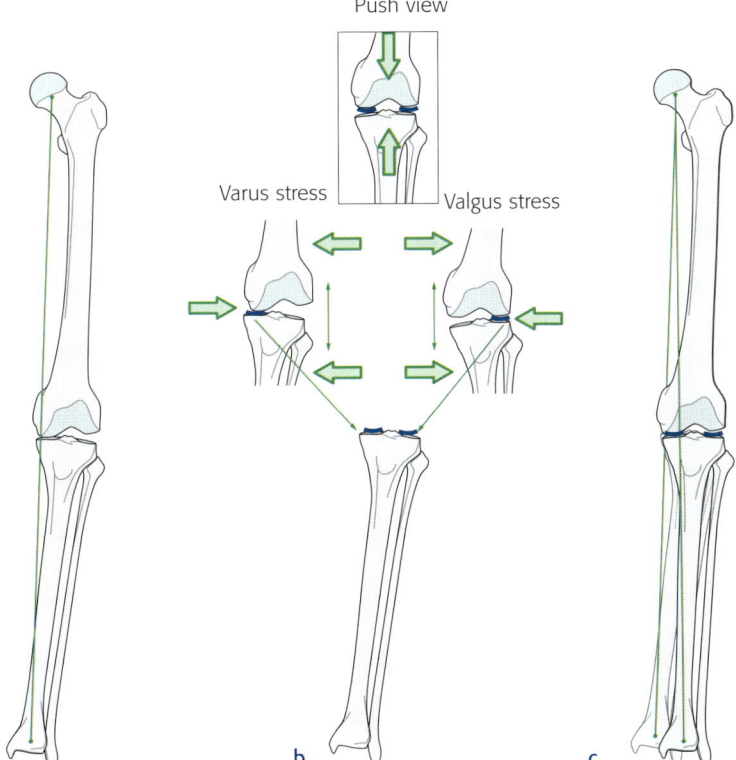

Push view

Varus stress   Valgus stress

Fig 4-3a–f

a–c The virtual "push view" helps to avoid overcorrection due to lateral instability. The joint spaces seen in the varus and valgus stress view (green arrows) are added to the tibial plateau. The tibia is superimposed on the weight-bearing x-ray of the leg in the corrected position with the joint spaces taken into account.

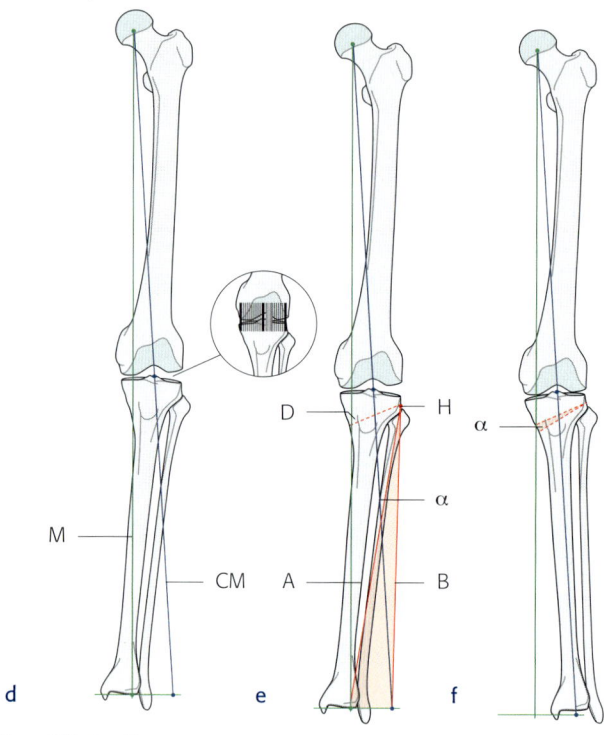

M   = Mikulicz line
CM = corrected mechanical axis
D   = mediolateral diameter of the osteotomy
H   = hinge
A   = line connecting hinge and preoperative center of ankle joint
B   = line connecting hinge and postoperative center of ankle joint
α   = correction angle

Fig 4-3a–f (cont)
d–f Determination of correction angle.

Step 2

In a valgization osteotomy, the mechanical axis is planned between 10 and 35% in the lateral compartment on the Fujisawa scale [6] (see Fig 4-2) depending on the severity of medial cartilage loss and between 0 and 20% in the medial compartment for varization osteotomy.

Step 3

The correction angle of the osteotomy and the height of the osteotomy gap are defined using the planning technique described by Miniaci [23]. The new weight-bearing line is drawn from the center of the femoral head, passing the knee at the point defined in step 2 to the height of the ankle joint line. The hinge of the osteotomy (H) is defined at the lateral cortex of the tibia and connected distally with the new and the old center of the ankle joint. The correction angle α can be measured between the two lines A and B (Fig 4-3d–f). The angle of correction at the proximal tibia corresponds to angle α between lines A and B.

Hernigou [28] developed a trigonometric chart which allows for determination of the opening of the osteotomy gap based on the mediolateral diameter of the osteotomy (D, Fig 4-3e) and the desired correction angle (see Table 4-1). Nevertheless, this should not replace preoperative radiographic planning.

Alternative planning algorithms for high-tibial osteotomy are described in the following chapter (see chapter 5 "Detailed planning algorithm for high-tibial osteotomies"). For planning of a supracondylar femoral varization osteotomy see chapter 13 "Supracondylar varization osteotomy of the femur with plate fixation".

Trigonometric chart

Mediolateral diameter (D) of the osteotomy (mm)	Correction angle	4°	5°	6°	7°	8°	9°	10°	11°	12°	13°	14°	15°	16°	17°	18°	19°
50 mm		3	4	5	6	7	8	9	10	10	11	12	13	14	15	16	16
55 mm		4	5	6	7	8	9	10	10	11	12	13	14	15	16	17	18
60 mm		4	5	6	7	8	9	10	11	12	14	15	16	17	18	19	20
65 mm		5	6	7	8	9	10	11	12	14	15	16	17	18	19	20	21
70 mm		5	6	7	8	10	11	12	13	15	16	17	18	20	21	22	23
75 mm		5	6	8	9	10	12	13	14	16	17	18	20	21	22	24	25
80 mm		6	7	8	10	11	13	14	15	17	18	19	21	22	24	25	26

Table 4-2   Trigonometric chart by Hernigou [27]. The osteotomy gap opening (in mm) depends on the mediolateral width of the osteotomy (in mm) and the planned correction angle, eg, if a correction of 11° is necessary in a horizontal osteotomy with a mediolateral diameter of 65 mm (line D) (see Fig 4-2), the opening of the osteotomy is 12 mm.

5 Formation of a surgical plan

The preparation for deformity corrections around the knee using diagnostics and planning of deformity correction will only lead to a predictable good result if this information is part of a surgical plan [29]. The following questions, adapted from fracture treatment planning [30], will help the surgeon to make the final preparations for the surgery:

1. Is the proposed osteotomy site surgically accessible?
2. Can the plan be carried out using intraoperative guides (eg, K-wires, templates, saw guides, etc) to enhance accuracy?
3. Is the location of the cuts biologically viable (living bone, no infection, extreme scarring, neurovascular compromised status, previous musculocutaneous flap surgery)?
4. Is stable fixation possible and which fixation method should be choosen?
5. Can the soft tissues withstand the degree of bony correction anticipated (lengthening, shortening, straightening)?

Answering these questions leads to a specific surgical tactic, which is the last step in the formation of a surgical plan (Table 4-3).

Surgical plan for deformity correction of lower leg		
1 Physical examination	Frontal and sagittal plane	a. Weight-bearing line
		b. Mechanical axis of femur and tibia
		c. Joint orientation angles
		d. Location of deformity (CORA)
	Transversal plane	a. CT limb rotation measurements
		b. Patellar tracking analysis
	Multiplane analysis	
2 Radiological deformity analysis		
3 Correlation of physical examination and radiological deformity analysis		
4 Definition of deformity and aim of correction		
5 Planning of correction		
6 Implant selection		
7 Description of surgical tactic		

Table 4-3   Schematic overview of a surgical plan for deformity correction of the lower leg [29]

6   Bibliography

[1] **Jackson DW, Warkentine B** (2007) Technical aspects of computer-assisted opening wedge high tibial osteotomy. *J Knee Surg;* 20(2):134–141.

[2] **Paley D, Herzenberg JE, Tetsworth K, et al** (1994) Deformity planning for frontal and sagittal plane corrective osteotomies. *Orthop Clin North Am;* 25(3):425–465.

[3] **Paley D, Tetsworth K** (1992) Mechanical axis deviation of the lower limbs. Preoperative planning of multiapical frontal plane angular and bowing deformities of the femur and tibia. *Clin Orthop Relat Res;* 280:65–71.

[4] **Paley D, Tetsworth K** (1992) Mechanical axis deviation of the lower limbs. Preoperative planning of uniapical angular deformities of the tibia or femur. *Clin Orthop Relat Res;* 280:48–64.

[5] **Pape D, Seil R, Adam F, et al** (2004) [Imaging and preoperative planning of osteotomy of tibial head osteotomy.] *Orthopäde;* 33(2):122–134. German.

[6] **Fujisawa Y, Masuhara K, Shiomi S** (1979) The effect of high tibial osteotomy on osteoarthritis of the knee. An arthroscopic study of 54 knee joints. *Orthop Clin North Am;* 10(3):585–608.

[7] **Staubli AE, De Simoni C, Babst R, et al** (2003) TomoFix: a new LCP-concept for open wedge osteotomy of the medial proximal tibia—early results in 92 cases. *Injury;* 34 Suppl 2:B55–B62.

[8] **Lobenhoffer P, Agneskirchner JD** (2003) Improvements in surgical technique of valgus high tibial osteotomy. *Knee Surg Sports Traumatol Arthrosc;* 11(3):132–138.

[9] **Aglietti P, Buzzi R, Vena LM, et al** (2003) High tibial valgus osteotomy for medial gonarthrosis: a 10- to 21-year study. *J Knee Surg;* 16(1):21–26.

[10] **Insall JN, Joseph DM, Msika C** (1984) High tibial osteotomy for varus gonarthrosis: A long-term follow-up study. *J Bone Joint Surg Am;* 66(7):1040–1048.

[11] **Coventry MB, Ilstrup DM, Wallrichs SL** (1993) Proximal tibial osteotomy. A critical long-term study of eighty-seven cases. *J Bone Joint Surg Am;* 75(2):196–201.

[12] **Hernigou P** (1996) [A 20-year follow-up study of internal gonarthrosis after tibial valgus osteotomy. Single versus repeated osteotomy.] *Rev Chir Orthop Réparatrice Appar Mot;* 82(3):241–250. French.

[13] **Rinonapoli E, Mancini GB, Corvaglia A, et al** (1998) Tibial osteotomy for varus gonarthrosis. A 10- to 21-year follow-up study. *Clin Orthop Relat Res;* 353:185–193.

[14] **Flierl S, Sabo D, Hornig K, et al** (1996) Open wedge high tibial osteotomy using fractioned drill osteotomy: a surgical modification that lowers the complication rate. *Knee Surg Sports Traumatol Arthrosc;* 4(3):149–153.

[15] **Georgoulis AD, Makris CA, Papageorgiou CD, et al** (1999) Nerve and vessel injuries during high tibial osteotomy combined with distal fibular osteotomy: a clinically relevant anatomic study. *Knee Surg Sports Traumatol Arthrosc;* 7(1):15–19.

[16] **Spahn G, Kirschbaum S, Kahl E** (2006) Factors that influence high tibial osteotomy results in patients with medial gonarthritis: a score to predict the results. *Osteoarthritis Cartilage;* 14(2):190–195.

[17] **Hofman S, Pietsch M, van Heerwaarden R** (2007) [Biomechanical principles and planning for osteotomies around the knee joint.] *Orthopädische Praxis;* 43(3):109–115. German.

[18] **Marti CB, Gautier E, Wachtl SW, et al** (2004) Accuracy of frontal and sagittal plane correction in open-wedge high tibial osteotomy. *Arthroscopy;* 20(4):366–372.

[19] **Reichwein F, Nebelung W** (2007) [High tibial flexion osteotomy for revision of posterior cruciate ligament instability.] *Unfallchirurg;* 110(7):597–602. German.

[20] **Noyes FR, Barber-Westin SD, Hewett TE** (2000) High tibial osteotomy and ligament reconstruction for varus angulated anterior cruciate ligament-deficient knees. *Am J Sports Med;* 28(3):282–296.

[21] **Johnson F, Leitl S, Waugh W** (1980) The distribution of load across the knee. A comparison of static and dynamic measurements. *J Bone Joint Surg Br;* 62(3):346–349.

[22] **Coventry MB** (1985) Upper tibial osteotomy for osteoarthritis. *J Bone Joint Surg Am;* 67(7):1136–1140.

[23] **Miniaci A, Ballmer FT, Ballmer PM, et al** (1989) Proximal tibial osteotomy. A new fixation device. *Clin Orthop Relat Res;* 246:250–259.

[24] **Dugdale TW, Noyes FR, Styer D** (1992) Preoperative planning for high tibial osteotomy. The effect of lateral tibiofemoral separation and tibiofemoral length. *Clin Orthop Relat Res;* 274:248–264.

[25] **Gautier E, Jakob RP** (1996) [The value of corrective osteotomies—indications, technique, results.] *Ther Umsch;* 53(10):790–796. German.

[26] **Jakob RP, Jacobi M** (2004) [Closing wedge osteotomy of the tibial head in treatment of single compartment arthrosis.] *Orthopäde;* 33(2):143–152. German.

[27] **Jacobi M, Jakob RP** (2005) Open wedge osteotomy in the treatment of medial osteoarthritis of the knee. *Tech Knee Surg;* 4(2):70–78.

[28] **Hernigou P** (2002) Open wedge tibial osteotomy: combined coronal and sagittal correction. *Knee;* 9(1):15–20.

[29] **Marti RK, van Heerwaarden RJ** (2008) *Osteotomies for Posttraumatic Deformities.* 1st ed. AO Publishing, Switzerland. Stuttgart New York: Georg Thieme Verlag.

[30] **Mast J, Jakob R, Ganz R** (1989) *Planning and reduction technique in fracture surgery.* 1st ed. Berlin Heidelberg New York: Springer Verlag.

Authors Dietrich Pape, Philipp Lobenhoffer, Mellany Galla

5 Detailed planning algorithm for high-tibial osteotomy

1 Introduction

Valgization osteotomy of the proximal tibia remains the treatment of choice for the young active patient with a progressively symptomatic varus knee and mild to moderate osteoarthritis. Although the natural history of the varus knee is not well established, it is widely accepted that patients with varus malalignment are prone to develop more severe medial compartment osteoarthritis unless the normal mechanics of the knee are restored [1–3]. Careful preoperative planning is mandatory to avoid undercorrection or overcorrection, two factors held responsible for early failure of the procedure [4–6].

Different planning methods may use different definitions for joint center, axis, and weight-bearing line.

For the definitions of physiological axes and angles of the lower limb see chapter 1 "Physiological axes of the lower limb".

The following planning methods are applicable for deformities in and near the knee joint in the absence of gross angular deformities of the long bones due to fracture pseudarthrosis or osteomalacia.

2 Radiographic work-up

Preoperative radiographic evaluation for high-tibial osteotomy (HTO) includes bilateral weight-bearing AP views in full extension and bilateral weight-bearing (PA) tunnel views in 45° of flexion (Rosenberg view, [7]). These allow an assessment of both the extent of knee arthritis and lower extremity alignment. Lateral and skyline views of the involved knee are also obtained. The planning should be performed on a long-leg weight-bearing AP x-ray including the hip and ankle joint obtained in correct rotation of the knee with the patient loading both legs. The authors' preferred planning method is based on this long-leg x-ray.

In clinical settings where hip and ankle joint centers cannot be simultaneously radiographed ("short AP view"), the exposed part of the distal femur and proximal tibia should be as long as possible. This allows for accurate measurements using the anatomic axis of both femur and tibia. Proper rotation of the limb is important and requires the patella to be centered between the femoral condyles and directed forward in the AP projection. Standardized technique is mandatory to assure that the x-rays are reproducible. In cases with a significant extension deficit, separate x-rays of the femur and tibia need to be obtained to enable accurate planning. Soft-tissue laxity can be quantified by the amount of medial joint opening between the involved and contralateral legs on the Rosenberg view [7] (Fig 5-1).

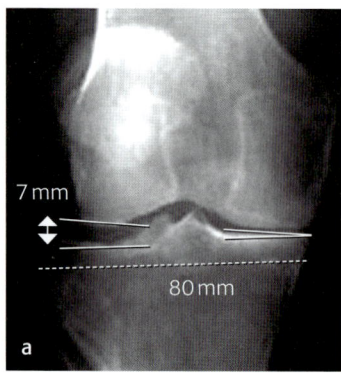
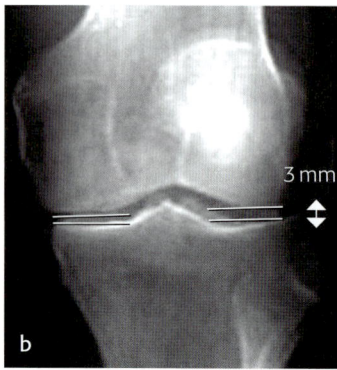

7 mm

3 mm

80 mm

a

b

Fig 5-1a–b   The Rosenberg view allows an assessment of the extent of knee arthritis [7] and helps to evaluate the amount of soft-tissue laxity contributing to the varus alignment.

3   Etiology of varus alignment

Total varus angulation of the knee is the sum of three potential components [8]:
1. The femorotibial geometric alignment
2. Narrowing of the medial joint space due to wear and tear of the meniscus and the osteocartilaginous complex
3. Separation of the lateral joint space due to lax lateral soft tissues and ligaments

The femorotibial alignment can be quantified by the mechanical or anatomical angle as mentioned above. Wear and tear of the medial compartment with consecutive joint-space narrowing on x-rays can be quantified by a number of different classification systems [9–11]. The amount of varus angular deformity caused by lateral joint opening must be compensated when planning an osteotomy to avoid an overcorrection.

3.1   Mathematical method
The side-to-side difference in lateral joint separation can be measured on the Rosenberg view (Fig 5-1). The following equation defines the amount of increased varus angulation resulting from a given separation of the lateral tibiofemoral joint due to slack lateral restraints (soft-tissue laxity) [8]:

$$\beta = \frac{c \times (\Delta S)}{TW}$$

Where ΔS equals the increments of lateral joint separation as a side-to-side difference, TW equals the tibial width, and c being a named constant of 76.4. The following case illustrates the equation: A 40-year-old male patient with progressive right medial knee pain has a lateral joint opening on varus testing following a twisting injury to his knee. A weight-bearing full-length x-ray shows a varus angular deformity of 7°. The Rosenberg view displays a 4 mm increase in lateral joint opening (Fig 5-1). The tibial plateau measures 80 mm in width. In this case, the calculated amount of varus angular deformity caused by slack lateral soft-tissue restraints is

$$\frac{76.4 \times (4\ mm)}{80\ mm} = 3.8°$$

Failure to account for the soft-tissue component of lateral joint opening would result in approximately 3.8° of valgus overcorrection [12].

3.2   Graphical method

In addition to the mathematical approach to quantify an eccentric joint space, there is a graphic alternative that might be more suitable for clinical practice. The tibia is redrawn and copied on glassine paper with the original x-ray underneath. After compensating the eccentric joint line the tibia is then fixed in the new position and the required degree of correction can easily be measured.

4   The aim of high-tibial osteotomy

The optimal correction and preoperative planning method recommended for varus knee deformities varies according to the author (Table 5-1). Both mechanical or anatomical femoro-tibial angles and the weight-bearing line can be used to plan the surgery. Coventry [13] recommended overcorrection of the varus alignment to at least 8° of anatomic femorotibial valgus based on regression analysis of the longevity of high-tibial osteotomies. Hernigou [14] used the mechanical limb axis and found good clinical results in patients with a mechanical valgus angle between 3–6°. Smaller (< 3°) or greater (> 6°) correction angles were associated with poorer clinical results. Recently, Dugdale and Noyes [12] showed that correcting an

Author	Preoperative planning using:	Desired postoperative angle of correction (valgus)	Desired postoperative position of the WBL as a percentage of the tibial plateau width
Coventry [13]	Anatomical axis	8–10°	–
Engel et al [4]	Anatomical axis	5–10°	–
Kettelkamp et al [5]	Anatomical axis	> 5°	–
Koshino et al [17]	Anatomical axis	6–15°	–
Hernigou et al [14]	Mechanical axis	3–6°	–
Ivarsson [18]	Mechanical axis	3–6°	–
Myrnerts [19]	Mechanical axis	3–6°	–
Miniaci et al [16]	WBL		60–70%
Noyes et al [20]	WBL		62%
Dugdale et al [8]	WBL		50–75%

Table 5-1   Recommended correction angles (weight-bearing line = WBL).

angular deformity based on the weight-bearing line (WBL) (Fig 5-2, Fig 5-3) accounts for tibial and femoral length and is more accurate than relying on the femorotibial angle as determined from limited x-rays. They recommended aiming for a postoperative WBL, cutting the proximal tibia on a point 62–66% of the tibial width in the frontal plane. This point usually corresponds to the lateral inclination of the lateral tibial spine and to a mechanical femorotibial valgus angle of 3–5°. The preference to use the WBL for planning an osteotomy is based on the study by Fujisawa [15] who demonstrated that cartilage ulceration did not further deteriorate after HTO in cases where the WBL passed through the optimum zone. He divided the tibia in two halves and defined this optimum zone as 30–40% width of the lateral half of the plateau. This corresponds to the recommendations of Miniaci [16] (60–70% width of the tibial plateau) and Noyes [9] (62% width of the plateau) since these authors based their calculations on the entire width of the tibia as 100% and not on the lateral half of the plateau as Fujisawa did (Fig 5-2).

- Use long-leg weight-bearing x-rays if possible.
  Assure symmetrical weight bearing and correct rotation for planning x-rays.
  Use weight-bearing line as base of planning, if possible.
  In valgization HTO the postoperative weight-bearing line should pass through a point 62% of the width of the tibial plateau on the lateral side, usually corresponding to the down slope of the lateral spine.
  In cases with asymmetric joint opening under weight bearing, the divergence of the femoral and tibial joint lines must be compensated either mathematically or graphically.

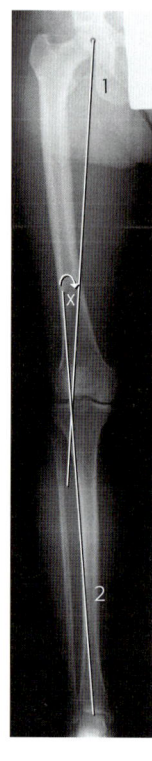

Fig 5-2 Bilateral weight-bearing AP x-ray in full extension for planning a high-tibial osteotomy according to the method by Noyes [8].

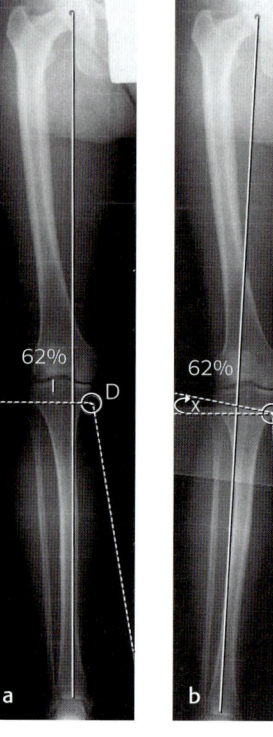

Fig 5-3a–b Using the method by Noyes [8], the template is cut through the osteotomy site and the tibia is rotated until the weight-bearing line (WBL) passes through the 62% coordinate.

5   Preoperative planning in the frontal plane

The preoperative planning methods outlined below can be applied to both closed- and open-wedge osteotomies.

5.1   Planning method according to Miniaci

Miniaci et al [16] recommend using the WBL to determine the frontal/coronal plane correction (Fig 5-4). Line 1 represents the planned WBL for the postoperative correction extending from the center of the hip through a coordinate 60–70% of the tibial plateau width past the ankle. Line 2 connects the osteotomy hinge point (H) with the center of the ankle. With the osteotomy hinge point as the center and the length of line 2 as the radius, an angular arc is drawn from the center of the ankle to the intersection of line 1. Line 3 connects the osteotomy hinge point with the arc intersection of line 1. The angle formed by lines 2 and 3 is the planned correction angle (x).

In closed-wedge osteotomies, the hinge point is located in the medial proximal tibial metaphysis, approximately 2.5 cm below the joint line. In open-wedge osteotomy, this hinge projects onto the lateral proximal metaphysis on the level of the proximal border of the tibiofibular joint, around 15 mm below the subchondral sclerosis zone of the lateral plateau (Fig 5-4). This angle (x) can now be drawn on the proximal tibia using the defined hinge point as tip of the triangle. In closed-wedge osteotomy, the two planes of the osteotomy are marked and the base of the triangle on the lateral cortex corresponds to the height of the wedge to be resected. In open-wedge osteotomy, the triangle should also be drawn and the base of the triangle on the medial cortex corresponds the opening of the osteotomy.

- The defect created by the saw blade must be considered when the surgery is performed.

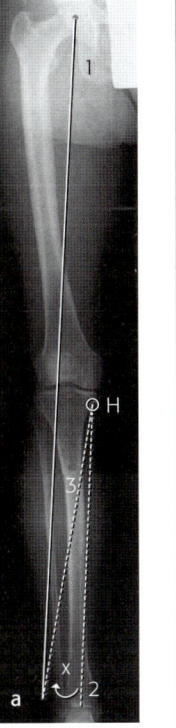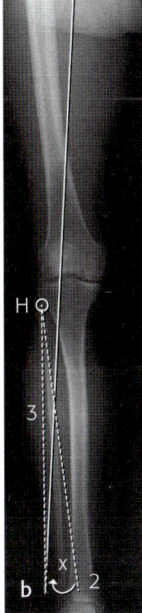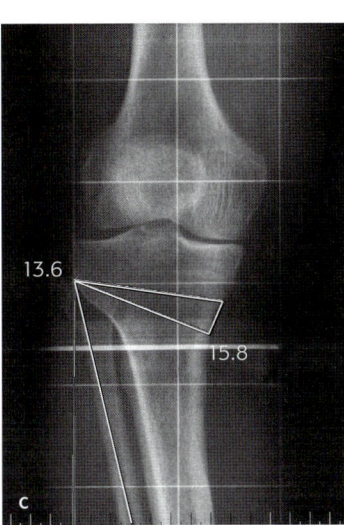

Fig 5-4a–c   Bilateral weight-bearing AP whole lower limb x-ray in full extension for planning a closed-wedge (a) and open-wedge (b and c) high-tibial osteotomy according to the method by Miniaci [16].

c   The correction angle determined in the first steps is now drawn on the prospective site of the osteotomy. The distance of the two lines at the cortex opposite to the hinge point equals the open wedge. A magnification factor of the x-ray must be corrected. Example: correction angle 13.6°, projected opening of the osteotomy 16.9 mm, corrected opening (magnification factor) 15.8 mm.

5.2 Planning method according to Dugdale and Noyes

Dugdale and Noyes [8] use the WBL for preoperative planning, and have described two planning methods. In the first method, line 1 is drawn from the center of the femoral head to the 62.5% of the tibial width. Line 2 is drawn from the center of the tibiotalar joint to the 62.5% coordinate. The angle formed by these two lines is the correction angle (x) (see Fig 5-2). In the second planning method, a line is drawn from the center of the hip to the 62.5% coordinate (see Fig 5-3a), the x-ray is cut in line with the osteotomy side and the distal tibia is rotated until the WBL passes through the 62% coordinate (see Fig 5-3b). The correction angle (x) corresponds to the lateral overlap for lateral closed-wedge osteotomies or the medial opening for medial open-wedge osteotomies.

5.3 Planning method according to Coventry

Coventry [13] based preoperative planning on the anatomic axis with the resected angular wedge (x) being the difference between the planned anatomic axis and the preoperative anatomic axis (Fig 5-5). This method is especially useful if only short AP view x-rays are available.

If the preoperative anatomic axis (AA pre OP) of 4° varus is to be corrected to a postoperative anatomic axis (AA post OP) the following equation can be used:

$$x = (AA_{\text{post OP}}) - (AA_{\text{pre OP}})$$
$$x = 8 - (-4) = 12°$$

The equation applies accordingly if the mechanical axis is used (Fig 5-6) [21] .

In summary, it appears that optimal postoperative alignment in the frontal plane is achieved with a weight-bearing line passing through 62–66% of (lateral) tibial width, a mechanical limb axis of 3–5° of valgus or an anatomical limb axis of 8–10° of valgus. Since all three suggested planning methods arrive at equivalent correction angles, all methods are equally suitable [21].

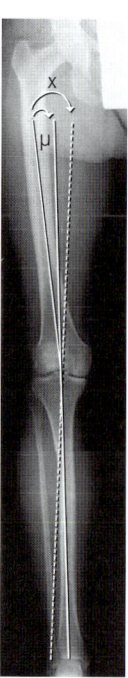
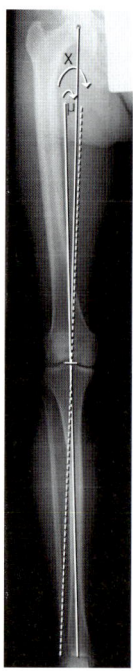

Fig 5-5   Bilateral weight-bearing AP x-ray in full extension for planning a high-tibial osteotomy according to the method by Coventry [13] using the anatomical axis with angle μ being the preoperative varus angle and angle x being the planned correction angle.

Fig 5-6   Bilateral weight-bearing AP x-ray in full extension for planning a high-tibial osteotomy according to the method by Coventry [13] using the mechanical axis with angle μ being the preoperative varus angle and angle x being the planned correction angle.

6   Size of the wedge

All planning methods have in common that the resected or opened size of the wedge influences the degree of correction. In high-tibial valgization osteotomies, the length of the lateral resected cortex (c) equals the true tibial width (TW) at the level of the osteotomy multiplied by the tangent of the resected wedge angle: $c = TW \times \tan \mu$ [21].

Current instrumentation sets for closed-wedge osteotomy allow resection of a predetermined angular wedge so that the length of c has not to be calculated. Tables relating the true tibial width at the height of the osteotomy to the correction angle are also available and are of interest especially in open-wedge osteotomies (see chapter 4 "Basic principles of osteotomies around the knee"). However, if the osteotomy is too oblique, the simple geometric relationship no longer applies. In cases with a significant extension gap, the degree of varus malalignment is overrated on the x-rays. In this case, separate x-rays of both tibia and femur are necessary to plan the osteotomy.

In order to check if the calculated wedge size is plausible, it should be noted that per centimeter wedge size the correction angle is changed by approximately 8–10°.

7   Prognostic factors

There are various risk factors associated with a poor clinical outcome after osteotomy, such as loss of correction, imprecise osteotomy, age, body weight, and patellofemoral osteoarthritis [22–24]. The differentiation between a constitutional and an acquired tibial varus is an important prognostic concept which has been introduced by Levigne in 1991 [25]. The malalignment of the varus knee can be either due to a constitutional or an acquired varus (wear and tear). In the former case, the valgization osteotomy cures the tibial malalignment. In the latter case, the HTO creates an unphysiological tibial valgus position with a poorer clinical outcome over time according to Levigne [25]. To differentiate between these two entities, the so-called "epiphyseal axis" of the proximal tibia has been defined. This axis runs perpendicular to the tibial plateau with a standard deviation of ± 2° and seems to be unaffected by bony wear (Fig 5-7) [26]. The angle between the epiphyseal axis and the mechanical tibial axis reflects the tibial bone varus angle (TBVA) which is 2.8° ± 2.7° on average. In Levigne's study [25], knees with a constitutional tibial varus had a TBVA > 5° and resulted in good clinical outcomes after high-tibial osteotomy. In knees with osteoarthritis-induced wear of the medial tibial plateau the TBVA was close to 0°. These patients showed rather poor results [26]. However, in severe osteoarthritis it can be difficult to determine the epiphyseal axis on plain x-rays [27].

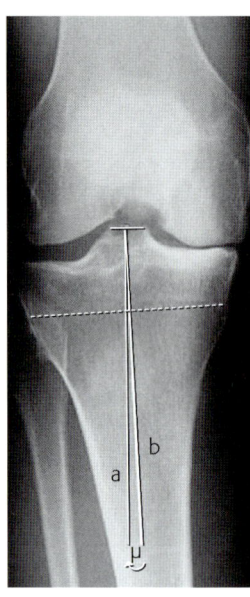

Fig 5-7   AP projection of the right tibia to determine the epiphyseal axis. A line is drawn (a) connecting the center of the tibial spines with the midpoint of a line connecting the two endpoints of the physis (dotted line). The epiphyseal axis is perpendicular to the tibial plateau with a standard deviation of 2°. The angle between the epiphyseal axis (a) and the mechanical axis (b) of the tibia determines the tibial bone varus angle (TBVA).

8   Preoperative planning in sagittal plane

The deformity in the sagittal plane can be assessed on the true lateral view of the knee (Fig 5-8). The physiologic range of the posterior tibial slope is presented in Table 5-2. However, the true tibial slope including the cartilaginous and meniscal elements is less than the bony tibial slope. Jenny et al studied 19 human tibias and noted mean average of 6° less slope when comparing bony slope with meniscal slope [28]. In cruciate ligament deficiencies the sagittal plane deformity should be considered. Dejour and Bonnin noted that increasing the tibial slope caused an increase in anterior tibial translation and hypothesized that tibial translation increases the tensile loads on the ACL [29]. Giffin et al reported that increasing the tibial slope by approximately 5° caused only a 2 mm anterior shift in the tibiofemoral resting position under 200 N axial compression without any changes in ACL computed forces [30].

However, it is widely accepted that increasing the posterior tibial slope increases the AP component of the joint contact force and reduces the posterior subluxation of the tibia in relation to the femur as seen in posterior cruciate ligament deficiencies. Decreasing the posterior slope decreases the AP component of the joint contact force and reduces the anterior subluxation of the tibia in relation to the femur as seen in anterior cruciate ligament deficiencies [21]. Altering the posterior tibial slope can also affect flexion contractures and hyperextension/recurvatum deformities (see chapter 11 "Osteotomy and ligament instability: tibial slope corrections and combined procedures around the knee joint").

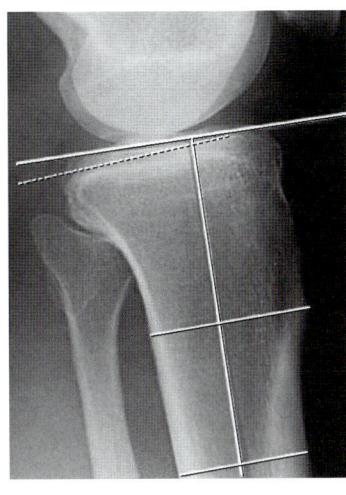

Fig 5-8   A true lateral x-ray of the left tibia showing the tibial slope measurement.

Author	Tibial slope angle
Lecuire et al, 1980 [31]	6°
Paley et al, 1992 [32]	10°
Insall, 1993 [33]	10°
Dejour et al, 1994 [29]	10° ± 3.1°
Matsuda et al, 1999 [34]	10.7°
Chiu et al, 2000 [35]	11.5°

Table 5-2   Physiologic range of the slope (inclination) of the tibial plateau.

9   Bibliography

[1]   **Aglietti P, Rinonapoli E, Stringa G, et al** (1983) Tibial osteotomy for the varus osteoarthritic knee. *Clin Orthop Relat Res;* 176:239–251.

[2]   **Coventry MB** (1965) Osteotomy of the upper portion of the tibia for degenerative arthritis of the knee. A preliminary report. *J Bone Joint Surg Am;* 47:984–990.

[3]   **Tjörnstrand B, Egund N, Hagstedt B, et al** (1981) Tibial osteotomy in medial gonarthrosis. The importance of over-correction of varus deformity. *Arch Orthop Trauma Surg;* 99(2):83–89.

[4]   **Engel GM, Lippert FG 3rd** (1981) Valgus tibial osteotomy: avoiding the pitfalls. *Clin Orthop Relat Res;* 160:137–143.

[5]   **Kettelkamp DB, Wenger DR, Chao EY, et al** (1976) Results of proximal tibial osteotomy. The effects of tibiofemoral angle, stanc-ephase flexion-extension, and medial plateau force. *J Bone Joint Surg Am;* 58(7):952–960.

[6]   **Tjörnstrand B, Selvik G, Egund N, et al** (1981) Roentgen stereophotogrammetry in high tibial osteotomy for gonarthrosis. Arch Orthop Trauma Surg; 99(2):73–81.

[7]   **Rosenberg TD, Paulos LE, Parker RD, et al** (1988) The forty-five-degree posteroanterior flexion weight-bearing radiograph of the knee. *J Bone Joint Surg Am;* 70(10):1479–1483.

[8]   **Dugdale TW, Noyes FR, Styer D** (1992) Preoperative planning for high tibial osteotomy. The effect of lateral tibiofemoral separation and tibiofemoral length. *Clin Orthop Relat Res;* 274:248–264.

[9]   **Ahlbäck S** (1968) Osteonecrosis of the knee—radiographic observations. *Calcif Tissue Res;* Suppl:36–36b.

[10]   **Benedetto KP** (1992) [Score of the IKDC.] (International Knee Documentation Committee). *Communication of the German Speaking Working Group for Arthroscopy.* (AGA), Nr 4. German.

[11]   **Kellgren JH, Lawrence JS** (1957) Radiological assessment of osteoarthrosis. *Ann Rheum Dis;* 16(4):494–502.

[12] **Pape D, Seil R, Adam F, et al** (2004) [Imaging and preoperative planning of osteotomy of tibial head osteotomy.] *Orthopäde;* 33(2):122–134. German.

[13] **Coventry MB** (1985) Upper tibial osteotomy for osteoarthritis. *J Bone Joint Surg Am;* 67(7):1136–1140.

[14] **Hernigou P, Medevielle D, Debeyre J, et al** (1987) Proximal tibial osteotomy for osteoarthritis with varus deformity: A ten to thirteen-year follow-up study. *J Bone Joint Surg Am;* 69(3):332–354.

[15] **Fujisawa Y, Masuhara K, Shiomi S** (1979) The effect of high tibial osteotomy on osteoarthritis of the knee. An arthroscopic study of 54 knee joints. *Orthop Clin North Am;* 10(3):585–608.

[16] **Miniaci A, Ballmer FT, Ballmer PM, et al** (1989) Proximal tibial osteotomy. A new fixation device. *Clin Orthop Relat Res;* 246:250–259.

[17] **Koshino T, Morii T, Wada J, et al** (1989) High tibial osteotomy with fixation by a blade plate for medial compartment osteoarthritis of the knee. *Orthop Clin North Am;* 20(2):227–243.

[18] **Ivarsson I, Myrnerts R, Gillquist J** (1990) High tibial osteotomy for medial osteoarthritis of the knee. A 5 to 7 and 11 year follow-up. *J Bone Joint Surg Br;* 72(2):238–244.

[19] **Myrnerts R** (1980) Failure of the correction of varus deformity obtained by high tibial osteotomy. *Acta Orthop Scand;* 51(3):569–573.

[20] **Noyes FR, Barber SD, Simon R** (1993) High tibial osteotomy and ligament reconstruction in varus angulated, anterior cruciate ligament-deficient knees. A two- to seven-year follow-up study. *Am J Sports Med;* 21(1):2–12.

[21] **Brown G, Amendola A** (2000) Radiographic evaluation and preoperative planning for high tibial osteotomies. *Operative Techn Sports Med;* 8:2–14.

[22] **Pape D, Adam F, Seil R, et al** (2005) Fixation stability following high tibial osteotomy: a radiostereometric analysis. *J Knee Surg;* 18(2):108–115.

[23] **Coventry MB, Ilstrup DM, Wallrichs SL** (1993) Proximal tibial osteotomy. A critical long-term study of eighty-seven cases. *J Bone Joint Surg Am;* 75(2):196–201.

[24] **Naudie D, Bourne RB, Rorabeck CH, et al** (1999) The Install Award. Survivorship of the high tibial valgus osteotomy. A 10- to 22-year followup study. *Clin Orthop Relat Res;* 367:18–27.

[25] **Levigne C** (1991) [Interest of the epiphyseal axes in arthroses. Analyses of the witnesses. The gonarthroses.] *Journées Lyonnaises de Chirurgie du genou;* 7:127–141. French.

[26] **Bonnin M, Chambat P** (2004) [Current Status of valgus angle, tibial head closing wedge osteotomy in medial gonarthrosis.] *Orthopäde;* 33(2):135–142. German.

[27] **Jenny JY, Boéri C, Ballonzoli L, et al** (2005) [Difficulties and reproducibility of radiological measurement of the proximal tibial axis according to Lévigne.] *Rev Chir Orthop Réparatrice Appar Mot;* 91(7):658–663. French.

[28] **Jenny JY, Rapp E, Kehr P** (1997) [Proximal tibial meniscal slope: a comparison with the bone slope.] *Rev Chir Orthop Réparatrice Appar Mot;* 84(5):435–438. French.

[29] **Dejour H, Bonnin M** (1994) Tibial translation after anterior cruciate ligament rupture. Two radiological tests compared. *J Bone Joint Surg Br;* 76(5):745–749.

[30] **Giffin JR, Vogrin TM, Zantop T, et al** (2004) Effects of increasing tibial slope on the biomechanics of the knee. *Am J Sports Med;* 32(2):376–382.

[31] **Lecuire L, Lerat JL, Bousquet G, et al** (1980) [The treatment of genu recurvatum (author's transl).] *Rev Chir Orthop Réparatric Appar Mot;* 66(2):95–103. French.

[32] **Paley D, Herzenberg JE, Tetsworth K, et al** (1994) Deformity planning for frontal and sagittal plane corrective osteotomies. *Orthop Clin North Am;* 25(3):425–465.

[33] **Insall JN** (1993) Total knee arthroplasty in rheumatoid arthritis. *Ryumachi;* 33(6):472.

[34] **Matsuda S, Miura H, Nagamine R, et al** (1999) Posterior tibial slope in the normal and varus knee. *Am J Knee Surg;* 12(3):165–168.

[35] **Chiu KY, Zhang SD, Zhang GH** (2000) Posterior slope of tibial plateau in Chinese. *J Arthroplasty;* 15(2):224–227.

All pictures in this chapter [12] are reprinted with permission from Springer Science+Business Media Deutschland GmbH.

Clinical applications

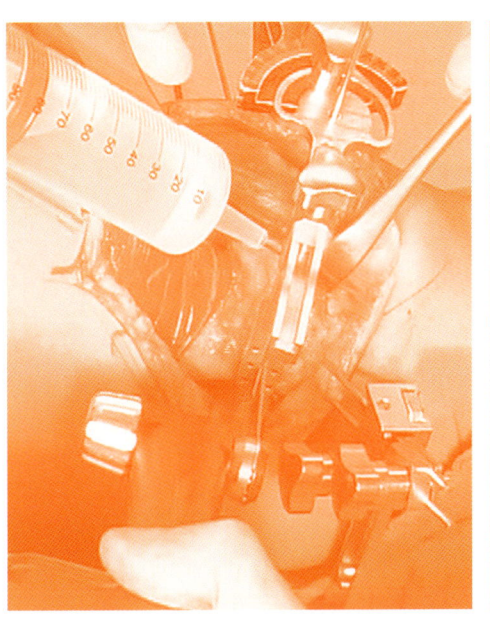 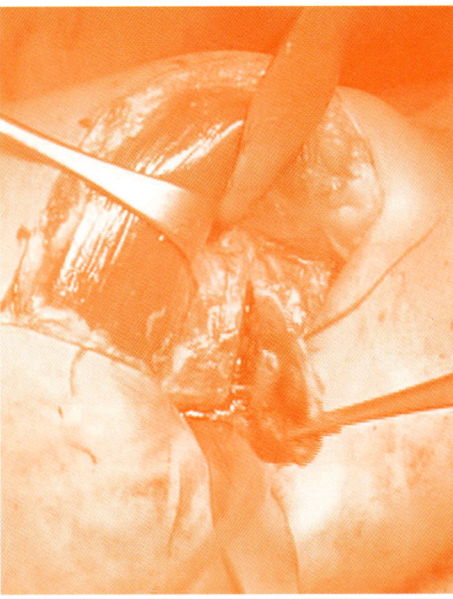 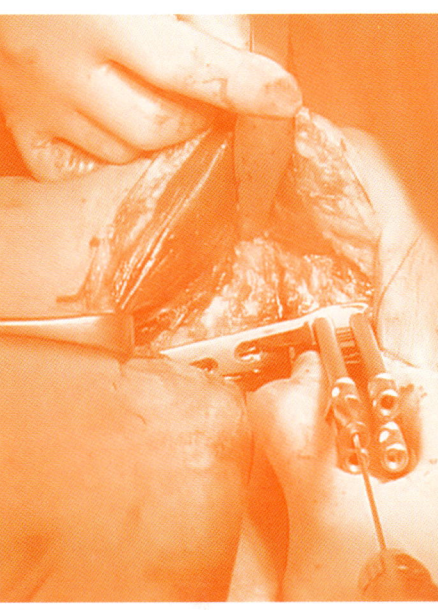

Ronald J van Heerwaarden, Paul Koning, Ibo B van der Haven

Koen C Defoort, Gijs G van Hellemondt, Ronald J van Heerwaarden, Alex E Staubli

6   High-tibial closed-wedge osteotomy

1   Introduction

The classical valgization closed-wedge high-tibial osteotomy (HTO) technique performed proximal to the tuberosity was inaugurated and propagated by Coventry in 1965 [1]. For a long time the closed-wedge procedure was a common and widespread method in treatment of medial gonarthritis, until the open-wedge technique gained new popularity. This development was favored by the introduction of new implant designs, especially plate fixators with angular stable locking head screws during the last years [2–6]. The medial open-wedge technique with these implants offers many advantages: the surgical technique is faster, the correction is more precise, and the risk of peroneal nerve lesion during fibula osteotomy is avoided. Open-wedge and closed-wedge osteotomies have similar indications [7, 8] and have demonstrated good results [9–13], although currently no long-term results with modern angular locked plates are available.

Despite the advantages of open-wedge HTO there are still certain indications for the closed-wedge osteotomy.

1. Patella baja is a relative contraindication for open-wedge HTO since this procedure significantly lowers the patella and can cause problems especially in patients with preexisting femoropatellar symptoms [14].
2. If a lateral arthrotomy is planned or scars exist at the lateral aspect of the knee, it might be wise to use a lateral approach again instead of performing a second medial incision.

Table 6-1 summarizes the differences between open- and closed-wedge valgization HTO with its indications, advantages, and disadvantages.

Indications

Open-wedge HTO	Closed-wedge HTO
Patella alta	Patella baja
Insufficient medial collateral ligament (open-wedge technique allows tensioning)	Intact medial collateral ligament
Associated anterior cruciate ligament (ACL) reconstruction	Associated anterior cruciate ligament (ACL) reconstruction
Simultaneous medial arthrotomy	Simultaneous lateral arthrotomy

Advantages/disadvantages

Open-wedge HTO	Closed-wedge HTO
Faster surgery	Longer surgery
Bone graft necessary in case of high correction	No graft necessary
Higher precision	Lower precision
Risk of saphenus nerve lesion	Risk of peroneus nerve lesion

Table 6-1   Summary of the differences between open- and closed-wedge valgization HTO with its indications, advantages, and disadvantages.

2 Surgical technique

2.1 Preparation

Standard desinfection and draping is performed. A single-shot antibiotic is applied. A tourniquet is placed on the thigh and is inflated.

2.2 Arthroscopy

A routine arthroscopy is performed prior to the osteotomy in every case to confirm the intactness of the lateral compartment. If necessary, an abrasion arthroplasty combined with microfracturing of the medial compartment is performed and intercondylar osteophytes are removed. Meniscal tears are treated. If an anterior cruciate ligament reconstruction is planned, it is preformed after the osteotomy procedure or as a secondary intervention.

2.3 Osteotomy

A straight longitudinal incision on the anterolateral aspect of the proximal tibia is performed, maintaining the option for a total knee arthroplasty in the future. The extensor muscles are carefully detached from the tibia and fibula. The peroneal nerve is exposed, the neck of the fibula is prepared, and a stepwise osteotomy of the fibula is performed: at the proximal aspect the anterior cortex of the fibula is osteotomized, and the fibula is subsequently, completely osteotomized 1 cm more distally. This approach avoids pressure to the peroneal nerve. The level of the oblique tibial osteotomy is now determined under fluoroscopic control. The sagittal slope should also be respected at this point. The osteotomy is guided by K-wires which are placed using the osteotomy guiding device which has a precision of 0.5°. This device allows the maintenance of a 5–10 mm bone bridge at the medial cortex, which is important for stability, especially if no angular stable implants are used. A partial osteotomy of the tuberosity is performed in the frontal plane, leaving the chisel in place to protect the tuberosity during the horizontal osteotomy, which is now performed

between the K-wires with a saw blade. After this, the bone wedge is removed and the angular stable plate fixator (ie, TomoFix lateral proximal tibia = TomoFix LPT) is fixed proximally with locking head screws (**Fig 6-1a**). The distal part of the plate is kept about 10 mm distant from the tibia. The plate tensioning device is mounted distally. The gap is slowly and carefully closed with the tensioning device. During this step attention must be paid to the correct displacement of the fibula osteotomy. Finally, the plate is fixed distally with locking head screws (**Fig 6-1b**). The extensor muscles are reattached and the wound is closed in layers.

2.4 Postoperative management

Partial weight bearing (15 kg) on crutches with the knee extended in a removable splint is allowed from the first postoperative day. Passive physical therapy of the knee also begins on the first postoperative day. Radiographic follow-up is performed postoperatively at 6 and 12 weeks (**Fig 6-2**). If bone consolidation is visible on the x-rays 6 weeks postoperatively, full weight bearing is allowed.

2.5 Complications

Many complications are described in association with closed-wedge HTO procedure:

- Damages to the peroneal nerve or the popliteal artery
- Intraarticular fractures
- Compartment syndrome
- Infection
- Deep vein thrombosis or pulmonary embolism
- Delayed union or nonunion of the osteotomy

Nevertheless, proper selection of patients, good preoperative planning, accurate operative technique, and correct postoperative management can limit the complication rate to a minimum [15].

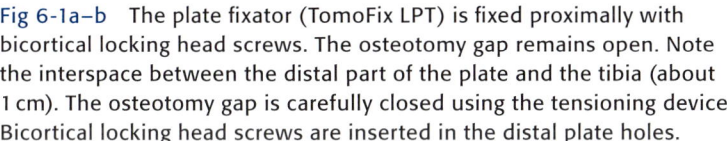

Fig 6-1a–b   The plate fixator (TomoFix LPT) is fixed proximally with bicortical locking head screws. The osteotomy gap remains open. Note the interspace between the distal part of the plate and the tibia (about 1 cm). The osteotomy gap is carefully closed using the tensioning device. Bicortical locking head screws are inserted in the distal plate holes.

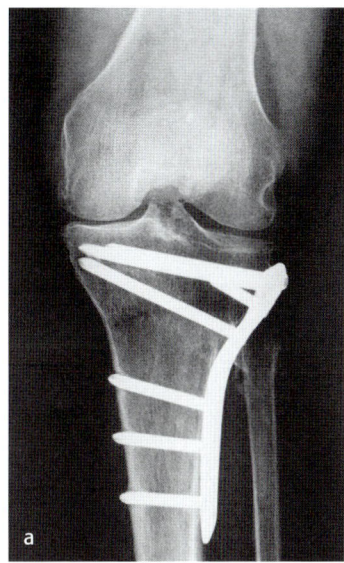
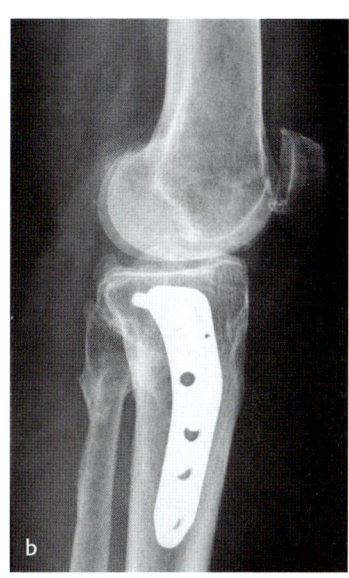

Fig 6-2a–b   Postoperative AP and lateral x-rays. Result after lateral closed-wedge high-tibial osteotomy.

3   Discussion

Closed-wedge osteotomy is a widespread method to perform valgization high-tibial osteotomy for medial varus osteoarthritis of the knee. The majority of studies with long-term follow up have investigated this technique. Good results are reported during the first years of follow-up with deterioration over the time. Insall showed in his study that at the 2-year follow-up 97 % of patients show good results, whereas after 5 years patient satisfaction decreases to 85 %, and after 9 years to 63 % [12]. Only two Japanese studies show very high survival rates after 15 years (90 %, respectively 93 %) [16, 17]. Unsatisfactory results are normally due to inadequate patient selection or planning or due to loss of correction especially if less stable implants have been applied.

Closed-wedge osteotomy has lost importance during the last years whereas open-wedge osteotomy is performed more frequently. This newer technique is easier, faster, and more precise, and avoids the risk of peroneal nerve lesion. Nevertheless, there are some remaining indications for the closed-wedge technique:

- In case of patella baja
- If the posterior slope needs to be decreased
- If a lateral arthrotomy is planned

4   Bibliography

[1]   **Coventry MB** (1965) Osteotomy of the upper portion of the tibia for degenerative arthritis of the knee. A preliminary report. *J Bone Joint Surg Am;* 47:984–990.

[2]   **Franco V, Cerullo G, Cipolla M, et al** (2002) Open wedge high tibial osteotomy. Tech Knee Surg; 1(1):43–53.

[3]   **Jacobi M, Jakob RP** (2005) Open wedge osteotomy in the treatment of medial osteoarthritis of the knee. *Tech Knee Surg;* 4(2):70–78.

[4]   **Lobenhoffer P, Agneskirchner JD** (2003) Improvements in surgical technique of valgus high tibial osteotomy. *Knee Surg Sports Traumatol Arthrosc;* 11(3):132–138.

[5]   **Staubli AE, De Simoni C, Babst R, et al** (2003) TomoFix: a new LCP-concept for open wedge osteotomy of the medial proximal tibia—early results in 92 cases. *Injury;* 34 Suppl 2:B55–B62.

[6]   **Stoffel K, Stachowiak G, Kuster M** (2004) Open wedge high tibial osteotomy: biomechanical investigation of the modified Arthrex Osteotomy Plate (Puddu Plate) and the TomoFix Plate. *Clin Biomech (Bristol, Avon);* 19(9):944–950.

[7]   **Brouwer RW, Bierma-Zeinstra SM, van Raaij TM, et al** (2006) Osteotomy for medial compartment arthritis of the knee using a closing wedge or an opening wedge controlled by a Puddu plate. A one-year randomised, controlled study. *J Bone Joint Surg Br;* 88(11):1454–1459.

[8]   **Höll S, Suttmöller J, Stoll V, et al** (2005) The high tibial osteotomy, open versus closed wedge, a comparison of methods in 108 patients. *Arch Orthop Trauma Surg;* 125(9):638–643.

[9]   **Billings A, Scott DF, Camargo MP, et al** (2000) High tibial osteotomy with a calibrated osteotomy guide, rigid internal fixation, and early motion. Long-term follow-up. J Bone Joint Surg Am; 82(1):70–79. Erratum in: *J Bone Joint Surg Am;* 82(3):450.

[10] **Coventry MB, Bowman PW** (1982) Long-term results of upper tibial osteotomy for degenerative arthritis of the knee. *Acta Orthop Belg;* 48(1):139–156.

[11] **Hernigou P, Medevielle D, Debeyre J, et al** (1987) Proximal tibial osteotomy for osteoarthritis with varus deformity. A ten to thirteen-year follow-up study. *J Bone Joint Surg Am;* 69(3):332–354.

[12] **Insall JN, Joseph DM, Msika C** (1984) High tibial osteotomy for varus gonarthrosis. A long-term follow-up study. *J Bone Joint Surg Am;* 66(7):1040–1048.

[13] **Rinonapoli E, Mancini GB, Corvaglia A, et al** (1998) Tibial osteotomy for varus gonarthrosis. A 10- to 21-year followup study. *Clin Orthop Relat Res;* 353:185–193.

[14] **Brouwer RW, Bierma-Zeinstra SM, van Koeveringe AJ, et al** (2005) Patellar height and the inclination of the tibial plateau after high tibial osteotomy. The open versus the closed-wedge technique. *J Bone Joint Surg Br;* 87(9):1227–1232.

[15] **Coventry MB** (1985) Upper tibial osteotomy for osteoarthritis. *J Bone Joint Surg Am;* 67(7):1136–1140.

[16] **Akizuki S, Shibakawa A, Takizawa T, et al** (2008) The long-term outcome of high tibial osteotomy: A ten- to 20-year follow-up. *J Bone Joint Surg Br;* 90(5):592–596.

[17] **Koshino T, Yoshida T, Ara Y, et al** (2004) Fifteen to twenty-eight years' follow-up results of high tibial valgus osteotomy for osteoarthritic knee. *Knee;* 11(6):439–444.

7 Principles of angular stable fixators

1 Surgical principles

In recent years there has been rapid development of the so-called "biological" internal fixation of metadiaphyseal multifragmentary and comminuted fractures and of techniques in osteotomies around the joints. The term "biological" refers to the preservation of bone and soft-tissue vitality that, combined with biomechanical stability, is essential for bone healing [1]. Titanium plates were introduced about 30 years ago [2], and due to their biomechanical properties and good biocompatibility, became standard devices in addition to the existing steel implants [2].

For a long time exact reduction and interfragmentary compression were considered the main principles of internal fixation to stabilize bone fragments in the diaphyseal and metaphyseal region of long bones. Osteosynthesis with an internal plate fixator is based on the so-called "splinting principle", ie, bridging of unstable fracture and osteotomy zones. This stimulates the consolidation of loose fragments. Within this concept, the "splinting" in comminuted diaphyseal and metaphyseal zones, and preservation of tissue vitality have priority over interfragmentary compression. Furthermore, bone healing is stimulated in this type of osteosynthesis by alternating load induced by functional postoperative exercises leading to micromotion in the fracture and/or osteotomy zone [3]. On the basis of mechanical testing of the "splinting principle", the relevant fixation techniques and implants were further developed in biomechanical studies at the AO Research Institute in Davos [1]. Principles of internal fixation apply equally to fracture healing and healing of osteotomies around the joints (see chapter 12 "Radiological examination of bone healing after open-wedge tibial osteotomy"). Exceptions to the treatment concept of "splinting" are intraarticular fractures, for which interfragmentary reduction without step-off and stable fixation remain the basic principles of fixation.

2 Development of open-wedge valgization osteotomy of the proximal tibia

The aim of valgization correction osteotomy of the proximal tibia is to unload a degenerated medial compartment, whereby the correction should heal without secondary loss of correction.

The following procedures are commonly performed in tibial head osteotomy:

- Open-wedge (additive) osteotomies
- Closed-wedge (subtractive) osteotomies
- Focal dome or gable-shaped osteotomies

The afore mentioned procedures differ in size and shape of the osseous contact zones. The largest bone interface is achieved in closed-wedge technique with removal of a lateral-based bone wedge, a technique that is still practised very frequently world-wide [4].

Open-wedge high-tibial osteotomy (HTO) was rather unpopular at first because common implants could not counteract the high axial compression and torsional forces at the proximal tibia. Complications due to failure of fixation often occured [5–7].

However, this surgical procedure gained greater acceptance as new implants were developed. The method of open-wedge tibial valgization osteotomy commonly performed now, creates a wedge-shaped gap with a medial base between the two main fragments, which results in an unstable situation. The size and volume of the gap depend on the amount of correction required.

The first results of open-wedge tibial correction osteotomy were published approximately 25 years ago. These cases were immobilized in a plaster until the bone has completely healed. In subsequent years, the osteotomy was stabilized by interposition of two or three bicortical iliac crest bone grafts that were transplanted into the osteotomy gap [6]. This procedure was suboptimal regarding precision and mechanical stability, not to mention significant morbidity at the iliac crest donor site. Far better results were obtained by combining internal fixation with the interposition of cement blocks [5, 6].

In recent years, various implants have been designed for internal stabilization of open-wedge tibial osteotomies, whereby a particular spacer plate (Puddu plate) [8] gained the most popularity. Nevertheless, a high failure rate was recorded, especially in osteotomy gaps greater than 10 mm, severely obese patients, and patients with manifest osteoporosis. Lobenhoffer et al reported a failure rate of 6% with corresponding loss of correction in 101 open-wedge osteotomies stabilized with this implant [9, 10]. Spahn conducted a study to compare this so-called spacer plate with the angular locking C-plate that he had developed himself [11]. The overall complication rate for the spacer plate was 43.6%. 11.7% of the patients required an additional lateral fixation. In this study, loss of correction was only observed with the Puddu plate.

At the end of the 1990s the author was using the 95° titanium angled blade plate at his hospital for closed- and open-wedge osteotomies of the tibia. Even corrections greater than 10° were easily achieved with this implant without filling the osteotomy gap (Fig 7-1).

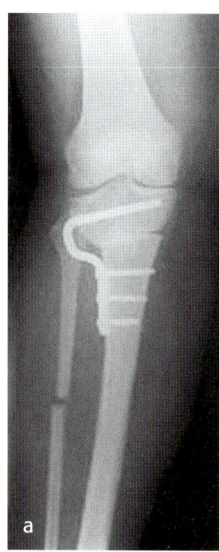 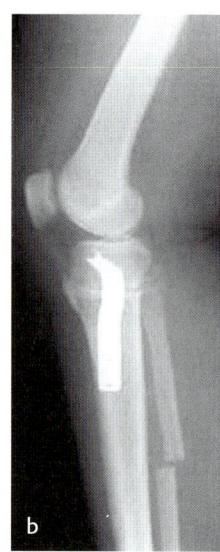 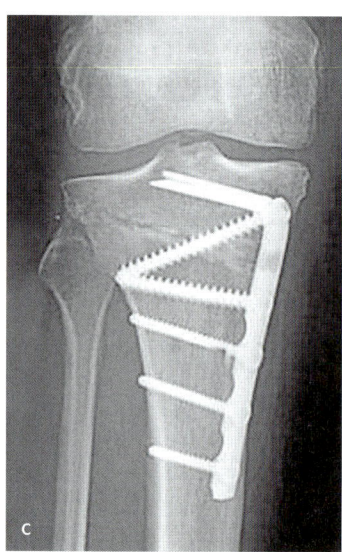 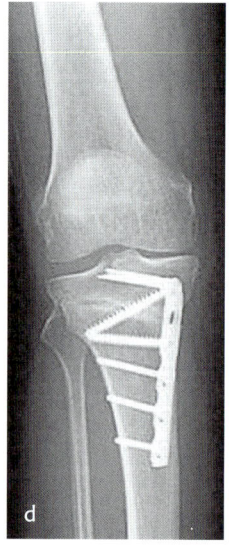

Fig 7-1a–d Proximal correction osteotomy of the tibia with an angled blade plate.
a–b Closed-wedge tibial head osteotomy of the right leg with osteotomy of the fibular diaphysis.
c–d Open-wedge tibial head osteotomy with a 95° titanium angled blade plate without bone graft in the osteotomy gap.

Hemicallotasis is another suitable procedure for unilateral and unidirectional correction. The medial distraction is achieved by applying a unilateral or ring fixator over several weeks or months. This method is frequently applied in Eastern Europe, in Anglo-Saxon and Scandinavian countries, and in Italy [12].

The advantages of the hemicallotasis method are nonextensive surgery, the possibility of secondary axial correction, and good applicability even for complex deformities. The disadvantages include the long wearing time, patient discomfort, pain during distraction, and, above all, the high rate of pin-track infections.

3   Application of angular stable plate fixators in open-wedge tibial osteotomy

3.1   The internal plate fixator TomoFix

The locking compression plates (LCPs) that have been developed over the past 20 years, eg, PC-Fix and the less invasive stabilization system (LISS), consist of an angular stable plate and a locking screw system, whereby the screw head locks into the threaded plate hole [13–15]. This internal fixation technique has become well established in fracture treatment [16, 17].

Early in the year 2000, the LCP system for the fixation of open- and closed-wedge correction osteotomies around the knee was first integrated into the new generation of plates and introduced to the market as the TomoFix (Fig 7-2). The idea behind the development of this implant was the adaptation of the LISS plate for the lower extremity to meet the demands of proximal tibial osteotomy [18]. The results were critically analyzed by the members of the Knee Expert Group (KNEG) of the AO in multicenter studies [9, 10]. Experience over the past 3 years has shown that the application of this implant offers great potential for the correction of both uniplanar and multiplanar deformities. Good results are also achieved with this implant in revision surgery for failed osteosynthesis with other implant systems. These good results did not depend on the application of bone graft in the osteotomy gap.

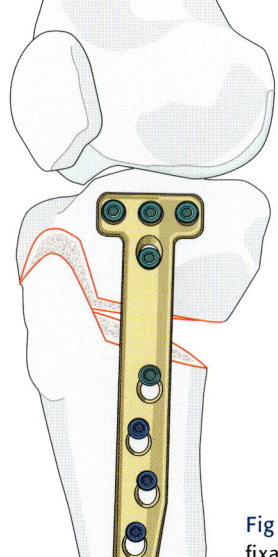

Fig 7-2   The TomoFix angular stable plate fixator applied to stabilize a proximal medial open-wedge tibial osteotomy.

3.1.1 Implant design

The design and construction of the plate fixator are shown in Fig 7-3. For a better and consistent understanding of plate design and surgical technique, the four plate holes in the proximal segment are marked A, B, C, and D and the four combination holes in the distal segment are marked 1, 2, 3, and 4. The plate design described here has proven to be of value over the last 8 years and is still applied in unmodified form today.

The T-plates are manufactured from pure titanium and are identical for the right and left side. The TomoFix plate fixator cannot be substituted by the proximal tibial fracture plate LCP 4.0/4.5 which is unsuitable for open-wedge HTO. The plate is made from a punched blank, whereby the shape of the plate is matched to the anatomy of the proximal tibia to correspond to an average valgus correction of 10°. The 38° curvature of this plate is equivalent to that of the average radius of the proximal tibia. The T-shape (T-arm = 32 mm) of the implant and its buttress, with three angular stable bolts oriented from antero-medial towards posterolateral and the continuous plate thickness of 2.8 mm over a length of 11.5 cm, ensure best possible elastic adaptation to the proximal tibial epiphysis, metaphysis, and diaphysis. This construction distributes bending forces over a long distance and neutralizes torsion avoiding punctual stress concentration (Fig 7-4).

The conical screw holes with their 2.5 double threads in the T-arm (holes A, B, and C) have an inclination of 4° caudally to prevent perforation of the tibial articular surface. The holes are aligned convergently and stabilize the lateral hinge by spring suspension of applied forces. Plate holes 1, 2, 3, and 4 in the longitudinal arm are arranged in staggered alignment to avoid longitudinal diaphyseal fissures. Holes A, B, and C are 360° threaded holes, whereas hole D and holes 1, 2, 3, and 4 are 270° combination holes.

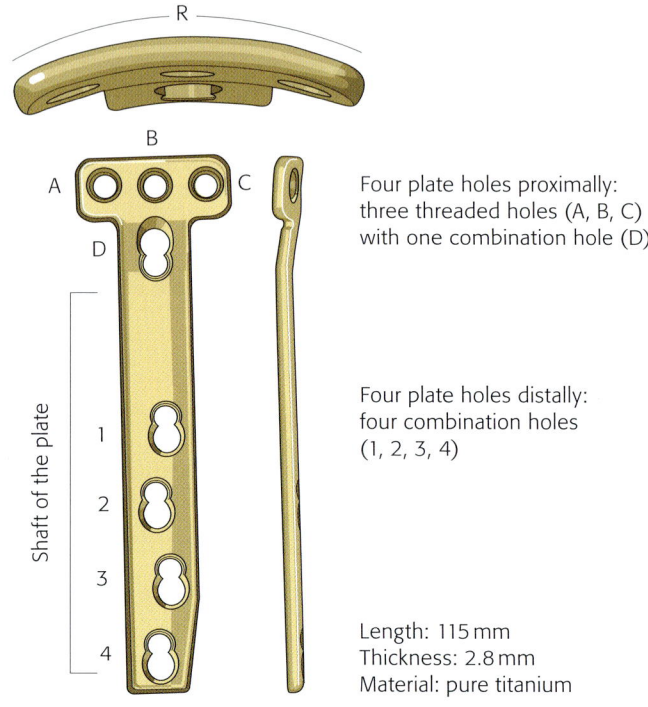

Four plate holes proximally: three threaded holes (A, B, C) with one combination hole (D)

Four plate holes distally: four combination holes (1, 2, 3, 4)

Length: 115 mm
Thickness: 2.8 mm
Material: pure titanium

Fig 7-3 Design of the TomoFix internal plate fixator with three threaded holes in the T-arm and 5 combination holes on the longitudinal arm.

The 5.0 mm locking head screws are self-cutting (green) and self-tapping/self-drilling (blue). The two 3 mm distance plugs for holes D and 3 or 4 act as spacers (see chapter 9 "High-tibial open-wedge valgization osteotomy with plate fixator", Fig 9-2d–e, and chapter 12 "Radiological examination of bone healing after tibial open-wedge osteotomy"). The screw heads all have a low profile and are locked with the torque screwdriver of 4 Nm limitation.

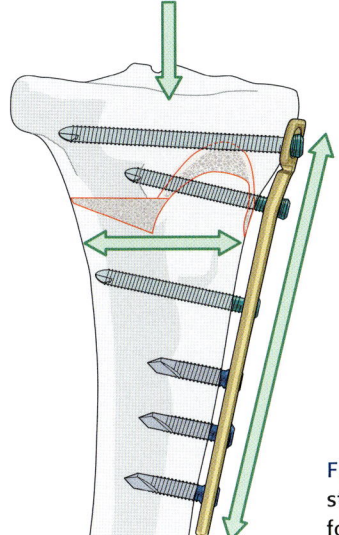

Fig 7-4 Balanced biomechanical stress distribution. The bending forces are distributed over a long distance during axial loading.

3.1.2   Implant length

Long plates ensure adequate axial stiffness. If a plate fixator stabilized with at least two locking head screws in each main fragment is loaded, plastic deformation will occur before the locking head screws start to move or bend. The torsional stiffness of an internal fixation is determined mainly by the plate's cross section and length, that is, by the spring deflection of the implant. Implant deformation caused by the application of force is distributed across a larger area reducing the risk of punctual stress concentration. Furthermore, stress distribution over a long distance reduces biomechanical stress at the screw-to-bone interface. The plate becomes more elastic with a long screw-free distance as a bridging element; however, in open-wedge osteotomy, prevention of secondary loss of correction by primary stability is essential. It is important to insert the screws as near as possible to the osteotomy.

The author has experienced only two fixation failures after open-wedge osteotomy with the TomoFix implant. Both cases were attributed to an overambitious indication. The implants failed at hole D in both instances, which corresponds to the biomechanical plate testing the author conducted. He was able to confirm by finite element analysis (FEA) that hole D was exposed to the greatest mechanical stress.

3.1.3   Screw insertion

In this type of internal fixation the number of screws inserted effects the stability significantly [19]. The axial stiffness of the implant correlates with the number of screws per osteotomy segment. The screws increase the torsional stiffness only if they are inserted bicortically or monocortically over a long distance. The closer a screw is positioned to the fracture or osteotomy gap, the greater the stiffness of the whole construct. The TomoFix plate is positioned at the proximal tibia allowing four screws to be inserted into the proximal and distal osteotomy segment in order to counteract rotational forces in the metadiaphyseal regions. In this way, biomechanical stiffness under torsional loading is determined by the number and lengths of the screws. Thus, in the cancellous bone of the tibial head all monocortical screws should be as long as possible to support the tibial plateau over a wide area (Fig 7-5). To increase the axial retention force of the locking head screws, the threads for holes A, B, C, and D of the TomoFix implant are slightly convergent in their orientation.

This explains why the author has not yet observed screw pull-out for the medially applied TomoFix plate.

3.1.4 Angular stable locking

In the design of the TomoFix plate, the spherical gliding principle of the conventional plate-to-screw head interface was abandoned in favor of a locking mechanism between the thread of the screw head and the corresponding thread of the plate hole. The green self-cutting and the blue self-tapping/self-drilling 5.0 mm locking head screws act as threaded bolts (Fig 7-6).

It is especially important to insert the threaded drill sleeves very precisely into the screw hole because the plate thickness only permits 2.5 double thread turns for fixation of the screw heads. Precise perpendicular insertion is vital to prevent tilting and subsequent incorrect or insufficient interlocking of the two threads. If the threads of the screw head and the plate hole are diverted due to nonperpendicular insertion, loss of stability during the consolidation process may occur. The torque screwdriver with its 4 Nm limitation must be used correctly, ie, only one "clicking sound" should be heard during tightening so that a "scouring effect" (cold welding) is not produced.

The LCP combination holes in the longitudinal arm (Fig 7-7) combine the options of compression osteosynthesis and splinting in one implant [13, 15, 16, 20].

3.1.5 Distance from the cortical surface

The insertion of angular stable locking head screws and the temporary application of 3 mm distance plugs creates a minor interspace between the implant and the tibial cortex (Fig 7-8a) so that the periosteal blood supply is not compromised (Fig 7-8b–c). Minimal implant contact limits the amount of pressure of the undersurface of the plate on the bone and prevents pressure necroses and compression of the structures beneath.

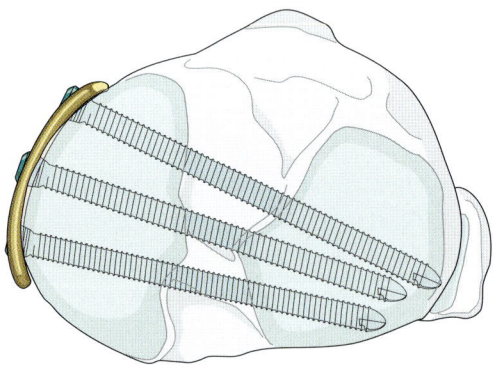

Fig 7-5   Transverse plane. The screws in the proximal segment should be as long as possible. The screws are slightly convergent in their alignment to increase axial retention force and ensure secure buttressing of the tibial plateau as far over as the lateral hinge.

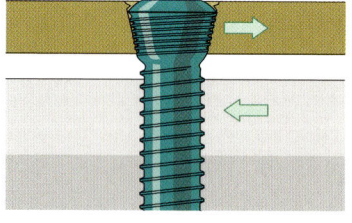

Fig 7-6   Threaded hole and locking screw with corresponding threaded screw head.

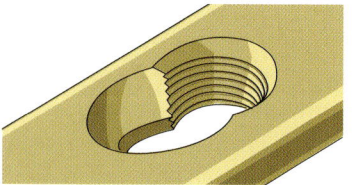

Fig 7-7   The combination holes in the longitudinal arm of the plate fixator allow for compression or locked fixation.

3.1.6   Minimally-invasive procedure

Wide exposure of the bone is not required when performing HTO according to the technique described in chapter 9 "Hightibial open-wedge valgization osteotomy with plate fixator". A 6–8 cm oblique incision is sufficient for the osteotomy and for correct positioning of the plate fixator. After preparation of a subcutaneous tunnel, the implant is inserted in a distal direction (Fig 7-9). During positioning it is necessary to ensure that the proximal end of the plate lies as posteriorly as possible parallel to the tibial joint surface and that the longitudinal arm lies midshaft. The screws are locked into the longitudinal arm of the plate fixator via a small additional incision. It is advisable to use an image intensifier to check position of the plate, the screws, and the preliminary K-wires.

3.1.7   Compression of the hinge and pretensioning of the plate

To stabilize the implant a temporary lag screw is inserted into combination hole 1 distal to the osteotomy after having tightened the screws A–C. The osteotomy gap must be closely observed during tightening of this lag screw. This procedure brings the lateral cortical bridge (lateral hinge) under compression and the TomoFix plate under pretension (Fig 7-10). In addition, the use of a lag screw combined with distance plugs draws the plate fixator closer to the bone surface of the proximal tibia without compromising the pes anserinus, the long fibers of the medial collateral ligament, or the periosteum (Fig 7-8b).

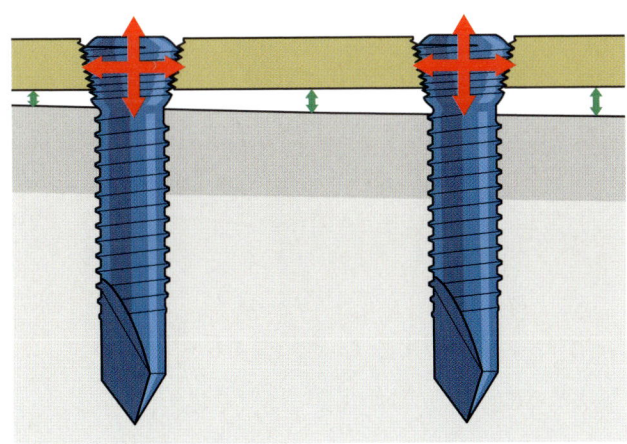

a

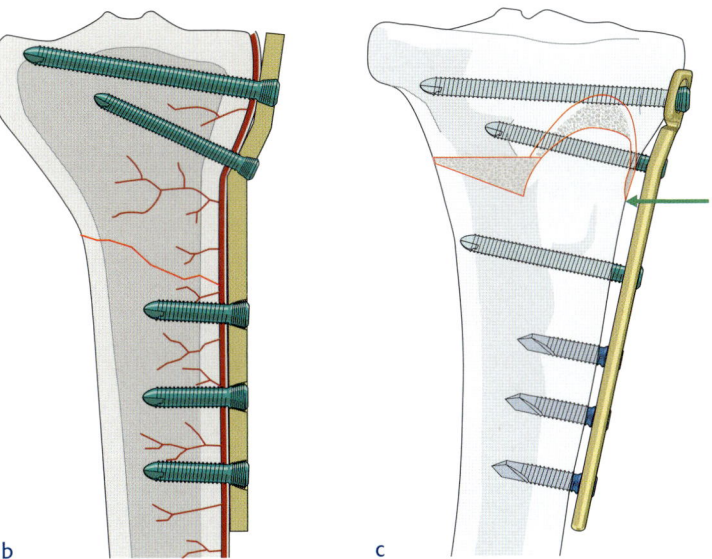

b   c

Fig 7-8a–c   Distance between the implant and the cortex.
a   Application of angular locking head screws and temporary spacers ensures a minimal interspace (green arrows) between the undersurface of the plate fixator and the bone.

b–c   The periosteal blood supply (red) is not impaired (b); the pes anserinus and the medial collateral ligament are preserved (arrow) (c).

3.1.8 Primary biomechanical stability

The 10 mm lateral bone bridge is the center of rotation in open-wedge HTO (Fig 7-11). The center of rotational angulation (CORA) [21] is located at the proximal end of the tibiofibular joint. This point facilitates the highest correction potential, and good compression can be achieved with the temporary lag screw through hole 1. Nevertheless, disruption of the lateral hinge may occur in severe deformities requiring a wide correction angle and in multiplanar correction procedures. This difficulty is resolved, however, by the angular stable principle of the TomoFix. The tension band effect of the quadriceps tendon and the tendons of the pes anserinus, the laterally preserved periosteum, and the ligamentotaxis of the tibiofibular joint increase the inherent stability including the internal fixation.

Biplanar osteotomy with the anterior saw cut ascending 110°, as described in chapter 9 "High-tibial open-wedge valgization osteotomy with plate fixator", contributes greatly to high primary stability. The anterior part of the tuberosity blocks tilting in the sagittal plane and torsional forces (Fig 7-12). In a comparative biomechanical study, Agneskirchner et al were able to confirm the biomechanical advantages of the construction principles of the TomoFix implant compared to other osteotomy plates [22].

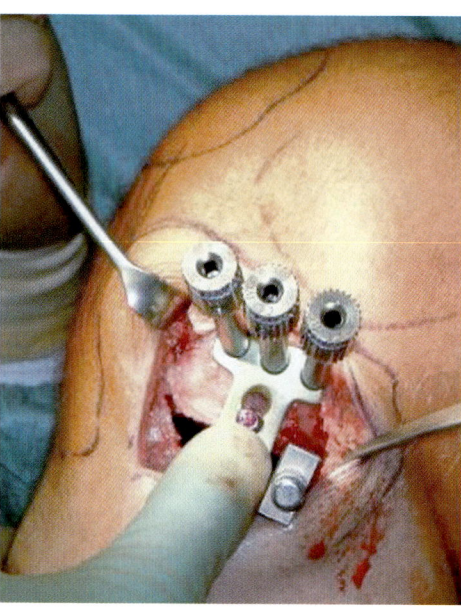

Fig 7-9   Insertion of the plate fixator in a distal direction through a subcutaneous tunnel.

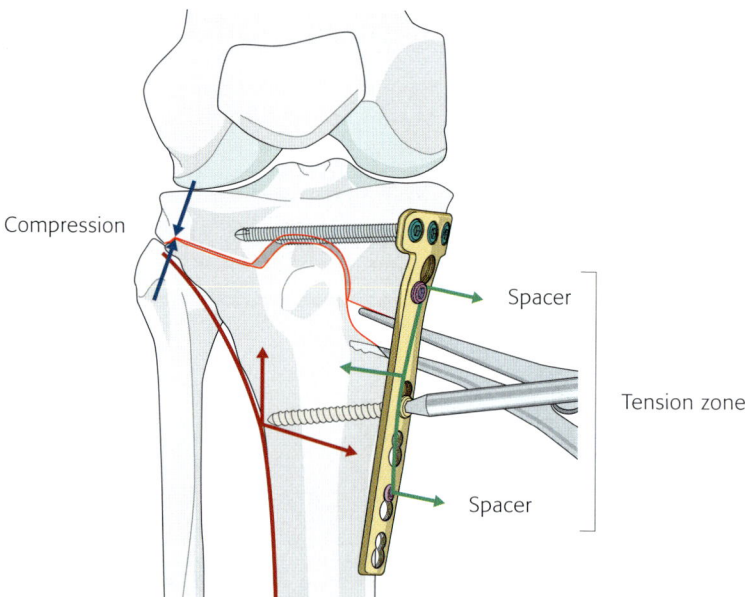

Fig 7-10   Principle of pretensioning by insertion of a temporary lag screw into the first plate hole distal to the osteotomy. The distal osteotomy segment is pulled towards the plate fixator (red and green arrows) and the lateral hinge is placed under compression (blue arrows).

3.2   The internal plate fixator SurFix

The angular stable plate fixator for correction osteotomy of the proximal tibia from SurFix (Fig 7-13) is not used very widely. This system is available in titanium and in steel and is stabilized by four 6.5 mm cancellous screws and four 4.5 mm cortex screws. Fixation is achieved by utilizing a polyaxial threaded sleeve and a lock screw. Internal fixation with this implant is generally combined with bone grafting of the osteotomy gap [7].

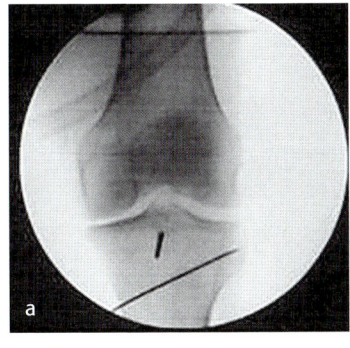 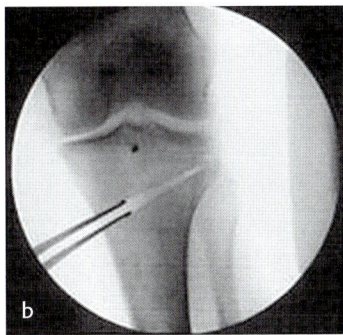 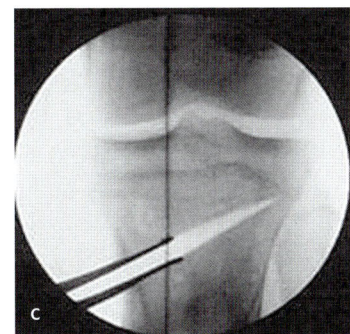

a   b   c

Fig 7-11a–c   A 10 mm wide lateral bone hinge is maintained when sawing the osteotomy. The center of rotation for open-wedge osteotomy is located in the intact lateral hinge.

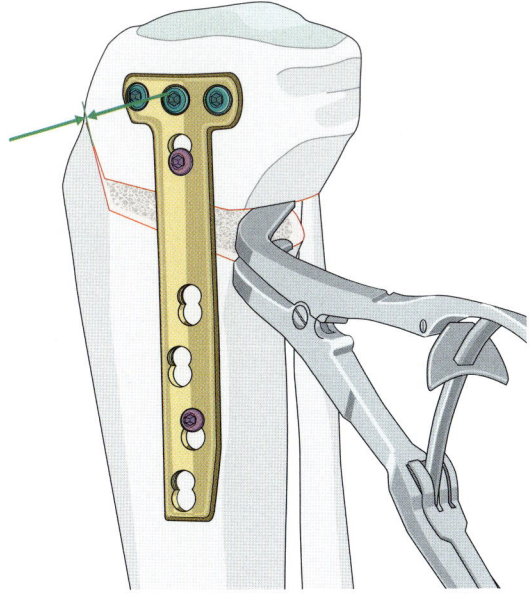

Fig 7-12   During spreading of the osteotomy the two bone surfaces of the anterior osteotomy behind the tibial tuberosity stay in contact and ensure greater mechanical stability against tilting in the sagittal plane (green arrows).

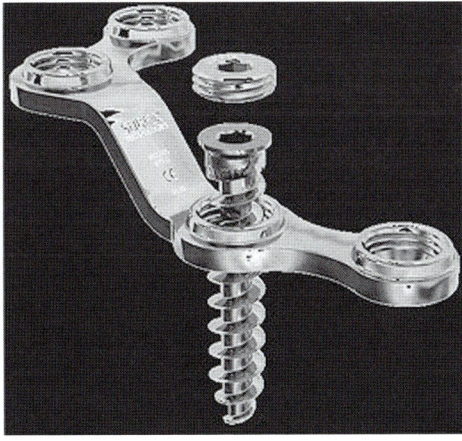

Fig 7-13   The SurFix internal plate fixator with a locking head screw.

4   Clinical results

Clinical results for fracture treatment with the locking compression implants [16, 17] and for open-wedge tibial osteotomies with TomoFix implants indicate easy handling, user-friendliness, and good reproducibility.

Short- and mid-term results (6 years follow-up) of open-wedge technique with the TomoFix plate fixator are convincing. The author's own investigations have shown that in 317 patients only 12 required secondary total knee replacement [23]. This mainly affected patients who had been treated in the first 2 years after introduction of this surgical method. We attribute this to our learning curve with regard to appropriate indications and improved surgical technique. Having gained this experience, we exclude patients with a body mass index (BMI) greater than 30 and severe nicotine abuse from treatment with this method.

In 2002 the author conducted a retrospective study of 92 of our patients and was able to prove that pain measured on the visual analog scale (VAS) had improved from an average preoperative value of 4 (3.5–5) to an average postoperative value of 2 (1.5–3) [23]. The patients attended further follow-up assessments and were found to be pain free on full weight bearing (VAS values of 0.5 to 1.5). They could ambulate without crutches, and pain-free full weight bearing was achieved on average after 10 weeks (6–12 weeks). No neurological complications were observed. In three patients, a total knee prosthesis was implanted within the first year after the correction osteotomy for the treatment of progressive degenerative joint disease and persistent pain. There were no surgical or technical difficulties during implantation of the prosthesis.

- The angular stable internal plate fixator, TomoFix, is a technically sophisticated implant. The biomechanical stability of open-wedge valgization HTO is based on the following concept:
    - Leaving a lateral cortical bridge of 10 mm as a lateral hinge
    - Biplanar osteotomy
    - Elastic fixation (splinting) with the TomoFix plate
    The fixation preserves the soft tissues and periosteal blood supply.
    A remaining disadvantage is the relatively large dimension of the implant, which has to remain in situ until bone consolidation has been completed to avoid secondary loss of correction. However, newer and smaller implant designs have been developed which are used in smaller patients (see chapter 20 "Development of plate fixators: current status and perspectives").

5   Bibliography

[1]   **Perren SM** (2002) Evolution of the internal fixation of long bone fractures. The scientific basis of biological internal fixation: choosing a new balance between stability and biology. *J Bone Joint Surg Br;* 84(8):1093–1110.

[2]   **Staubli AE, Matter P, Allgöwer M** (1978) [Analysis of documented osteosyntheses done with the titanium dynamic compression plate.] Thesis. German.

[3]   **Tepic SS, Perren M** (1995) The biomechanics of the PC-Fix internal fixator. *Injury;* 26:5–10.

[4]   **Coventry MB, Ilstrup DM, Wallrichs SL** (1993) Proximal tibial osteotomy. A critical long-term study of eighty-seven cases. *J Bone Joint Surg Am;* 75(2):196–201.

[5]   **Goutallier D, Julieron A, Hernigou P** (1992) [Cement wedge replacing iliac graft in tibial wedge osteotomy.] *Rev Chir Orthop Réparatrice Appar Mot;* 78(2):138–144. French.

[6]   **Hernigou P** (1996) [A 20-year follow-up study of internal gonarthrosis after tibia valgus osteotomy. Single versus repeated osteotomy.] *Rev Chir Orthop Réparatrice Appar Mot;* 82(3):241–250. French.

[7]   **Jarry A, Hulet C, Jambou S** (2004) [Morphological modifications of the tibia after valgization osteotomy.] *Ann Orthop Ouest;* 36:92–106. French.

[8]   **Puddu GC, Cerullo G, Cipolla M, et al** (1998) [Usage of a plate for open-wedge osteotomies of the tibia.] *Rodilly;* 6:33–37. Italian.

[9]   **Lobenhoffer P, De Simoni C, Staubli AE** (2002) Open-wedge high tibial osteotomy with rigid plate fixation. *Tech Knee Surg;* 1:93–105.

[10]   **Lobenhoffer P, Agneskirchner JD** (2003) Improvements in surgical technique of valgus high tibial osteotomy. *Knee Surg Sport Traumatol Arthrosc;* 11(3):132–138.

[11]   **Spahn G** (2003) Complications in high tibial (medial opening wedge) osteotomy. *Arch Orthop Trauma Surg;* 124(10):649–653.

[12]   **Catagni MA, Guerreschi F, Ahmad TS, et al** (1994) Treatment of genu varum in medical compartment osteoarthritis of the knee using the Ilizarov method. *Orthop Clin North Am;* 25(3):509–514.

[13]   **Frigg R** (2001) Locking compression plate (LCP). An osteosynthesis plate based on the dynamic compression plate and the Point Contact Fixator (PC-Fix) *Injury;* 32:63–66.

[14]   **Frigg R** (2003) Development of the Locking Compression Plate. *Injury;* 34 Suppl 2:B6–B10.

[15]   **Wagner M** (2003) General principles for the clinical use of the LCP. *Injury;* 34 Suppl 2:B31–B42.

[16]   **Gautier E, Sommer C** (2003) Guidelines for the clinical application of the LCP. *Injury;* 34 Suppl 2:B63–B76.

[17]   **Sommer C** (2003) Editorial. *Injury;* 34 Suppl 2:B4–B5.

[18]   **De Simoni C, Staubli AE** (2000) [New fixation technique for the medial open-wedge osteotomy of the proximal tibia.] *Schweiz Med Wochenschrift;* 119:130–142. German.

[19]   **Stoffel K, Dieter U, Stachowiak G, et al** (2003) Biomechanical testing of the LCP—how can stability in locked internal fixators be controlled? *Injury;* 34 Suppl 2:B11–B19.

[20]   **Babst R, Rosenkranz J, Rikli D** (2002) [Treatment of distal articular femoral fractures: treatment with the LISS.] *Trauma Berufskrankh;* 4:44–50. German.

[21]   **Paley D, Pfeil J** (2000) [Principles of deformity corrections around the knee.] *Orthopäde;* 29(1):18–38. German.

[22]   **Agneskirchner JD, Freiling D, Hurschler C, et al** (2006) Primary stability of four different implants for opening wedge high tibial osteotomy. *Knee Surg Sports Traumatol Arthrosc;* 14(3):291–300.

[23]   **Staubli AE, De Simoni C, Babst R, et al** (2003) TomoFix: A new LCP-concept for open wedge osteotomy of the medial proximal tibia—early results in 92 cases. *Injury;* 34 Suppl 2:B55–B62.

Authors   Jens D Agneskirchner, Christiane D Wrann, Denise Freiling, Christof Hurschler, Philipp Lobenhoffer

8   Biomechanical testing of different plates

1   Introduction

Adequate stable fixation is mandatory for safe healing of both additive and subtractive osteotomies around the knee, in order to minimize the risk of nonunion and loss of correction. It has been shown that for open-wedge high-tibial osteotomy (HTO), short spacer plates (Puddu plates) have a large failure rate and a high risk of implant or screw breakage and loss of correction.

Angular stable implants (internal fixators) have replaced conventional plate systems in operative fracture management to a large extent. The highly improved stability of these plates and the possibility of to use them as a "biologic" osteosynthesis with only a minimal approach (MIPO) has made them superior to the non-angular stable plates in many applications.

Due to the long lever arms of the lower extremity and the risk of nonunion, osteotomies around the knee always have been problematic [1–3]. The established system of angular stable osteosynthesis was therefore applied to the concept of osteotomies around the knee, and the plates were specially adapted and precontoured to fit the lateral and medial anatomy of the proximal tibia and distal femur.

This chapter describes a set of experiments that were carried out to test the primary fixation strength of the implants of the TomoFix group for the medial proximal tibia.

In a first series the original TomoFix plate (TomoFix standard implant) was comparatively tested against three other implants (spacer plates), which are available on the market for fixation of HTO [4]. In two following series a modified TomoFix plate (TomoFix next generation, NG), which was developed and designed by the Knee Expert Group (KNEG) of the AO and by Synthes, and a special new small plate of TomoFix (TomoFix small version), designed for the Asian population and small patients, were tested. The results were compared to existing data for the implants.

2 Methods

2.1 Mechanical testing system (Fig 8-1)

Fifteen (n = 15) third generation large composite tibiae were used in this study (saw bones Europe AB, Malmö, Sweden). The tibiae have been reported to reproduce the structural mechanical properties of healthy young adult tibiae [5, 6]. They were embedded in a two component polyurethane casting resin (UREOL FC 53, Vantico GmbH, Wehr, Germany) at their proximal and distal ends, and mounted in a specially designed fixture which was attached to a materials testing machine (MiniBionx 858, MTS Systems Corporation, Eden Prairie, MN,

USA). The fixture was constructed to allow standardized axial loading at a 62% lateral offset from the center of the joint as recommended for clinical use [7] (Fig 8-2). The tibial plateau was embedded in a shallow mold so that force could be applied and different osteosynthesis plates attached without interference. Load was applied to the tibial plateau by means of a ball joint which allowed complete rotational freedom of motion. The distal end of the tibia was potted in a cylinder attached to a universal joint which allowed frontal and sagittal plane rotation but constrained axial rotation.

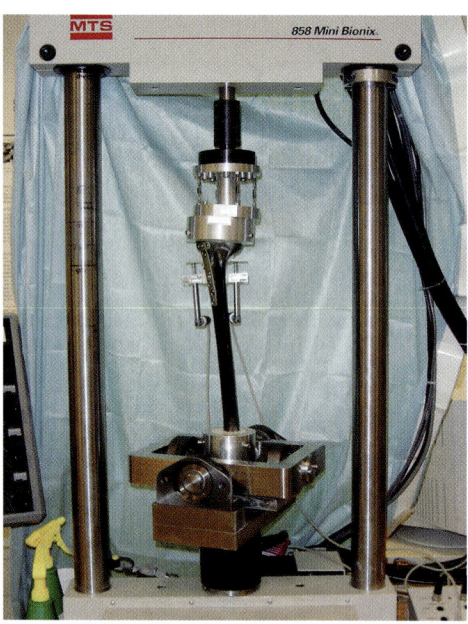

Fig 8-1 Testing set-up with axial loading of 3rd generation composite tibiae (saw bones) using a mechanical testing system (MTS) and a specially designed mounting fixture.

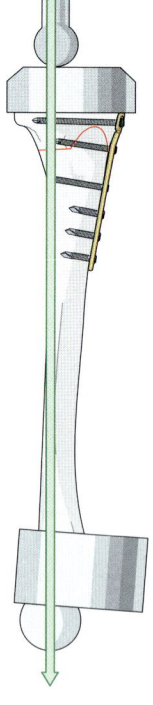

Fig 8-2 Standardized loading at the 62%-point of mediolateral diameter of proximal tibia.

2.2   Implants tested in first series (Fig 8-3)

Four different fixation devices were compared (Table 8-1, Fig 8-3): a short spacer plate without locking bolts (open-wedge osteotomy plate, OWO) (n=4), a short spacer plate with multidirectionally insertable locking bolts (multidirectional angular stable osteotomy plate, MSO) (n=5), a long spacer plate with multidirectionally insertable locking bolts (MSOnew) (n=2), and the TomoFix standard fixator (n=4).

Plate	Single-load to failure tests (n)	Dynamic staircase load to failure tests (n)	
OWO	2	2	
MSO	2	3	First series
MSOnew	Not tested	2	
TomoFix standard	2	2	
TomoFix next generation (NG)	4	5	Second series
TomoFix small version	5	5	Third series

Table 8-1   Types of plates, tested numbers (n), and loading protocol.

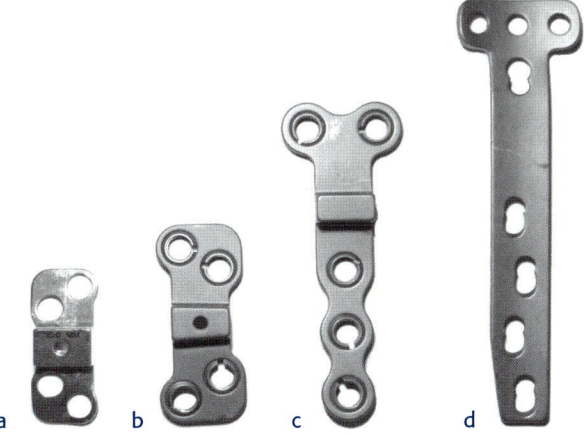

Fig 8-3a–d   Tested implants of first series.
a   Short spacer plate without locking bolts (OWO).
b   Short spacer plate with multidirectionally insertable locking bolts (MSO).
c   Long spacer plate with multidirectionally insertable locking bolts (MSOnew).
d   TomoFix standard.

a   b   c   d

2.3 Osteotomy (Fig 8-4)

All osteotomies were performed using exactly the same technique and by the senior author according to the standardized technique recommended by the KNEG of the AO (described in chapter 9 "High-tibial open-wedge valgization osteotomy with plate fixator") [8]. This comprised a biplanar osteotomy with a horizontal cut of the posterior 2/3 of the tibia. This cut was incomplete leaving 10 mm of lateral bone intact (lateral hinge), which served as the pivot-point during the opening of the osteotomy. The second and complete cut was carried out in the anterior third of the tibia in the frontal plane, ascending 110° behind the tibial tuberosity. The surface areas of this frontal-plane cut maintained direct contact during the opening of the osteotomy ensuring correct axial and rotational alignment of the osteotomized bone. The opening was carried out slowly and carefully over several minutes using the 3-chisel technique in order to avoid microfractures in the lateral cortex during the process of bending around the hinge. A standardized opening of 10 mm was created in all tested saw bones.

2.4 Mounting of the implants (Fig 8-4, Fig 8-5, Fig 8-6)

After opening the osteotomies, all plates were mounted according to the manufacturers' guidelines using the original operative instruments. In the three types of plates with spacer blocks (OWO, MSO, MSOnew), a direct contact of the spacer blocks with the adjacent surface of the osteotomy gap was assured, so that loading was transmitted through the bearing surface of the spacer. The distal cortical screws of OWO, MSO, and MSOnew were inserted bicortically, and the proximal cancellous screws were inserted at an angle of 90° to the plate. The screws of the MSO and MSOnew plates were locked into place using the instruments designed by the manufacturer for that purpose. The TomoFix standard plate was attached to the bones using the original small gap spacers as well as the drilling guides to ensure appropriate locking of all bolts within the plate. The three most proximal screws, as well as the screw distal to the osteotomy, were inserted bicortically. The three most distal screws were inserted monocortically.

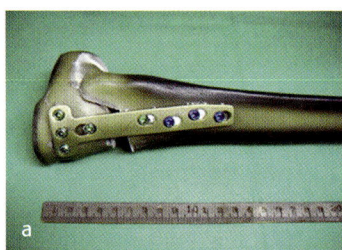
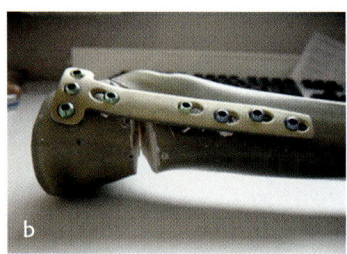
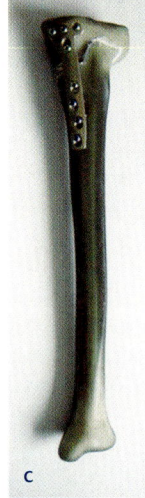

Fig 8-4a–c 3rd generation saw bones mounted with TomoFix standard after biplanar medial open-wedge osteotomy (10 mm).

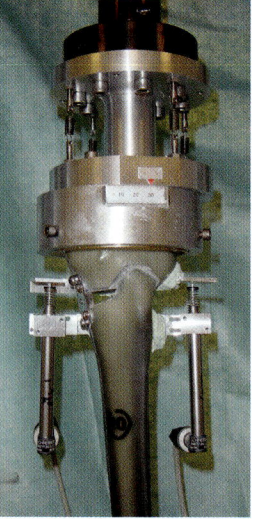

Fig 8-5 Linear displacement transducers mounted medially and laterally between the proximal and distal segment of the osteotomy, used for continuous measuring of the motion at the osteotomy gap during the loading (specimen with OWO).

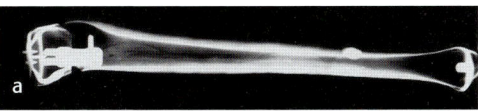

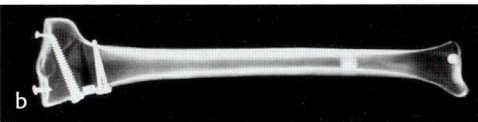

Fig 8-6a–b X-rays of specimen after osteotomy and mounting of a testing plate (OWO), which was carried out to ensure an intact lateral cortex.

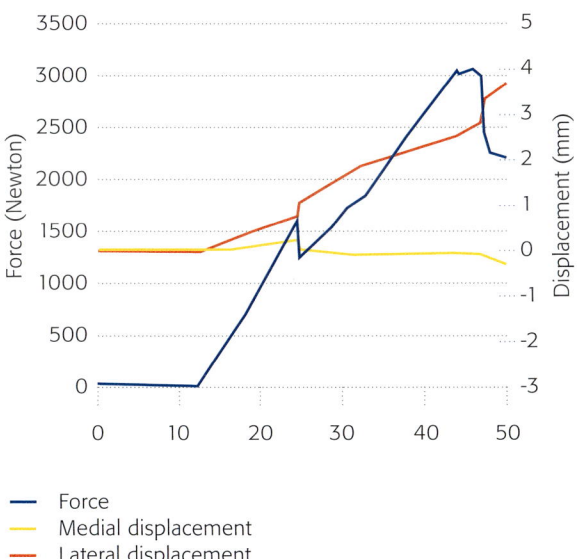

— Force
— Medial displacement
— Lateral displacement

Fig 8-7 Single-load to failure curve in a saw bone with TomoFix standard. Failure typically occurred in two steps, first a microfracture (PF1), then total failure of the lateral cortex (PF2) was seen.

2.5   Displacement at osteotomy gap (Fig 8-5)

After attachment of the plates, the tibiae were embedded in the mounting fixtures and inductive linear displacement transducers (SM277, Schreiber Messtechnik, GmbH, Oberhaching, Germany) were attached at the medial and lateral sides of the osteotomy gap using bone cement in a reproducible manner with a small alignment fixture. The displacement transducers allowed measurement of the motion between the proximal and distal segment of the osteotomy with a spatial resolution of 0.01 mm.

2.6   Testing protocol (Fig 8-7)

The specimens were tested according to two protocols (see Table 8-1); the first consisted of two nondestructive low-load cyclical preloading cycles followed by a displacement-controlled single-load to failure, the second of a load-controlled cyclical staircase fatigue loading protocol to failure. The prefailure loadings at low load were intended to simulate a patient either partially or fully weight bearing immediately after surgery. Two sinusoidal loadings were thus applied for 60 cycles at 0.25 Hz and a loading level of 150 N and 800 N. The specimens were subsequently destructively loaded to failure at 1 mm/s and the displacement across the osteosynthesis gap during failure was measured. The first point of failure (PF1) and its corresponding loading were defined as the point at which the first reduction in loading occurred (first peak, Fig 8-7), the second point at which the maximum loading occurred (PF2, Fig 8-7). For the specimens loaded to fatigue failure, a staircase dynamic loading protocol was defined based on the average ultimate load of the specimens subjected to a single-load to failure (~ 1600 N). The initial loading level was set to 50 % of that load (800 N), and loading was increased in 10 % steps after the successful completion of each loading step of 20,000 cycles (loading levels: 800N (LL1), 960 N (LL2), 1120 N (LL3), 1280 N (LL4), etc; loading frequency = 2 Hz). Loading was terminated after actuator displacements of more than 2 mm were observed during one loading cycle, which was defined as failure of the construct, and the total number of cycles as well as the loading step were recorded.

2.7 Residual stability after failure

The stiffness of the different bone-implant constructs after failure was tested comparatively in order to determine the residual stability after breakage of the lateral cortex. The proximal and distal segment of the osteotomy with the plates still in place, but with failed lateral cortex, were manually twisted and bent, and the resulting displacements at the lateral cortex were measured with a ruler.

3 Results of first series with TomoFix standard

3.1 Low-load cyclical tests

Axial cyclical loading with 150 N and 800 N was tolerated by all implants without failure. No visible damage to saw bone, implant, or the saw-bone implant interface was found. Sinusoidal steady state displacements were measured at both the medial and lateral osteotomy gap secondary to the force which was cyclically applied by the testing machine at 0.25 Hz for 60 cycles. Loading with 800 N created a displacement with a maximum amplitude of 0.13 mm medially and 0.44 mm laterally. These displacements were constant over all 60 cycles in all tested bones and in all implants.

3.2 Destructive single-load to failure tests

3.2.1 Mode of failure (Fig 8-7, Fig 8-8)

All tested bone-implant constructs in the single-load to failure tests (n = 6) failed at the lateral cortex of the saw bone with an identical failure mode (see Fig 8-5). First a fissure in the lateral cortex was observed creating a sudden drop in the applied loading force measured (see Fig 8-6). Another major drop-off of the loading force was typically observed as total failure of the lateral cortex with manifest breaking of the entire lateral bone hinge occurred (see Fig 8-6). Apart from MSO, where additional fissures in the bone around the distal and anterior screw were noted at the time of PF2 (see Fig 8-7), no fractures

or breakages in any other area of the saw bone were noted in any of the tested bone-implant constructs. In OWO and MSO, an additional flexion displacement of the proximal segment of the osteotomy in the sagittal plane was observed at PF2 (Fig 8-8), which was not observed in TomoFix standard.

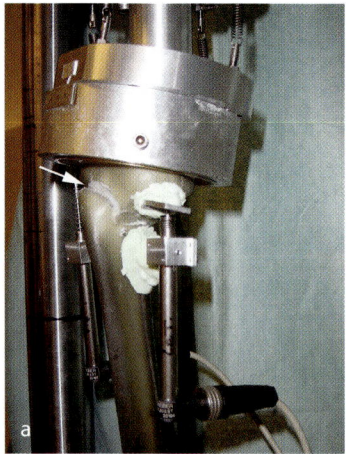
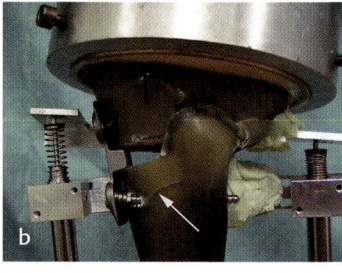

Fig 8-8a–b   Modes of failure: in both short implants the proximal segment was tilted posteriorly with a consequential off-set (arrow) at the osteotomy cut behind the tibial tuberosity. Additional fissure (arrow) in saw bone around anterior, distal screw, which was seen in the bones stabilized with MSO (single-load to failure test).

3.2.2   Force at failure (Fig 8-9)

At PF1 the average of the force was highest in OWO, the lowest in MSO. At PF2 the highest force leading to failure was measured for TomoFix standard, the lowest for OWO.

3.2.3   Displacement at failure

At the medial osteotomy gap the lowest displacement at PF1 and PF2 was measured in the saw bones with the TomoFix standard, the highest displacements were found in MSO bones. At PF1 the TomoFix standard and MSO yielded the lowest displacements laterally. At PF2 the lowest values were measured in the OWO bones and the highest in MSO bones.

3.3   Destructive cyclical-load to failure tests
3.3.1   Cycles until failure (Fig 8-10)

Similar to the mode of failure observed in the specimens tested for a single-load to failure, all the tested bone-implant constructs (n = 9) failed in fatigue at the lateral cortex. The OWO failed at loading level (LL) 2 after an average of 31,834 cycles (4.45 hours), MSO at LL3 after 47,169 cycles (6.5 hours), both MSOnew and TomoFix standard failed at LL4 after 65,520 cycles (9.1 hours) with TomoFix standard having the lowest standard deviation.

3.3.2   Displacement at different loading levels (Fig 8-11)

The maximum displacements at the medial and lateral osteotomy gap during the loading levels were measured. At LL1 (800 N, 20,000 cycles at 2 Hz) the highest displacements both medially and laterally were found in the MSOnew constructs. The lowest displacements were observed in the bones with TomoFix standard. At LL2 (960 N) and LL3 (1120 N) MSOnew was again found to have the largest displacement across the osteotomy gap and TomoFix standard the lowest.

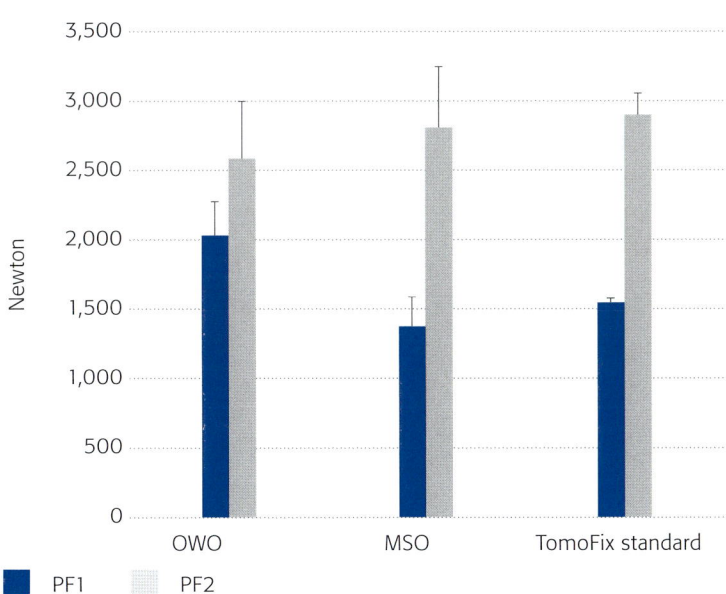

Fig 8-9   Average maximum loads at single-load to failure tests. TomoFix standard implant compared to short spacer plates.

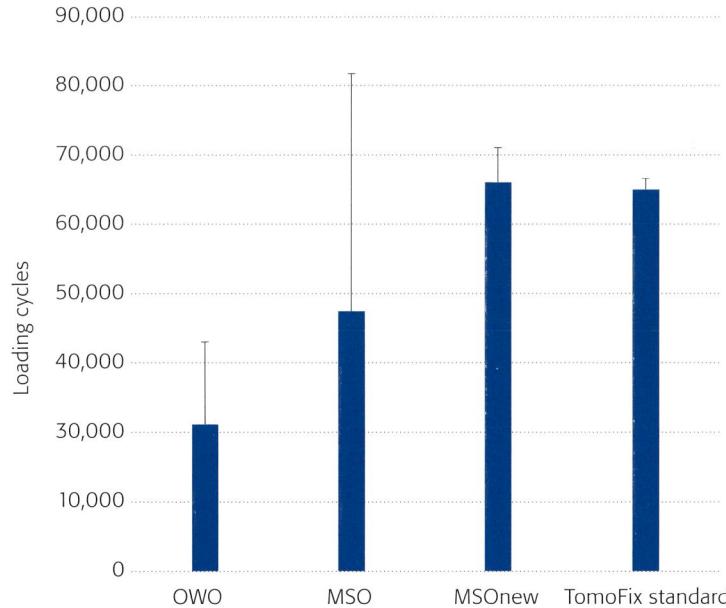

Fig 8-10   Average of loading cycles at time of failure (staircase long-term cyclical loading tests), TomoFix standard implant compared to spacer plates.

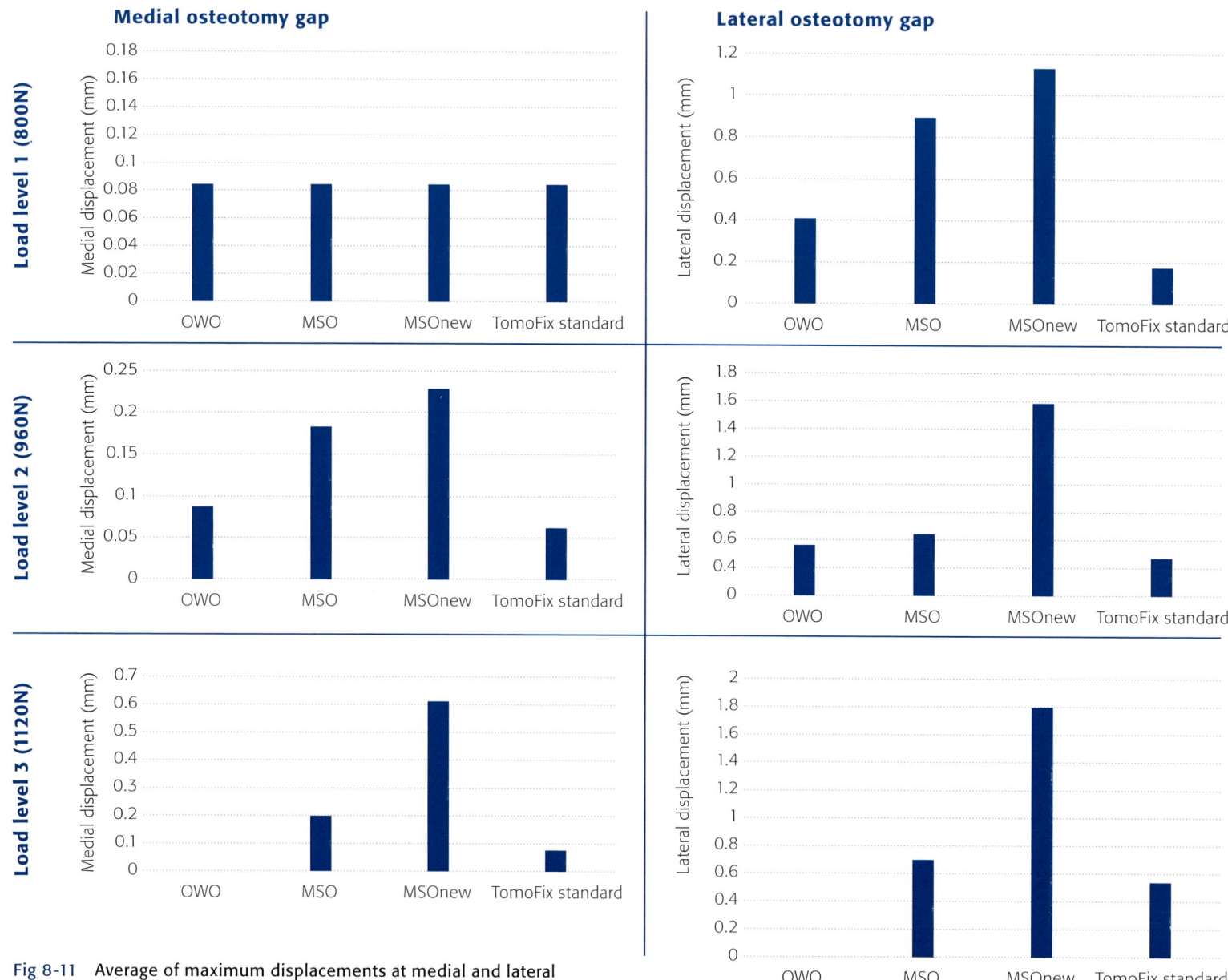

Fig 8-11 Average of maximum displacements at medial and lateral osteotomy gap at different loading levels during the cyclical load-to-failure tests. TomoFix standard implant compared to spacer plates.

3.3.3   Residual stability after failure (Fig 8-12, Fig 8-13)

Large differences were found in the remaining stability of the bone-implant constructs after termination of the tests with the lateral cortex being fractured. In the bones with the short implants (OWO and MSO), the proximal and distal segment of the osteotomy could be manually displaced by more than 10 mm with the undamaged plates still in place. In MSOnew, the segments could be displaced by 3–4 mm in the frontal plane and by 6–7 mm in the sagittal plane. In TomoFix standard, a maximum of approximately 1 mm of displacement was measured in both the frontal and sagittal plane after failure of the lateral bone bridge.

- **Results of TomoFix standard implant compared to three spacer plates**
  - Short cyclical loads of 800N (80 kg) were tolerated by all implants without problems, the lateral hinge remained intact.
  - In the destructive single-load to failure test TomoFix standard implant outperformed the spacer plates, the lateral cortex failed at 2,881 N, compared to approximately 2,500 N of the short spacer plates.

- There was no plate breakage. All constructs finally failed with a breakage of the saw bone.
- All constructs failed with a uniform failure mode: first a fissure in the lateral cortex was observed (PF1), which created a step off in the time-load diagram. Then the constructs failed with total breakage of the lateral cortex (PF2) with another step off in the time-load diagram.
- TomoFix outperformed all spacer plates in the cyclical-load to failure tests, and resisted more than 60,000 cycles of cyclical load.
- Displacement at the medial and lateral osteotomy gap was lowest in TomoFix standard, as compared to the spacer plates.
- After complete fracture of the lateral cortex the constructs with the small spacer plates were highly unstable. TomoFix standard saw bones remained stable against manual displacement forces.

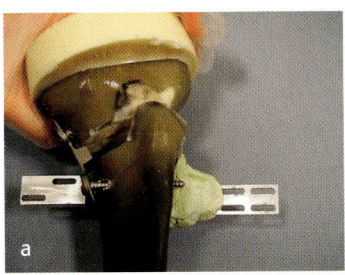 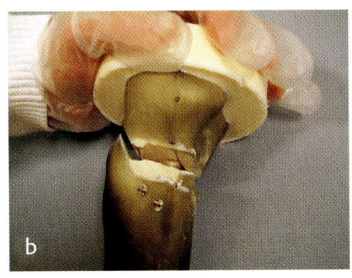 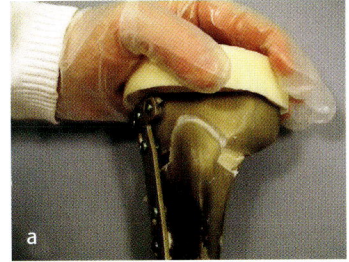 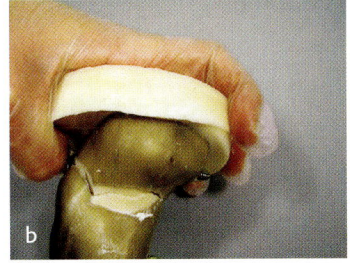

Fig 8-12a–b   Residual stability of saw bone plate construct after broken lateral cortex, stabilized with the short spacer implants: MSO (a), OWO (b). High instability between the proximal and distal segment with a large displacement of the lateral cortical edges was seen.

Fig 8-13a–b   Residual stability of saw boneplate construct after broken lateral cortex, stabilized with the TomoFix standard. Despite the fact, that the lateral cortical bridge was entirely broken the proximal and distal segment of the osteotomy could be displaced by less than 1 mm.

4 Results of TomoFix next generation (NG)

Using the same set-up and loading protocol in a second series the newly developed modified version of TomoFix (TomoFix next generation NG) was tested. Experiments with TomoFix standard implant were carried out as a reference and for the standardization in order to make sure that the same loading and measuring conditions were present as in the first testing series.

4.1 Low-load cyclical tests

Axial cyclic loading with 150 N and 800 N for 4 minutes was tolerated by all implants without failure. Only rhythmic oscillation of the implant was observed without irreversible displacement. These observations are consistent with the results of the previous study.

4.2 Destructive single-load to failure tests

4.2.1 Reference testing TomoFix standard implant

One reference testing was performed with a TomoFix standard implant. Very similar values in mode of failure and force to failure were obtained as in the former test series.

4.2.2 Mode of failure

Mode of failure was uniform in all implants tested, and was identical to the failure mode observed in the TomoFix standard implants, with first a fissure in the lateral cortex (PF1) followed by a breakage of the complete lateral cortex (PF2). No failure of the implant itself was observed.

4.2.3 Force at failure (Fig 8-14)

In the TomoFix NG the average force measured at PF1 was 2,383 N which was 50 x higher than in the TomoFix standard. Force at PF2 was in 3,365 N in average which was also higher that in the TomoFix standard. Even after complete fracture of the lateral cortical (PF2) remained the implant-bone construct stable against rotational forces.

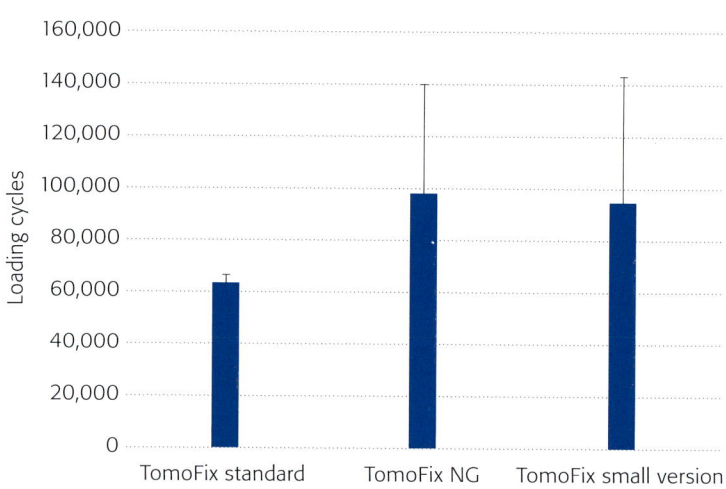

Fig 8-14 Average of loading cycles at time of failure (staircase long-term cyclical loading tests). TomoFix standard compared to TomoFix NG and TomoFix small version.

4.3   Destructive cyclical-load to failure tests

4.3.1   Reference testing TomoFix standard implant

In this test series the TomoFix standard implant reached one loading level (LL) less than in the previous study, and displacement was higher.

4.3.2   Cycles until failure (Fig 8-15)

In most cases the lateral cortex was fissured but not fractured at the end of the cyclical-load failure tests. On average the TomoFix NG implant failed after 97,598 cycles (13.6 hours) almost equalling LL 5. By comparison the TomoFix standard reached only LL 4 and failed after 9.1 hours.

4.3.3   Displacement at different loading levels

The maximum displacements at the medial and lateral osteotomy gap in the TomoFix NG were higher at all LL than in the TomoFix standard as measured in the previous study, but similar to the displacements measured with the reference testing of the TomoFix standard. This variation was explained by interinvestigator variability, as a different investigator performed the tests in the current study. In addition, more implants of the same type were tested this time, which could have resulted in a higher variation between implants and a higher standard deviation.

4.3.4   Residual stability after failure

The implant-bone constructs retained stability against rotational forces after fatigue failure in the cyclical-load test.

■ **Results of TomoFix NG**

▨ Short cyclical load up to 800 N (80 kg) was tolerated by the implant without problems, the lateral cortex remained intact.

▨ In the destructive single-load to failure test the implant resisted significantly higher forces than TomoFix standards before complete failure.

▨ In the destructive cyclical-load to failure tests the implant achieved higher loading levels and more cycles as compared to the TomoFix standard implant.

▨ After complete fracture of the lateral hinge (PF2) the implant-bone construct remained stable against rotational forces.

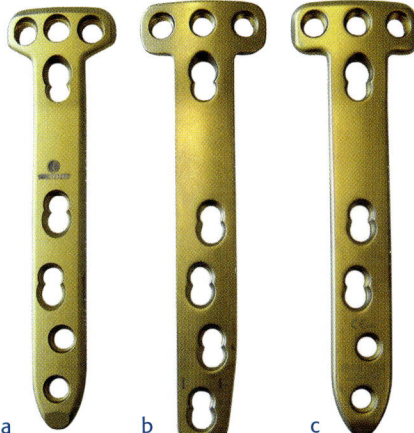

Fig 8-15a–c   Tested implants of second and third series.
a   TomoFix small version.
b   TomoFix standard.
c   TomoFix NG.

5   Results of TomoFix small version

The TomoFix small version was specially designed for smaller patients and the Asian population. This implant is shorter than TomoFix standard and TomoFix NG. It also has no combination holes at hole 3 and 4 and features a smaller radius at the proximal end (Fig 8-15, Table 8-2). Therefore, in this study only medium-sized saw bones instead of large-sized were used. 4th generation saw bones were used in this series. Besides those modifications the same set-up and protocols were used as in the previous studies. In all test cycles, five TomoFix small version implants and again one TomoFix standard implant were tested.

5.1   Low-load cyclical tests

Axial cyclical loading with 150 N and 800 N for 4 minutes was tolerated by all implants without failure. Only rhythmic oscillation of the implant was observed without irreversible displacement. These observations are consistent with the results of the previous study.

5.2   Destructive single-load to failure tests
5.2.1   Reference testing TomoFix standard implant

One reference testing was performed with a TomoFix standard implant applied to a medium-size saw bone. The TomoFix standard achieved lower values than in the previous studies. Testing results of the TomoFix small version implant were compared against this reference test.

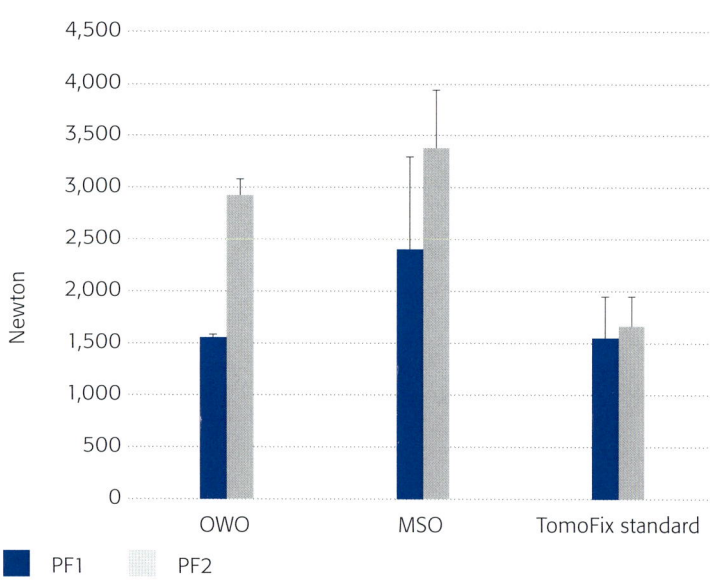

Fig 8-16   Average maximum loads at single-load to failure tests with TomoFix standard, TomoFix NG, and TomoFix small version.

	Standard and NG	Small version
Length (L)	115 mm	112 mm
Width (W)	16 mm	14 mm
Thickness (T)	3 mm	3 mm
Distance proximal holes A, B, C, (P)	11 mm	9 mm
Radius proximal part (R)	38 mm	30 mm
Sagittal angle proximal holes A, B, C (α)	4° caudally	4° caudally

Table 8-2   Dimensions of TomoFix standard, TomoFix NG, and TomoFix small version.

5.2.2 Mode of failure

Mode of failure was uniform in all implants tested and identical to the failure mode observed in the TomoFix implants in the previous studies. First fissuring of the lateral cortex was observed (PF1) followed by a complete fracture of lateral cortex (PF2). Again no breakage of the implants themselves occurred.

5.2.3 Force at failure (Fig 8-16)

In the TomoFix small version the average force measured at PF1 was 1,581 N, which was 43% higher than in the TomoFix standard. Force at PF2 was in 1,704 N in average which was 10% lower than the TomoFix standard. Despite a complete fracture of the lateral hinge (PF2) the implant-bone construct remained stable against manually applied forces.

5.2.4 Displacement at failure

The destructive single-load to failure tests demonstrated that the high forces required to damage the lateral cortex exert too much compression on the linear distance transducers. In this part of the experiment these transducers were not applied.

5.3 Destructive cyclical-load to failure tests

5.3.1 Reference testing of TomoFix standard

In this test series the TomoFix standard implant reached the same loading level (LL) as in the previous study and running time was longer than in the first study.

5.3.2 Cycles until failure (see Fig 8-14)

In all cases, the lateral cortex was fissured but not fractured by the end of the loading failure tests. On average the TomoFix small version implant failed after 96,365 cycles (13.4 hours) and almost equalled LL 5. By comparison the TomoFix standard fixator reached only LL 4 and running time was 10.2 hours.

5.3.3 Displacement at different loading levels

The maximum displacements at the medial and lateral osteotomy gap in the TomoFix small version at the end of LL 1–3 were comparable to that of the TomoFix standard fixator at the corresponding LL. Displacements in the TomoFix small version at the end of the test were clearly higher than in the TomoFix standard accompanied by a high-standard deviation. This high-standard deviation was caused by one implant-bone construct which had a significant shorter running time than the average.

5.3.4 Residual stability after failure

The implant-bone constructs retained stability against manually applied rotational forces.

- **Results of TomoFix small version**
  - Short cyclical load of up to 800 N (80 kg) was tolerated by the implant without problems, and the lateral cortex remained intact.
  - In the destructive single-load to failure test the implant obtained comparable forces to the the TomoFix standard and TomoFix NG.
  - In the destructive cyclical-load to failure tests the implant achieved loading levels and displacements in the lower loading levels, comparable to the TomoFix standard implant.
  - After complete fracture of the lateral hinge (PF2), the implant-bone construct remained stable against manually applied rotational forces.
  - Some increased displacements in the cyclical-load to failure tests were observed, which were caused by one single implant-bone construct with significantly shorter running time.

6   Discussion

In this biomechanical comparative study, the primary stability and fixation strength of specially designed implants for high-tibial open-wedge valgization osteotomy was tested. An axial loading model was used with the loading force transmitted at the 62%-point of the mediolateral diameter of the tibial plateau. This loading alignment was selected since the best results in treatment of unicompartimental osteotoarthritis can be expected if the mechanical axis (Mikulicz line) after valgization HTO runs exactly through this point of the knee joint line. This technique of correcting the mechanical axis has been applied in more than 500 patients in the authors' institution with excellent clinical results. Thus, the loading of an osteotomized tibia in a standing patient was simulated. The specially designed mounting fixture allowed for an exact and reproducable adjustment of the force vector in all tested specimens. Moreover, the design ensured that bending moments at the proximal and distal end were eliminated during the loading.

Third generation large composite tibiae saw bones were used for the tests and improved 4th generation saw bones for the tests with TomoFix small version. These models, which are commercially available, are specially designed and constructed for comparative biomechanical tests. The cortical wall is simulated by an E-glass-filled epoxy, the cancellous bone by a rigid polyurethane material. The compressive strength of these materials is claimed to be 120 Mpa (cortex) and 4.8 Mpa (cancellous) corresponding to the values of healthy adult tibiae. This has been validated in experiments where the structural properties of the composite bones and cadaveric specimens were comparatively investigated [5]. In bending and axial loading tests, the use of composite bones has been recommended since the interspecimen variability of these artificial bones among each other is much lower than in cadaveric specimens. The interspecimen variability of stiffness in cadavers might

outweigh the differences anticipated due to differences in the tested implants. Thus, by using the composite saw bones, the mechanical properties of the bone-implant constructs could be quantified realistically without any bias caused by intrinsic variances between cadaveric tibiae.

Osteotomy and opening of the gap was accomplished with maintenance of an intact lateral cortical bone bridge in all tested bones. All osteotomies were performed in the same manner by the senior author using the clinically established technique of the biplanar cut. This setup guaranteed that variances originating from a difference in the bone stiffness or the osteotomy technique were nearly eliminated. All measured data could therefore be directly attributed to the tested implants, since this was the only variable.

Four implants with different designs were tested in the first series. No direct failure of any implant such as breaking or bending was observed. Failure in all specimens occurred at the lateral cortex, indicating that this is the weakest point in an axial loading situation with the mechanical axis at the 62%-point of the mediolateral knee joint line. However, failure of the cortex did not take place in any implant in the prefailure tests with cyclical loading at 150 N and 800 N, which were performed to simulate a patient with partial and total weight bearing. Likewise, none of the constructs failed at LL 1 (800 N) in the cyclical loading tests.

In the single-load tests failure at the lateral cortex occurred in two steps in all specimens and all series: first a fissure in the cortical bridge was observed, which was accompanied by a sudden drop off in the applied load. This was followed by complete breaking of the saw bone at the lateral cortex with another major decrease in the transmitted load. Differences in the load of failure at these points were found between the implants, especially at PF2 where the rigid TomoFix standard resisted to failure the longest compared to the short implants (OWO, MSO). These differences were found in the single-load to failure tests, but especially also in the long-term cyclical tests, indicating the superior load resistance and rigidity of the plate fixator.

These data suggest that irrespective of the implant, at least short-term axial loading is well tolerated with an intact lateral cortical bridge. Caution is required in directly extrapolating the results of this study to the clinical setting, since traction forces and bending moments, caused by muscles and ligaments, play an important role and were not simulated in the authors' testing model.

The displacements at the medial and lateral osteotomy gap largely differed between the tested implants, in particular in the cyclical-load to failure tests. The plates fixators of the TomoFix group showed the lowest displacements in all specimens and at all load levels, whereas the short plates (OWO, MSO) provided better stability than the prototype long spacer plate (MSOnew). This suggests that the length of the implant does not determine the implant stability regarding the displacement. Nonetheless, the long spacer plate (MSOnew) withstood the cyclical load significantly longer than the short implants and in this parameter had equal results to the TomoFix standard.

Residual stability after failure of the lateral cortex was tested in all specimens. With all plates macroscopically intact and no loosening or breaking of screws detectable, large differences between the implants were found regarding motion between the two parts of the osteotomy. With the lateral bone hinge entirely broken, the short plates showed high instability between the fragments in all planes. In the long plates this

motion was significantly less, especially in the plate fixator, where almost no difference in the stiffness of the bones before failure and after damage of the lateral cortex could be noticed and only some micromotion at the broken lateral cortex was observed. These results suggest that in patients with failed lateral cortex a short implant design provides insufficient stability for safe bone healing and maintenance of the correction. In reality this disadvantage might be partially compensated by some stability given by the periosteum and the fibula, which were absent in our test model. However, it also underlines the importance of intact structures on the lateral side in the short implants. Furthermore, it suggests that the plate fixator provides enough stability for loading situations or normal gait even with a broken lateral cortex.

Apart from a study on the stability of different fixation techniques in closed-wedge valgization osteotomy [9], the present investigation is to our knowledge the first study comparing the stability and fixation strength of four different implants after valgization open-wedge osteotomy in a set-up comprising both single-load to failure as well as long-term cyclical failure tests. There are two other studie, which similarly tested the stability of some of these implants. In one examination the angular stable plate fixator (TomoFix standard) was tested against the non-angular stable short spacer plate (OWO) [10]. Although in this study axial as well as torsional stiffness were tested, only single-load to failure and no cyclical long-term failure tests were performed. Similar to the results of that study, significant better stability was found for the plate fixator compared to the spacer plate in the present study. Another study compared the stability of the non-angular stable spacer plate (OWO) to a C-plate and a tibial plate in an animal cadaver model [11]. A plate fixator was not tested. However, it was found that the resistance of the spacer plate to axial stress was lower than in C-plates.

▪ Conclusion

The results of this biomechanical testing shows that the implant design has a strong influence on the stability of the osteosynthesis after high-tibial open-wegde valgization osteotomy. Short implant designs are inferior to longer designs even if they are designed with angular stable locking head screws. In long plates the thickness and rigidity of the material plays an important role, with a thin and more flexible plate providing less stability than a thick and rigid plate. The TomoFix standard implant outperformed the spacer plates in almost all parameters of stability and displacement both in static single-load to failure testing as well as in dynamic long-lasting cyclical loading.

The new modified implants of TomoFix (TomoFix next generation and TomoFix small version) lead to very similar results compared to the TomoFix standard implant. The changes to the design have no significant influence on the biomechanical properties.

Reliable fixation with safe bone union and a long-term maintenance of the correction can best be achieved with a rigid, long plate fixator with locking head bolts, using either TomoFix standard, TomoFix NG, or TomoFix small version.

7   Bibliography

[1]   **Lobenhoffer P, Agneskirchner JD, Zoch W** (2004) [Open valgus alignment osteotomy of the proximal tibia with fixation by medial plate fixator.] Orthopäde; 33(2):153–160. German.

[2]   **Lobenhoffer P, Agneskirchner JD** (2003) Improvements in surgical technique of valgus high tibial osteotomy. *Knee Surg Sports Traumatol Arthrosc;* 11(3):132–138.

[3]   **Warden SJ, Morris HG, Crossley KM, et al** (2005) Delayed- and non-union following opening wedge high tibial osteotomy: surgeons' results from 182 completed cases. *Knee Surg Sports Traumatol Arthrosc;* 13(1):34–37.

[4]   **Agneskirchner JD, Freiling D, Hurschler C, et al** (2006) Primary stability of four different implants for opening wedge high tibial osteotomy. *Knee Surg Sports Traumatol Arthrosc;* 14(3):291–300.

[5]   **Cristofolini L, Viceconti M** (2000) Mechanical validation of whole bone com-posite tibia models. J Biomech; 33(3):279–288.

[6]   **Heiner AD, Brown TD** (2001) Structural properties of a new design of composite replicate femurs and tibias. *J Biomech;* 34(6):773–781.

[7]   **Fujisawa Y, Masuhara K, Shiomi S** (1979) The effect of high tibial osteotomy on osteoarthritis of the knee. An arthroscopic study of 54 knee joints. *Orthop Clin North Am;* 10(3):585–608.

[8]   **Lobenhoffer P, De Simoni C, Staubli AE** (2002) Open wedge high-tibial osteotomy with rigid plate fixation. *Techn Knee Surg;* 1(2):93–105.

[9]   **Flamme CH, Kohn D, Kirsch L, et al** (1999) Primary stability of different implants used in conjunction with high tibial osteotomy. *Arch Orthop Trauma Surg;* 119(7–8):450–455.

[10] **Stoffel K, Stachowiak G, Kuster M** (2004) Open wedge high tibial osteot-omy: biomechanical investigation of the modified Arthrex Osteotomy Plate (Puddu Plate) and the TomoFix Plate. *Clin Biomech (Bristol, Avon);* 19(9):944–950.

[11] **Spahn G, Wittig R** (2002) Primary stability of various implants in tibial opening wedge osteotomy: a biomechanical study. *J Orthop Sci;* 7(6):683–687.

Authors   Mellany Galla, Philipp Lobenhoffer, Alex E Staubli

9   High-tibial open-wedge valgization osteotomy with plate fixator

1   Surgical principles

The purpose of valgization osteotomy of the proximal tibia is treatment of medial unicompartmental osteoarthritis with varus deformity [1, 2] by shifting the mechanical weight-bearing axis (Mikulicz line) laterally to relieve the medial compartment. High-tibial osteotomy may delay the need for arthroplasty in young and physically active patients. It is regarded as an established procedure for medial osteoarthritis, showing good results [3]. The operation is frequently performed in so-called closed-wedge technique from a lateral approach by removal of a bone wedge as described by Coventry [1] and Maquet [4] (Fig 9-1).

The lateral approach necessitates fibular osteotomy or release of the proximal tibiofibular joint and internal fixation of the tibial head laterally. The need to detach the extensor muscles at the lateral aspect of the tibial head is associated with the risk of damage to the peroneal nerve, which has been reported in the literature at between 3.3% and 11.9% for closed-wedge procedures [3]. Electromyographic data even indicate a nerve lesion in 27% of cases [5].

In contrast to the lateral closed-wedge method, the medial open-wedge technique offers certain advantages:

▧   Only one osteotomy is required.
▧   Fibular osteotomy, dissection of the peroneal nerve, and detachment of the extensor muscles can be avoided.
▧   No shortening of the lower extremity.

The correction of the mechanical axis can be adjusted intra-operatively by gradual opening of the osteotomy gap ("fine-tuning"), whereby ligament instabilities can be treated at the same time by alteration of the caudal inclination of the tibial plateau in the sagittal plane (tibial slope) (see chapter 11 "Osteotomy and ligament instability: tibial slope corrections and

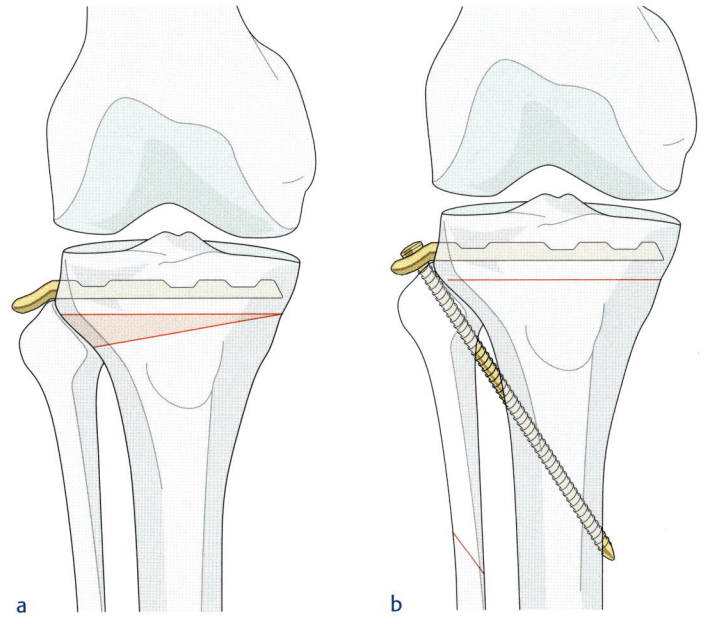

a   b

Fig 9-1a–b   Valgization osteotomy of the proximal tibial head in closed-wedge technique with excision of a lateral wedge and osteotomy of the fibula.

combined procedures around the knee joint"). Incomplete osteotomy, leaving a 10 mm bone bridge laterally and a biplanar cutting technique (see below), will increase postoperative stability. The application of a specially designed plate fixator (eg, TomoFix) allows opening of the osteotomy gaps of up to 13 mm without the need for autograft [2].

■ Medial open-wedge valgization osteotomy of the proximal tibia is performed as a biplanar osteotomy: horizontal osteotomy of the posterior 2/3 of the tibia leaving a lateral bone bridge of 10 mm as a hinge; anterior ascending complete osteotomy behind the tibial tuberosity at an angle of 110°. The osteotomy is opened slowly, ensuring that the lateral hinge remains intact. Stabilization of the correction with an angular locking system (eg, TomoFix). An osteotomy gap of 13 mm or more should be filled with autogenous cancellous bone graft. This method avoids fibular osteotomy, dissection of the peroneal nerve, release of the extensor muscles, and shortening of the lower extremity.

2 Implant design of the angular locking plate fixator TomoFix

The presented plate fixator (TomoFix) is a specially modified T-shaped locking compression plate (LCP) that has locking holes in the proximal part and combination holes in the longitudinal shaft of the plate (Fig 9-2a). The proximal locking holes are adapted to the anatomy of the proximal tibia. An LCP guide sleeve is utilized for drilling the screw holes and ensures

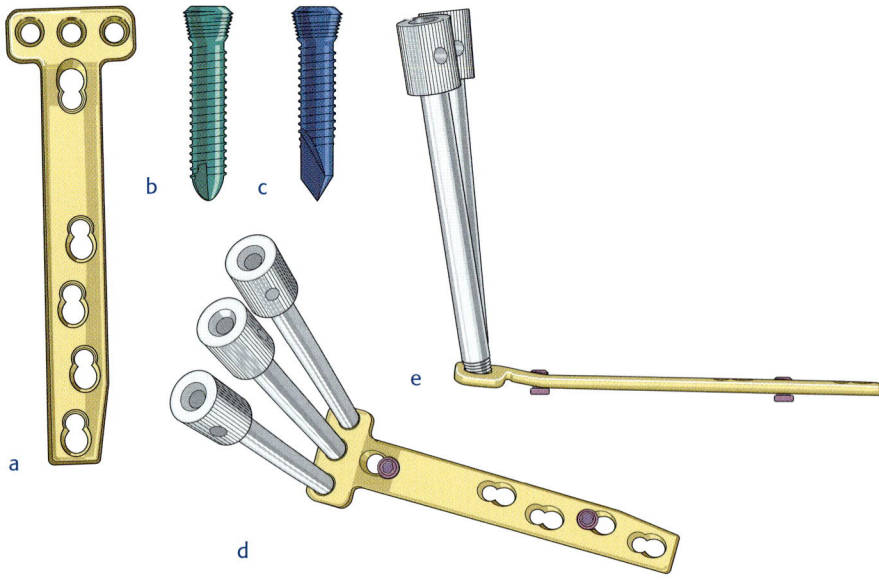

Fig 9-2a–e
a   T-shaped TomoFix plate fixator with threaded screw holes in the proximal arm and combination holes in the longitudinal arm.
b   Self-tapping bicortical locking screws (diameter 3.7 mm) with threaded head (diameter 5 mm) available in different lengths (green).
c   Self-drilling and self-tapping monocortical locking screws (diameter 3.7 mm) with threaded head (diameter 5 mm) available in lengths 18 mm and 26 mm (blue).
d–e TomoFix plate fixator with guide sleeves and two 3 mm distance holders (pink).

correct screw alignment. The locking screws are locked at a fixed angle in the conical threaded plate holes with the torque screwdriver. Self-drilling and self-tapping screws are available that can be inserted mono- or bicortically (Fig 9-2b–c). Since angular locking screws do not have a compressive effect, there is no risk of secondary loss of correction after locking the screws. The TomoFix plate guarantees a rigid fixation even in osteoporotic bone. The temporary insertion of 3 mm distances holders preserves the periosteal blood supply and prevents irritation of tendons and ligaments (Fig 9-2d–e).

3   Indications and contraindications

The indications for open-wedge valgization osteotomy of the proximal tibia (see Table 9-1) are unicompartmental medial osteoarthritis and varus deformity of the lower extremity in physically active patients. This operation can be performed simultaneously with other reconstructive procedures at the medial compartment of the knee to correct varus malalignment, eg,

- Osteochondral autograft transfer system (OATS)
- Autogenous chondrocyte transplantation (ACT)
- Matrix-associated chondrocyte implantation (MACI)
- Collagen meniscus implant (CMI)

In anterior cruciate ligament (ACL) reconstruction with pre-existing varus deformity, a valgization-extension osteotomy of the proximal tibia will lead to axial correction and reduction of anterior tibial shift. A valgization-flexion tibial head osteotomy stabilizes posterolateral knee joint instability in varus deformity (see chapter 11 "Osteotomy and ligament instability: tibial slope corrections and combined procedures around the knee joint"). The preoperative range of motion of the knee should be at least extension/flexion 0-10-120°. Extension deficits up to 10° can be corrected by altering the tibial slope during osteotomy. Patients should not be older than 65–70 years of age.

Contraindications are (see Table 9-2):
- Severe obesity
- Loss of lateral meniscus
- Degenerative joint disease or third or fourth degree cartilage damage in the lateral compartment according to the Outerbridge classification [6]
- Limited range of motion of the knee joint, especially extension deficits > 20° (see above)

The procedure should not be carried out in patients with poor soft-tissue conditions at the medial proximal tibia or in acute or chronic inflammation.

Indications
Unicompartmental medial osteoarthritis
Varus deformity of the lower extremity
Patient less than 65–70 years of age
Patients who are physically very active
As an adjuvant treatment for the correction of varus deformity at the following operations: 1. Osteochondral autograft transfer system (OATS)   2. Autogenous chondrocyte transplantation (ACT)   3. Matrix-associated chondrocyte implantation (MACI)   4. Collagen meniscus implant (CMI)
Valgization-extension osteotomy for anterior knee instability and varus deformity
Valgization-flexion osteotomy for posterior/posterolateral knee joint instability

Table 9-1   Indications for open-wedge valgization osteotomy.

Contraindications
Severe obesity
Loss of lateral meniscus
Degenerative joint disease or third or fourth degree cartilage damage in the lateral compartment according to the Outerbridge classification
Limited range of motion at the knee joint, especially extension deficits >20°
Poor soft-tissue condition at the proximal medial tibia
Systemic or local inflammation
Nicotine abuse

Table 9-2   Contraindications for open-wedge valgization osteotomy.

4   Preoperative planning

Correction of axial deformity by osteotomy of the proximal tibia requires careful preoperative planning. Any possible complications or risks must be explained fully to the patient.

4.1   Patient information

In addition to general surgical risks such as vessel and nerve injuries, thrombosis/embolism, complications in wound healing, and early and late infections, the patient must also be made aware of the possibility of delayed bone healing. Hematoma of the lower extremity often develops as well as swelling and lymph edema. It should be emphasized that at a gap width of 13 mm or more requires harvesting and transplantation of cancellous bone graft from the iliac crest. There may be minimal lengthening of the affected extremity (Table 9-3).

Patient information
General surgical risks such as vessel and nerve injuries, thrombosis/ embolism, disturbed wound healing, early and late infections
Delayed bone healing
Hematoma
Postoperative swelling and lymph edema
Possible need to harvest and transplant cancellous bone from the iliac crest for gaps >13 mm
Minimal lengthening of the corrected lower extremity
Partial weight bearing for 6 weeks postoperatively

Table 9-3   Information to the patient on open-wedge valgization osteotomy.

4.2   Preoperative diagnostics

Physical examination includes evaluation of the range of motion and the stability of the ligaments. The skin and soft tissues must also be inspected.

Radiological diagnostics include x-rays of the knee in three planes and a weight-bearing x-ray of the entire leg. A weight-bearing view of the knee in 45° flexion, a so-called Rosenberg view, and MRI may provide information on the extent of damage of the medial compartment, but are not mandatory.

Prior to the planned procedure, diagnostic knee joint arthroscopy is performed under the same anesthesia in standard technique via the anterolateral portal. The lateral compartment and the lateral meniscus must be intact. Cartilage damages in the medial joint are precisely documented, unstable cartilage flaps are debrided, and microfracturing can be performed. In cases of mechanically relevant tears, the medial meniscus is partially resected (Table 9-4).

Mandatory	Optional
Clinical examination of range of motion and ligament stability	Rosenberg view (weight-bearing view with the knee in 45° flexion)
Inspection of skin and soft-tissue condition	Magnetic resonance imaging (MRI)
Radiographic views of the knee joint in two planes, also tangential x-ray of the patella and weight-bearing film of the entire leg	
Diagnostic knee joint arthroscopy to evaluate the condition of the cartilage in the lateral compartment	

4.3   Radiological planning

The authors refer the reader to chapter 4 "Basic principles of osteotomies around the knee" where the planning procedure of the desired axial correction is presented in detail.

4.4   Positioning of patient and instruments

For open-wedge valgization osteotomy of the tibial head the patient is placed in supine position under general or spinal anesthesia. A lateral support and foot pad are attached to the operating table so that the leg can be easily positioned in 90° flexion and in full extension. The entire leg including the iliac crest is draped to allow harvesting of cancellous bone and intraoperative assessment of the leg axis. A thigh tourniquet is normally not required, but a sterile tourniquet can be used. Preoperative systemic single-shot antibiotic prophylaxis is applied. The image intensifier for intraoperative fluoroscopy is placed on the opposite side.

Instruments

- TomoFix plate fixator, mono- and bicortical locking screws
- Guide wires
- Oscillating saw with a wide saw blade approximately 90 mm long and a narrow saw blade approximately 50 mm long
- Several flat chisels (15–20 mm wide)
- Spreading chisel (optional)
- Calliper
- Arthrodesis spreader
- Measuring wedges

Table 9-4   Preoperative diagnostics.

5   Surgical technique

As described above, diagnostic arthroscopy of the knee is performed under the same anesthesia to evaluate and document the state of the cartilage in the lateral compartment. Unstable cartilage flaps in the medial joint are debrided and suitable areas are microfractured.

The operation begins with the knee in 90° flexion. First, the anatomical landmarks are drawn on the skin:

- Medial joint line
- Cranial border of the pes anserinus
- Superficial collateral medial ligament
- Tibial tuberosity

The skin incision runs from the insertion of the pes anserinus for about 6–8 cm ascending posterocranially aiming at the posteromedial corner of the tibial head (Fig 9-3). The infrapatellar branch of the saphenous nerve is preserved. After division of the subcutis and the fascia at the cranial border of the pes anserinus, the pes tendons are retracted distally with a hook. This exposes the anterior border of the superficial portion of the medial collateral ligament, which is elevated from the tibia with a raspatorium. The long fibers of the superficial medial collateral ligament are then carefully detached from the tibial insertion with a scalpel until the posteromedial cortex of the proximal tibia is exposed. A Hohmann retractor is inserted behind the tibial ridge. At the anterior edge of the incision, the insertion of the patellar tendon at the tibial tuberosity and the medial border of the patellar ligament are exposed (Fig 9-4). The cranial border of the patellar tendon insertion must be clearly visualized so that the destination of the ascending osteotomy can be defined later in the procedure.

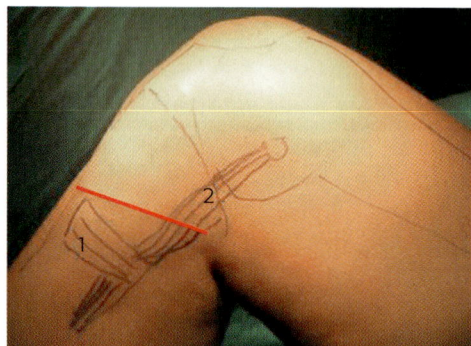

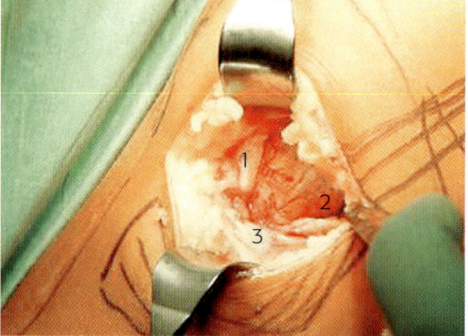

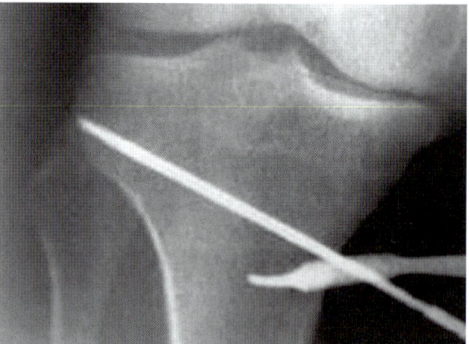

Fig 9-3   The landmarks are drawn on the skin: medial joint line, cranial margin of the pes anserinus (1), line of the superficial medial collateral ligament (2), and the tibial tuberosity. The skin incision (red) runs from the insertion of the pes anserinus about 6–8 cm ascending posterocranially aiming at posteromedial corner of the tibial head.

Fig 9-4   Operation site: medial border of the patellar tendon (1), superficial medial collateral ligament (2), cranial border of the pes anserinus (3).

Fig 9-5   Two 2.3 mm guide wires are drilled into the tibial head under image intensification to mark the direction of the osteotomy. The wires aim at the upper third of the proximal tibiofibular joint, the tips of the wires end exactly at the lateral tibial cortex.

The leg is now positioned in full extension and the knee joint adjusted in exact AP view under fluoroscopy. The medial and lateral compartments must be fully aligned in AP projection, and the leg should be held by the assistant in such a way that one third of the fibular head is covered by the tibia and the patella is located exactly anterior. While this position is maintained, two 2.3 mm guide wires are drilled into the tibial head under image intensification to mark the direction of the osteotomy. Both wires should run parallel and aim towards the upper third of the proximal tibiofibular joint (Fig 9-5).

When placing the two wires, it is important to ensure that there is sufficient space cranial to the saw cut for the three locking bolts in the T-arm and the first proximal screw in the longitudinal shaft of the plate fixator. The wires end exactly at the lateral tibial cortex. First, the posterior wire is inserted at the cranial border of the pes anserinus just in front of the posterior tibial ridge. The second wire is placed about 2 cm anterior and parallel to the first wire. Since both wires end at the lateral tibial cortex, the width of the tibial head can now be measured with reference to the two inserted wires. This is done by holding a third wire of the same length onto the cortex and measuring the excess length compared to the inserted wires (Fig 9-6). The tibial diameter is generally 5–10 mm smaller anteriorly than posteriorly. The measured values should be noted. The depth of the saw cut is 10 mm less than the value measured against the wires in order to leave a lateral bone hinge; the depth is marked on the saw blade.

The knee is positioned in 90° flexion again. The course of the anterior ascending osteotomy is marked with an electrocautery and runs at an angle of 110° to the horizontal saw cut ending behind the patellar tendon insertion (Fig 9-7). This tuberosity segment should be at least 15–20 mm wide.

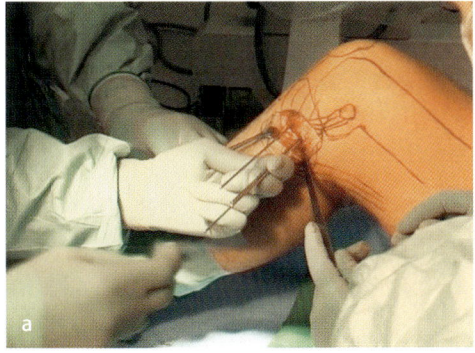 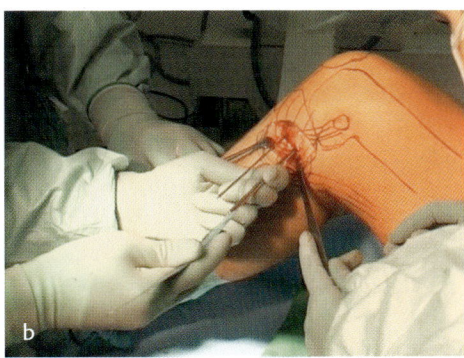

Fig 9-6a–b   Measuring the length of the wires. A third wire of the same length is placed on the cortex and the exceeding length is measured in comparison to the inserted wires.

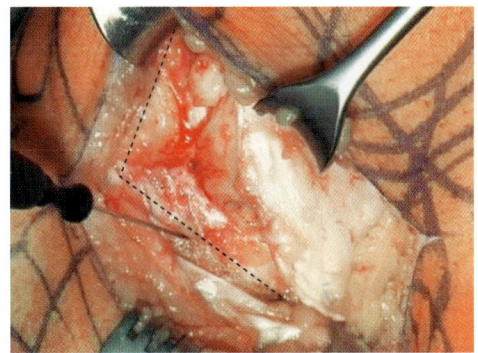

Fig 9-7   Marking the horizontal and the anterior osteotomy at an angle of 110° with an electrocautery.

The horizontal osteotomy is performed with the oscillating saw below the two guide wires that act as guide rails. Attention must be paid to complete the osteotomy of the hard posteromedial tibial cortex. The anatomical structures dorsal of the posterior tibial surface tibia are protected by a Hohmann retractor. The entire sawing procedure is performed slowly, with very little pressure, and under constant cooling of the saw blade by irrigation (Fig 9-8).

Transection of the posterior tibial cortex is noticeable due to a loss of resistance to the saw. Once the planned horizontal depth has been achieved in the posterior two thirds of the tibia, the anterior ascending saw cut can be made with a narrow saw blade. The ascending cut consists of a complete osteotomy including the lateral cortex. It is advisable to start the ascending cut with the saw perpendicular to the cortex with the saw blade pointing in posterolateral direction in order to avoid slippage. After transection of the medial cortex, the saw blade can be directed in the frontal plane. Fig 9-9 illustrates the principle of the biplanar osteotomy. When the osteotomy is opened, bone contact between the two surfaces of the anterior osteotomy is maintained, which guarantees better postoperative biomechanical stability in the sagittal plane.

Next, the depth of the osteotomy is marked on a broad flat chisel which is then inserted into the transverse osteotomy as far as the lateral bone bridge. Another broad flat chisel is placed between the first chisel and the guide wires; the depth of the second flat chisel is about 10 mm less than the first (Fig 9-10). The chisels are carefully driven into the osteotomy gap by light hammer blows. This will open the osteotomy.

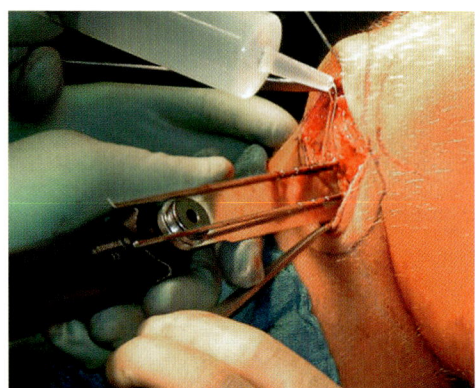

Fig 9-8   Sawing of the horizontal osteotomy with the oscillating saw below the two guide wires with minimal pressure and constant irrigation cooling of the saw blade. The structures posterior to the tibia are protected by a Hohmann retractor.

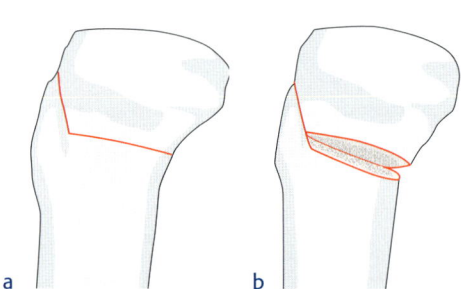

a   b

Fig 9-9a–b   Principle of the biplanar osteotomy. Horizontal osteotomy in the posterior 2/3 of the tibia and anterior osteotomy ascending at an angle of 110° behind the tibial tuberosity. During spreading osteotomy the two surfaces of the anterior ascending part stay in contact and ensure postoperative stability in the sagittal plane.

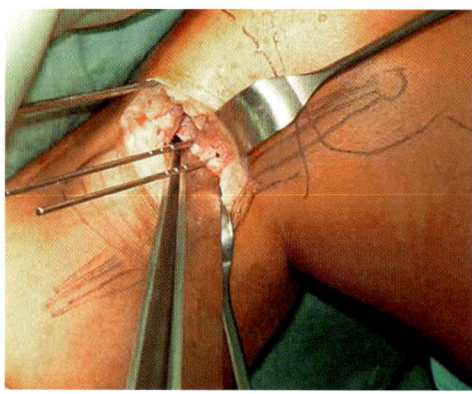

Fig 9-10   Insertion of the flat chisels to the measured depth of the osteotomy.

Two alternative techniques are available to open the osteotomy gap further. Additional flat chisels can be inserted between the ones already in place, whereby every additional chisel is inserted a little less than the previous one, or a spreader chisel (Fig 9-11a) is placed into the osteotomy gap created by the first two chisels, and the gap is opened to the desired width by opening the spreader with a large screwdriver (Fig 9-11b). The latter method is preferred by the authors.

The osteotomy should be opened slowly over a period of several minutes in order to prevent fracturing of the lateral cortex. Leaving the two guide wires in place while opening the gap leads to stiffening of the proximal segment and prevents fracture of the articular surface of the tibia. The width of the osteotomy gap is monitored during the opening procedure using a calliper. When the planned width has been achieved,

an arthrodesis spreader is placed in the posteromedial corner of the osteotomy (Fig 9-12). The chisels can now be removed.

Due to the medial collateral ligament complex the osteotomy tends to open more anteriorly during spreading, thus increasing the caudal inclination of the tibial plateau (tibial slope). Therefore, it is important to ensure sufficient release of the long superficial fibers of the medial collateral ligament and symmetrical opening of the horizontal osteotomy. When correcting an isolated varus deformity, the tibial slope (caudal inclination of the plateau) should not be altered (Fig 9-13). If ligament instabilities or extension deficits are being treated alongside the axial correction, an alteration of the tibial slope may be required [7, 8] (Fig 9-13). Asymmetrical opening of the osteotomy by insertion of additional measuring wedges into the osteotomy gap alters the caudal inclination of the tibial

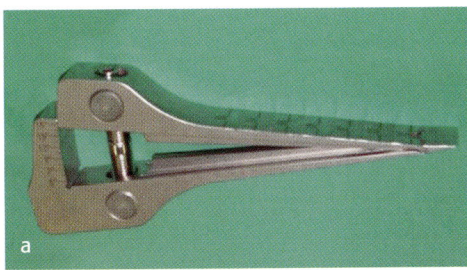

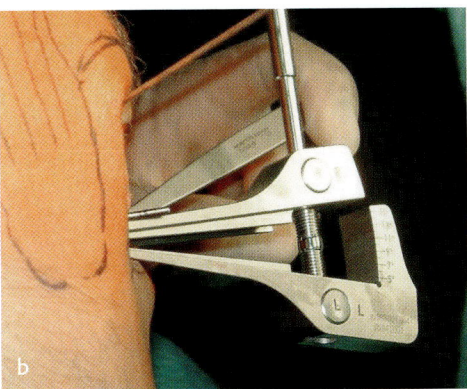

Fig 9-11a–b
a   Spreader chisel.
b   Using the screwdriver, the spreader chisel is opened in situ to the planned width of the osteotomy gap.

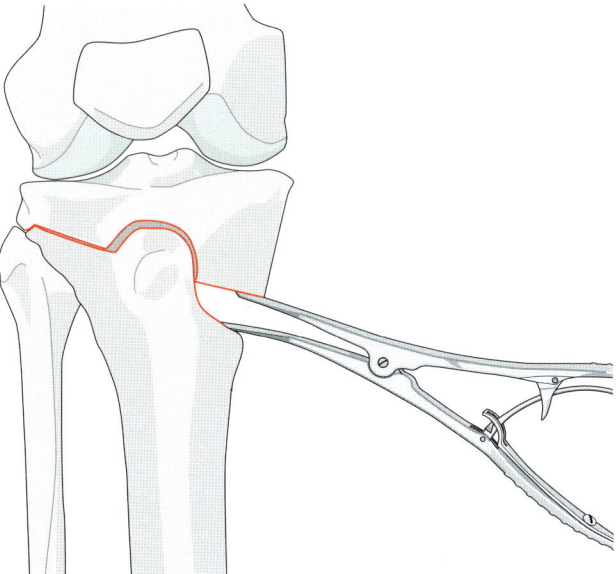

Fig 9-12   When the desired width has been achieved, an arthrodesis spreader is placed on the posteromedial cortex of the osteotomy.

plateau (see chapter 11 "Osteotomy and ligament instability: tibial slope corrections and combined procedures around the knee joint"). For example, the posterior subluxation tendency of the tibia in patients with posterior knee instability and hyperextension of the knee can be treated by increasing the tibial slope. This is achieved by opening the anterior part of the osteotomy more than the posterior part (so-called flexion osteotomy). The resulting translation of the tibia counteracts the posterior drawer sign [9]. Reduction of the slope is achieved by extension osteotomy (posterior opening greater than anterior opening) and can treat anterior knee instability (Fig 9-13). In addition, this method can improve range of motion in cases of extension deficit.

After spreading of the osteotomy gap to the desired width, the leg is again placed in extension. In this position, the leg axis can be evaluated clinically and radiologically. Under image intensification a long measuring rod is placed at the center of the femoral head and at the center of the upper ankle joint (Fig 9-14). The corrected weight-bearing line should now intersect with the tangent to the tibial plateau in the lateral compartment at the 62% point [10] (Fig 9-15). The axis can be adjusted by opening or closing the arthrodesis spreader as required. When the knee is extended, attention should be paid to the adaption of the surfaces of the anterior ascending part of the osteotomy.

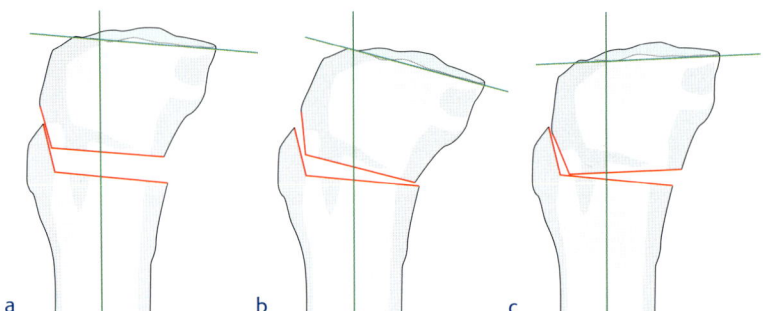

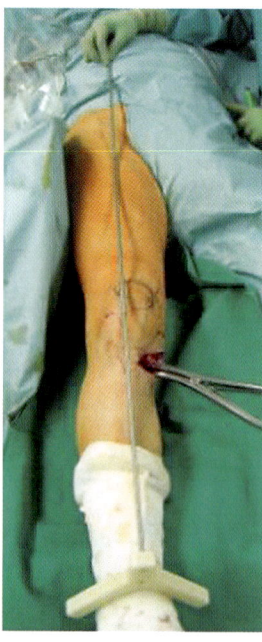

Fig 9-13a–c
a   If the tibial slope is to remain unchanged, the horizontal osteotomy gap must be opened symmetrically.
b   The caudal inclination of the tibial plateau may be altered by asymmetric opening of the osteotomy. Hyperextension of the knee and posterior subluxation of the tibia due to posterior knee instability can both be treated by increasing the tibial slope (so-called flexion osteotomy).
c   The slope can be reduced by extension osteotomy (opening the posterior part of the osteotomy more than the anterior part) and may produce stability in patients with anterior knee instability.

Fig 9-14   The leg axis is evaluated in extension with a long measuring rod that is placed at the center of the femoral head and at the center of the upper ankle joint under image intensification.

The plate fixator with its preassembled proximal drill sleeves and distance holders is slid into a subcutaneous tunnel (Fig 9-16). The longitudinal arm is aligned with the tibial diaphysis avoiding anterior or posterior cortical overhang, the solid mid-portion of the fixator lies over the osteotomy, and the proximal locking screws lie subchondral near the joint line. The implant is temporarily stabilized by insertion of a K-wire into the central drill sleeve. After predrilling with a 4.3 mm drill bit, the three proximal self-tapping locking screws of the T-arm are inserted one after the other. The locking screws are inserted with a power drill. The plate fixator should not rotate as the screws are locked into the thread of the plate hole ("helicopter effect"). Since bicortical fixation is not necessary for this implant, and to avoid soft-tissue irritation, the screw tips should not protrude beyond the lateral cortex, ie, the length of the screws should be a few millimeters less than the value actually measured. When all three proximal bolts have been inserted, they are tightened with a torque screwdriver and locked at a fixed angle in the plate holes.

Next, a temporary lag screw is inserted into the first plate hole distal to the osteotomy. This compresses the lateral hinge by pulling the distal osteotomy segment towards the plate fixator. Potential fissures within the lateral bone hinge are brought

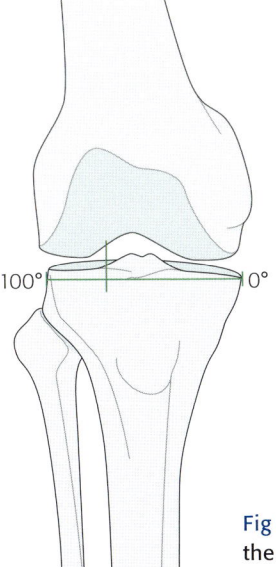

Fig 9-15 The mechanical axis should cross the tangent to the tibial plateau in the lateral compartment at the 62 % point after correction [10].

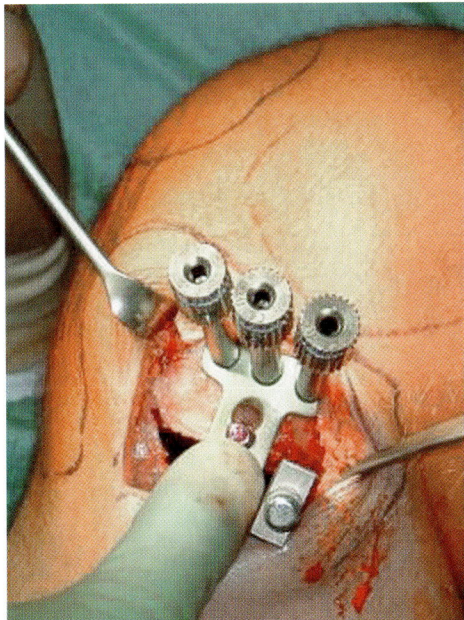

Fig 9-16 The plate fixator with its preassembled proximal drill sleeves and distance holders is slid into the subcutaneous tunnel. The proximal locking screws are situated about 1 cm below the joint line.

under elastic preload and distraction on the lateral side is eliminated (Fig 9-17). In addition, the plate fixator is drawn closer to the surface of the proximal medial tibia reducing soft-tissue irritation over the implant. The osteotomy gap is watched constantly while the lag screw is tightened slowly to avoid secondary loss of correction. In the last step of the operation this screw is replaced by a bicortical locking screw.

The screws in the longitudinal arm are inserted from the distal to proximal end. Two distance holders are inserted into the plate fixator before fixation to maintain a distance of 3 mm from the bone surface and prevent irritation of the pes

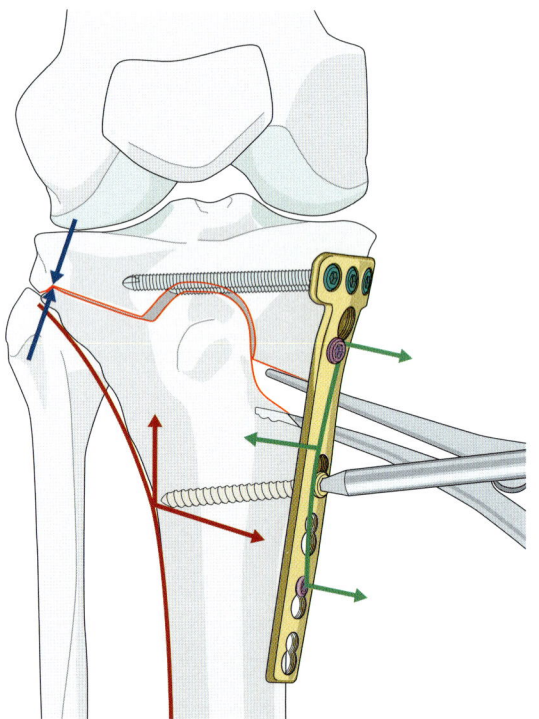

Fig 9-17 Principle of preloading by application of a temporary lag screw in the first plate hole distal to the osteotomy. The distal osteotomy segment is pulled towards the plate fixator.

anserinus and the medial collateral ligament. The preassembled distance holders are not removed until immediately before insertion of the definitive screw. The distal locking screws are introduced through a stab incision over the distal distance holder, which can be palpated easily through the skin. The plate holes distal and proximal to the distance holder can be exposed by retracting the skin with two small retractors. Since monocortical self-drilling and self-tapping locking screws are being utilized, only shallow drilling of the medial tibial cortex with the 4.3 mm drill bit through an LCP universal drill sleeve is required. In general, 26 mm locking screws are used, but 18 mm screws are available for patients with a narrow shaft diameter. The lag screw distal to the osteotomy gap is replaced by a bicortical locking screw, and a locking head screw is inserted proximal of the gap. After locking all screws at fixed angle with the torque screwdriver, the arthrodesis spreader is removed. To prevent secondary bleeding from the cancellous surface of the osteotomy, a collagen fleece is cut to size and placed between the bone and the internal fixator to cover the osteotomy gap. The long fibers of the medial collateral ligament are repositioned. If the gap width exceeds 13 mm, autogenous cancellous bone graft is harvested from the anterior iliac crest and is transplanted in the osteotomy gap before inserting the collagen fleece. It is not necessary to fill the gap with bone substitute.

Suction drainage is not necessary, but the authors recommend inserting an overflow drainage which exists proximally.

Image intensifier x-rays of the knee in two planes are taken for documentation before the subcutaneous tissue and the skin are closed. The soft tissue and especially the skin must be closed with extraordinary accuracy to ensure sufficient implant cover. Elastic bandaging of the leg is completed in the operating room.

■ **Operative steps**

1. Anatomical landmarks are drawn, skin incision from the insertion of the pes anserinus ascending 6–8 cm posterocranially.
2. Pes tendons are retracted distally.
3. Careful release of the superficial fibers of the medial collateral ligament and exposure of the entire medial border of the patellar ligament.
4. Level and direction of the osteotomy are marked with two 2.3 mm guide wires aiming at the upper third of the proximal tibiofibular joint; the wires end exactly at the lateral cortex.
5. Length is measured using the wires and osteotomy depth is marked on the saw blade.
6. Biplanar osteotomy is marked with electrocautery at an angle of 110°.
7. Horizontal osteotomy in the posterior 2/3 of the tibia beneath the guide wires leaving a lateral bone bridge of 10 mm as a hinge.
8. Complete anterior ascending osteotomy at an angle of 110°.
9. Opening of the osteotomy with the broad flat chisels.
10. Spreading of the osteotomy and insertion of an arthrodesis spreader on the cortical surface of the posteromedial corner of the osteotomy.
11. Attention must be paid to the tibial slope.
12. Clinical and radiographical evaluation of the leg axis in extension.
13. Insertion of the plate fixator and locking of proximal screws.
14. Insertion of a temporary lag screw into the first plate hole distal to the osteotomy.
15. Insertion of screws into the remaining plate holes from distal to proximal after removing the distance holders.
16. Lag screw is replaced by a bicortical locking screw.
17. For an osteotomy gap of 13 mm or more, the gap is filled with autogenous cancellous bone graft.
18. Collagen fleece placed over the osteotomy gap.
19. Radiological documentation in both planes and wound closure.

6   Postoperative management

Cryotherapy begins immediately after the operation (eg, Cryo/ Cuff System). The use of an intermittent vein compression pump (eg, VenaFlow System) in the primary phase is strongly recommended. The bandage is changed on the first post-operative day to assess the soft-tissue condition. Ambulation with 15–20 kg body weight (checked on a weighing scale) with underarm crutches begins on the first postoperative day and continues for 4 weeks. In weeks 5–6, weight bearing is increased, and full weight bearing is permitted from the 7th postoperative week.

Since the range of motion of the knee is not restricted, an orthesis or brace is not required. Thromboembolism prophylaxis with low-molecular weight heparin under regular testing of the thrombocyte count should be continued until full weight bearing is reached. Physical therapy includes active and passive exercises. Daily manual lymph drainage is recommended since postoperative lymph edema occurs relatively frequently. Electrotherapy for muscle stimulation (EMS device) is optional.

Skin sutures are removed on day 10–12 postoperatively.

Follow-up x-rays in two planes are taken on the 3rd post-operative day and 6 weeks postoperatively.

- Postoperative weeks 1–4: partial weight bearing with 15–20 kg with underarm crutches.
  Postoperative weeks 5–6: increased weight bearing.
  Full weight bearing from the 7th postoperative week.
  No limit to range of motion.
  Thromboembolism prophylaxis and manual lymph drainage.

7   Errors, hazards, and complications

Application of the TomoFix plate fixator requires detailed knowledge of the implant and its specific locking technique. Angular locking must be precise, whereby the alignment of the locking screws as predetermined by the plate holes must be strictly observed. Correct positioning of the TomoFix implant is essential. The longitudinal plate arm must be exactly aligned with the tibial diaphysis. The proximal part should not be positioned too high or too low, otherwise the locking screws cannot be inserted correctly (Table 9-5).

In order to avoid over- or undercorrection of the mechanical axis exact preoperative planning is mandatory. Potential planning errors can be recognized and corrected in time by intraoperative verification of the axis prior to internal fixation.

Transection of the posterior tibial cortex risks damage to the popliteal vessels in the third segment. This would become immediately apparent during surgery without a tourniquet by severe bleeding from the osteotomy gap. In such a case, the popliteal vessel and nerve bundle can be easily reached by extending the medial skin incision distally. The fascia parallel to the posterior tibial border is dissected longitudinally distal to the pes anerinus. The vessel and nerve bundle is exposed between the medial portion of the gastrocnemius muscle and the tibial diaphysis. The artery runs medially and the vein and tibial nerve more laterally. If the popliteal vessels are damaged, they can be clamped and sutured according to common vascular surgery techniques. If the tibial nerve is damaged, two-stage suture or reconstruction is indicated.

Postoperative swelling of the soft tissues and lymph edema can be treated with oral antiphlogistic therapy, manual lymph drainage, and intermittent vein compression pumps.

Errors, hazards, and complications

Incorrect positioning of the implant: it must be remembered that the orientation of the locking screws is predetermined by the plate holes and that the longitudinal arm must be exactly aligned with the tibial diaphysis.

Over- and undercorrection of the mechanical axis as a result of inadequate preoperative planning and insufficient intraoperative assessment of the axis.

Damage to the bone surface due to excessive pressure and heat during sawing.

Injury to the popliteal vessel and nerve bundle during transection of the posterior tibial cortex.

Hematoma.

Postoperative soft-tissue swelling and lymph edema.

Deep crural thrombosis and/or pulmonary embolism.

Compartment syndrome.

Superficial and deep infections.

Delayed consolidation of the osteotomy gap.

Table 9-5   Errors, hazards, and complications in open-wedge valgization osteotomy.

Manifestation of deep crural thrombosis and/or pulmonary embolism require special internal treatment.

The clinical symptoms of imminent compartment syndrome (elastic swelling of the extremity, impaired sensitivity of the lower extremity, especially in the area of the superficial peroneal nerve) must be recognized early, possibly evaluated with a compartment measuring device. The tolerable compartment pressure depends on the clinical symptoms (pain, neurological status) and the difference of the compartment pressure compared to the patient's diastolic blood pressure. Incision of the fascia is indicated if the difference is less than 30 mm Hg.

In case of postoperative hematoma, evacuation and drainage are required. Postoperative infection is treated by early revision with debridement, systemic antibiosis, and insertion of antibiotic carriers, if necessary. If the internal fixation is stable and the soft-tissue cover intact, the plate fixator can be left in situ, otherwise change of management to an external fixator is advised (see chapter 17 "Management of complications after high-tibial open-wedge osteotomy").

Delayed consolidation of the osteotomy gap is often expressed as persistent pain on ambulation after 6–9 weeks postoperatively. In these cases, the AP x-ray reveals a small micromotion callus at the lateral cortex of the osteotomy. Treatment consists of secondary cancellous bone grafting.

8   Results

From October 2000 to February 2006 the authors performed high-tibial valgization osteotomy according to the described technique in a total of 707 patients. Average patient age was 40 years.

The mean width of the osteotomy gap was 10.6 mm. All patients attended follow-up until they were capable of full weight bearing and consolidation of the osteotomy gap had been confirmed radiologically. Secondary loss of correction did not occur in any of these cases.

Eleven patients received secondary cancellous bone graft to treat delayed bone healing.

Hematoma was evacuated during hospital stay in twelve cases.

Revision surgery was needed for two patients a few days after the first operation due to overcorrection. In these cases the distal locking screws were removed from the plate fixator, the mechanical axis was corrected and the plate was restabilized by insertion of new bicortical locking screws in the distal part of the longitudinal arm. The further course for these patients was uneventful.

In three other cases late infection with irritation of the soft tissues over the implant became manifest 4 months postoperatively. After removal of the plate fixator and insertion of antibiotic carriers, there were no further healing disturbances in these patients.

Fig 9-18 and Fig 9-19 show follow-up x-rays after valgization osteotomy in open-wedge technique with an osteotomy gap of 10 mm. The x-rays on the third postoperative day show the intact lateral hinge and the osteotomy gap in both planes (Fig 9-18). Consolidation of the osteotomy gap, especially posteromedially, can be seen on the follow-up x-rays after 24 months (Fig 9-19).

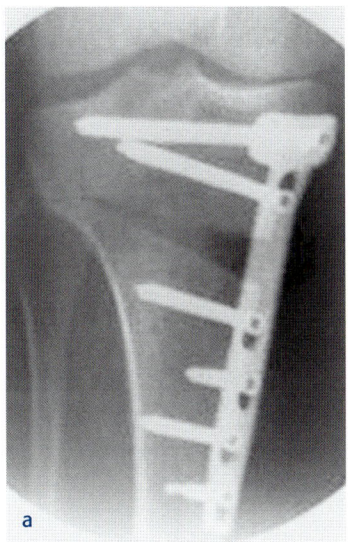
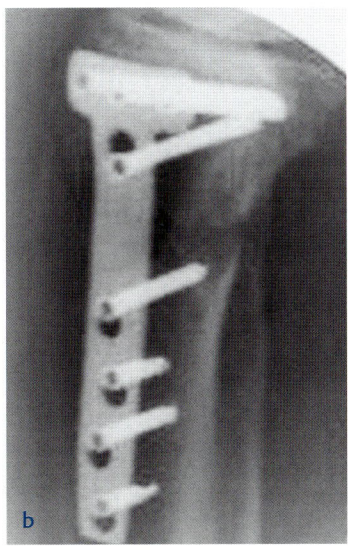
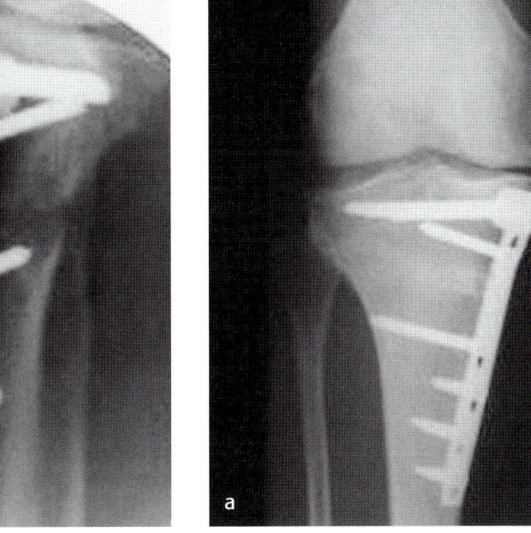
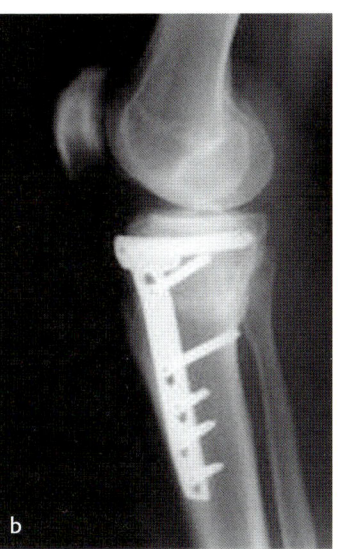

Fig 9-18a–b   The immediate postoperative x-rays show an intact lateral bone bridge and the osteotomy gap (10 mm) in both planes.

Fig 9-19a–b   Follow-up x-ray after 24 months showing consolidation of the osteotomy gap especially posteromedially.

9 Bibliography

[1] **Coventry MB** (1979) Upper tibial osteotomy for gonarthrosis. The evolution of the operation in the last 18 years and long term results. *Orthop Clin North Am;* 10(1):191–210.

[2] **Lobenhoffer P, de Simoni C, Staubli AE** (2002) Opening wedge high-tibial osteotomy with rigid plate fixation. *Tech Knee Surg;* 1:93–105.

[3] **Coventry MB** (1984) Upper tibial osteotomy. *Clin Orthop Relat Res;* 182:46–52.

[4] **Maquet P** (1976) Valgus osteotomy for osteoarthritis of the knee. *Clin Orthop Relat Res;* 120:143–148.

[5] **Aydogdu S, Cullu E, Araç N, et al** (2000) Prolonged peroneal nerve dysfunction after high tibial osteotomy: pre- and postoperative electrophysiological study. *Knee Surg Sports Traumatol Arthrosc;* 8(5):305–308.

[6] **Outerbridge RE** (1961) The etiology of chondromalcia patellae. *J Bone Joint Surg Br;* 43:752–757.

[7] **Lobenhoffer P, Agneskirchner JD** (2003) Improvements in surgical technique of valgus high tibial osteotomy. *Knee Surg Sports Traumatol Arthrosc;* 11(3):132–138.

[8] **Lobenhoffer P, Agneskirchner JD, Zoch W** (2004) [Open valgus osteotomy of the proximal tibia with fixation by medial plate fixator.] *Orthopäde;* 33(2):153–160. German.

[9] **Lobenhoffer P** (1999) [Chronic instability after posterior cruciate ligament injury: tactics, technique, and results.] *Unfallchirurg;* 102(11):824–838. German.

[10] **Fujisawa Y, Masuhara K, Shiomi S** (1979) The effect of high tibial osteotomy on osteoarthritis of the knee. An arthroscopic study of 54 knee joints. *Orthop Clin North Am;* 10(3):585–608.

Authors   Christiane D Wrann, Christof Hurschler, Philipp Lobenhoffer, Jens D Agneskirchner

10   Effect of osteotomies on cartilage pressure in the knee

1   Introduction

The aim of correction osteotomies is the transfer of mechanical load from diseased, arthritic areas of the joint to areas with intact, healthy cartilage. The open-wedge high-tibial valgization osteotomy (HTO) is a treatment method for medial varus osteoarthritis of the knee aiming for a shift of the weight-bearing axis by a correction of the leg axis. The degenerated medial compartment cartilage is thus decompressed resulting in a relief of pain and a delay of cartilage damage.

Good clinical short- and mid-term results have been reported [1–8]. However, favorable results seem to be strongly dependent on a precisely performed correction of the mechanical axis [9]. Undercorrection with a persisting varus usually leads to poor results. Overcorrection into large valgus may result in medial joint opening and rapid development of lateral osteoarthritis [10]. Various recommendations on the precise amount of the valgus alignment achieved postoperatively have been published. Some authors refer to the anatomical axes of the femur and tibia and recommend a postoperative alignment of 8–10° valgus [11–14]. Others focus on the mechanical axes of the femur and tibia and suggest a postoperative alignment of 3–5° valgus [5, 10, 15]. However, these recommendations are based on individual clinical experiences and only a few retrospective studies.

- **Principles of correction osteotomy**
  - The aim of open-wedge high-tibial valgization osteotomy is the redistribution of pressure on the tibiofemoral joint cartilage.
  - Good results are achieved with high-tibial osteotomy if correction is precisely performed.
  - Different recommendations regarding the amount of correction are found in the literature.

Probably the most commonly applied concept in preoperative planning is based on the work of Fujisawa et al [16]. In this retrospective clinical study, arthroscopy was performed in 54 knee joints before and after closed-wedge HTO evaluating the tibiofemoral joint cartilage with a follow-up of 4 months to 6 years. The postoperative weight-bearing axis was correlated with cartilage damages. The correction achieved postoperatively was evaluated by measuring the intersection of the corrected weight bearing axis with the tibial plateau. The tibial plateau was divided into four sections and the point of intersection was assigned to the corresponding section. Fujisawa et al [16] concluded from their findings that for ideal correction the postoperative axis should lie within the lateral 30% of the tibial plateau as measured from its midpoint. From this study emerged the recommendation that the weight-bearing axis should postoperatively pass through the so-called "Fujisawa point", ie, it should intersect with the knee joint line at 62% of the tibial plateau entire width measured from its medial cortex [17–19].

Despite an enormous increase of interest in osteotomies, so far no results have been published that quantify the load-transfer effect of shifting the weight-bearing axis on tibiofemoral joint contact pressure with reliable implication for the right amount of correction. The work of Fujisawa et al was published in 1979, when knee arthroscopy, the only parameter used in the study to evaluate outcomes, was still developing. Further weaknesses of the mentioned study are the relatively small patient groups (approximately twelve knee joints per group) and the complete lack of postoperative clinical data such as pain or joint effusion.

Because of the discrepancy between the high number of osteotomy procedures being performed and the lack of experimental data on the actual intraarticular effects of correction osteotomies of the knee, the authors undertook a literature search on this subject and carried out a biomechanical study that will be presented in this chapter.

2   Literature overview: experimental studies of the effect of different load axes on tibiofemoral pressure distribution

The effect of different loading axes in the frontal plane on the distribution of pressure in the tibiofemoral compartments has already been the subject of several experimental studies with different measuring techniques and experimental designs. Before direct measurement of joint cartilage pressure was technically possible, indirect methods were employed based on evaluation of x-rays, eventually combined with gait analysis and measurements of ground reaction forces with force plates [20–22]. The first direct measurement of transferred joint forces and contact pressure was obtained by application of strain gauges [23, 24]. Next, pressure sensitive films (Fuji films) were used, indicating the applied pressure by change of colour [25, 26]. The current techniques employ pressure-sensitive film that measures changes in electromechanical resistance (Tekscan system). These sensors offer highest accuracy and best reproducibility and have provided the basis for the most recent studies on this subject [27, 28].

In the past, the majority of studies were based on test cycles under static conditions and rarely under dynamic conditions, ie, simulation of gait cycle with an increase and decrease in loading. Nevertheless, all the studies were basically able to demonstrate that alterations of the axial alignment resulted in redistribution of load within the compartments of the tibio-femoral joint. Varus deformity resulted in greater loading of the medial compartment and valgus deformity in greater loading of the lateral compartment. This inequality in the distribution increased with the degree of axis deviation and the amount of applied force [24, 25].

In addition to those studies describing tibiofemoral pressure distribution under the influence of different loading axes in the frontal plane, only two experimental studies have been published on the effect of high-tibial correction osteotomy on contact pressure distribution within the knee joint. One of these studies employed the closed-wedge technique for correction of deformities in the frontal plane (valgus-varus) [26]. The other study, published by the authors, focused on contact pressure changes after correction osteotomy in the sagittal plane [27]. Measurements of the contact pressure in the knee joint after correction osteotomy in the varus-valgus plane in open-wedge technique have not yet been published. Furthermore, data correlating the degree of valgus with the desired changes in intraarticular contact pressure distribution are currently not available.

In a biomechanical study with knee joint specimens, Riegger-Krugh et al [26] examined the effect of closed-wedge HTO on contact pressure distribution in the tibiofemoral joint using Fuji films. However, in this study measurements were only possible under static conditions. Both varus and valgus malalignment were simulated and a closed-wedge osteotomy of 5° was performed. The authors found differences in contact pressure distribution as expected, with higher contact pressure in the medial compartment in varus malalignment and higher contact pressure in the lateral compartment in valgus malalignment. Surprisingly, with neutral loading axis less contact pressure was recorded medial than lateral. After valgization HTO the contact pressure distribution was similar to that of a neutral leg axis. The authors concluded that because of those minimal changes in the contact pressure distribution a closed-wedge HTO of 5° would result in an undercorrection in most patients.

Since the used mounting device for the specimens allowed only for limited adaptations to the different preexisting anatomical axes and did not simulate in vivo conditions, general conclusions for the degree of correction in the clinical situation can only be drawn to a limited extent.

In a biomechanical study conducted by the authors tibiofemoral contact pressure was measured after flexion HTO, ie, after altering the mechanical axes in the sagittal plane [27]. In a dynamic experimental model involving a knee joint kinemator, contact pressure was measured with the Tekscan system. Flexion osteotomy was performed as a supratuberositous open-wedge osteotomy parallel to the slope of the tibial plateau and then the tibial slope was gradually increased from its original position in 5°-steps to 20°. This osteotomy addressed the alignment in the sagittal plane. The alignment in the frontal plane (varus-valgus) was not changed.

The flexion osteotomy significantly altered the tibiofemoral contact pressure distribution: as the tibial slope increased, the tibiofemoral contact area in the medial compartment shifted anteriorly, whereas the posterior joint area was unloaded. This effect was most prominent in extension (see chapter 11 "Osteotomy and ligament instability: tibial slope corrections and combined procedures around the knee joint").

In addition to these biomechanical studies on cadaveric specimens, two other studies that measured tibiofemoral contact pressure intraoperatively in vivo have been published. One study measured pressure distribution with an implemented telemetric pressure measurement device during implantation of a total knee replacement. The patient was supine under general anesthesia, testing was performed in normal alignment and under varus and valgus stress [29]. The second study measured tibiofemoral contact pressure during diagnostic arthroscopy with the patient under local anesthesia. F-scan pressure measurement sensors from the Tekscan system were inserted into the medial and lateral compartments and contact pressure was recorded during two-leg and single-leg stance and after application of a valgus splint [30].

■ **Literature overview of cartilage pressure measurements**
Early studies: indirect measurement of intraarticular pressure by analysis of x-rays, gait analysis, and measurement of ground reaction forces.
Direct measurement of pressure on the cartilage for the first time with color-coded films (Fuji): different contact pressure distribution due to different mechanical axes.
Only one study published on cartilage pressure measurement after high-tibial valgization osteotomy in **closed-wedge technique** [26].
No study published on valgization osteotomy in **open-wedge technique**.

3   Biomechanical investigation of tibiofemoral pressure distribution after tibial head valgization osteotomy in open-wedge technique

As explained in the previous paragraphs there is currently no data available that quantifies the effects of open-wedge HTO on contact pressure distribution of the tibiofemoral joint. Therefore the authors conducted the study as presented in this chapter.

3.1   Materials and methods

Seven knee joints were tested in full extension under axial loading according to a standardized loading protocol (peak load 1000 N) in a material testing system (Minibionix 858, MTS Systems Corporation, Minneapolis) (Fig 10-1). Different loading axes of the lower leg were simulated by varying the anatomic alignment angles of the distal femur and the proximal tibia using a specially designed and constructed fixation device. The fixture compensated different preexisting anatomical femoral and tibial angles and guaranteed a standardized and reproducible intersection between the mechanical loading axis and the knee base line for each testing cycle. The distal end of the tibia and the proximal end of the femur were potted in cylinders attached to universal clamps, which allowed frontal and sagittal plane movement but constrained axial rotation (Fig 10-2).

The knee base line was measured as the width of the tibial plateau and divided into sections (measured in percent) beginning from the medial margin of the cortex. Correct positioning was determined by a vertical laser beam indicating the direction of the axial load application (Fig 10-1). The intersection of the load axis with the joint line at the medial cortex of the tibial plateau was defined as 0% (varus alignment). Further tests were performed with the axis at the 25% point, 50% point (neutral axis), 62% (Fujisawa point), and 75% point. Subsequently, an intraligamentous medial open-wedge

HTO was performed in standard technique (see chapter 7 "Principles of angular stable fixators") (Fig 10-3, Fig 10-4). The opening of the gap was standardized at 9 mm, the medial collateral ligament initially was left intact, and the loading axis again adjusted to 62%. Finally, the distal superficial part of the medial collateral ligament bridging the osteotomy was dissected from anterior to posterior in two steps (Fig 10-5).

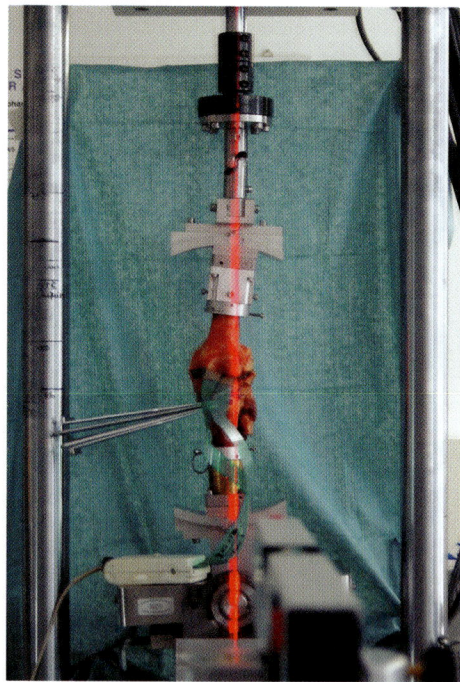

Fig 10-1   Experimental design for pressure measurement in the mechanical testing system (MTS).
A knee specimen is mounted in a special holding device. The mechanical axis is simulated by a perpendicular laser beam. Several flat chisels have been inserted into the osteotomy gap to open the osteotomy at the medial tibial head.

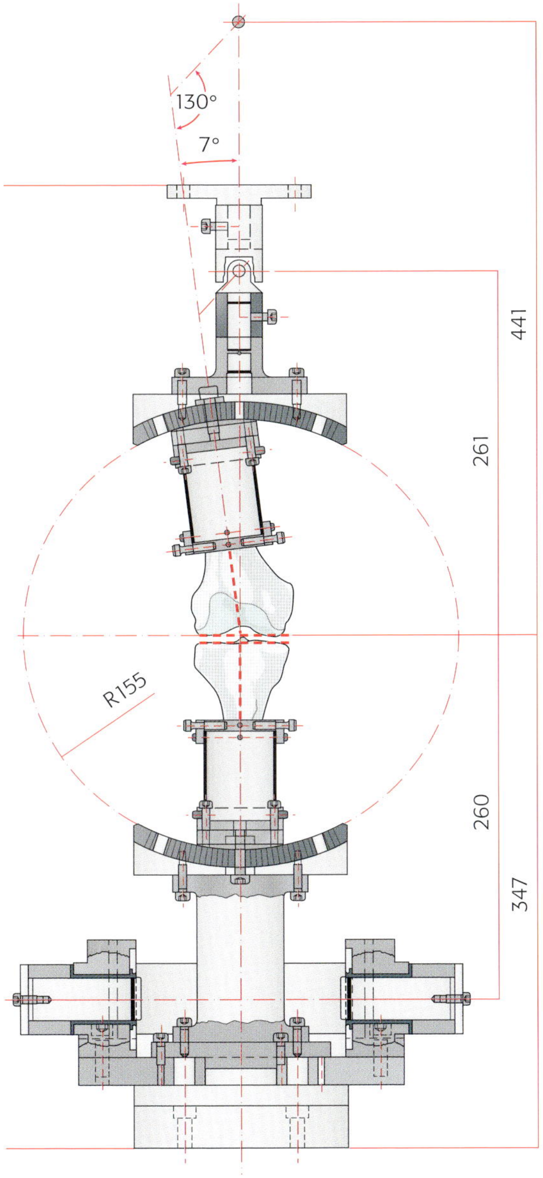

Fig 10-2   Custom-made fixation device for simulation of different axes in a specimen knee.
The loading axes can be modified and adjusted.

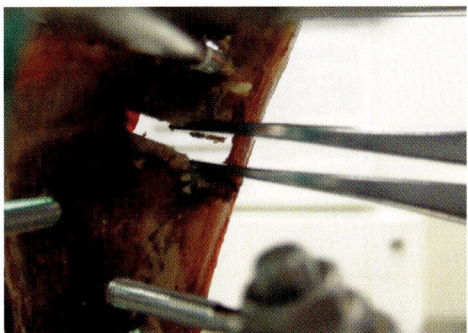

Fig 10-3   Intraligamentous open-wedge valgization osteotomy is performed. An osteotomy spreader opens the osteotomy gap.

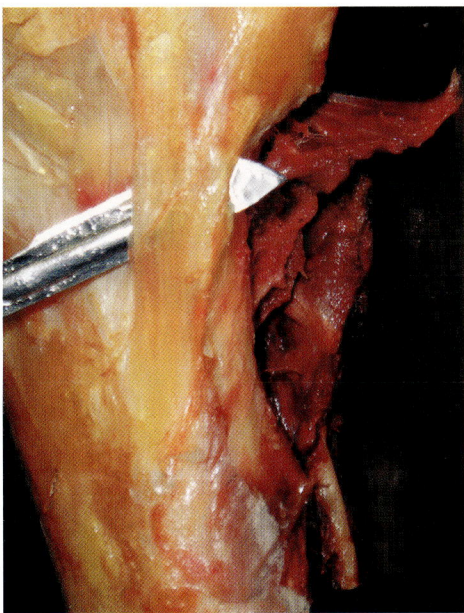

Fig 10-4   Knife under superficial portion of the medial collateral ligament which is subsequently released stepwise.

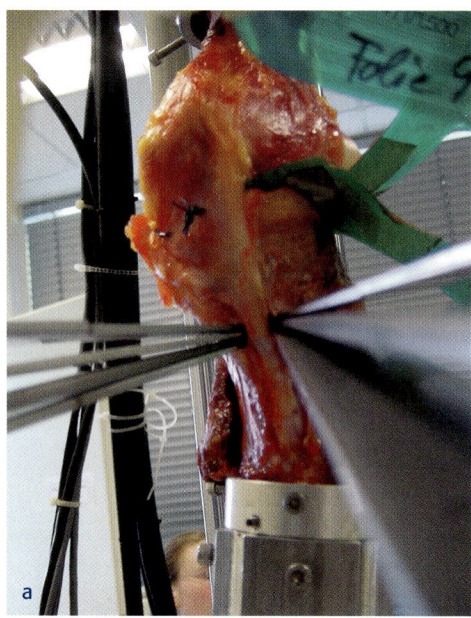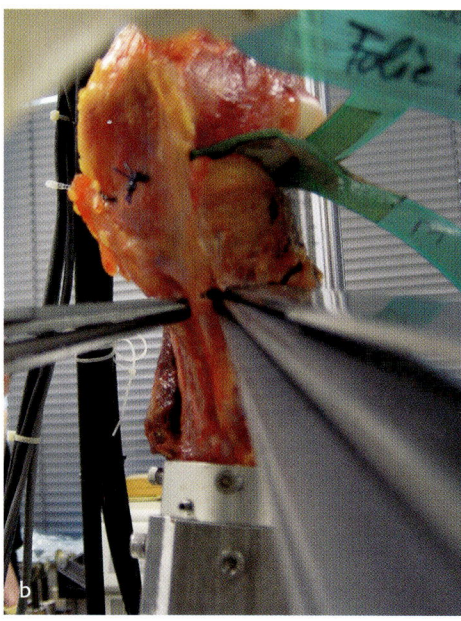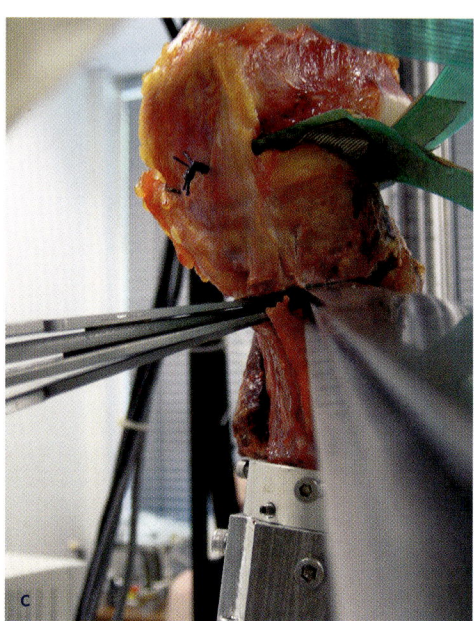

Fig 10-5a–c   Gradual release of the superficial distal portion of the medial collateral ligament.
a   Ligament intact, flat chisel in the osteotomy gap.
b   Anterior half of the superficial portion of the medial collateral ligament is released.
c   Complete release of the superficial portion of the medial collateral ligament.

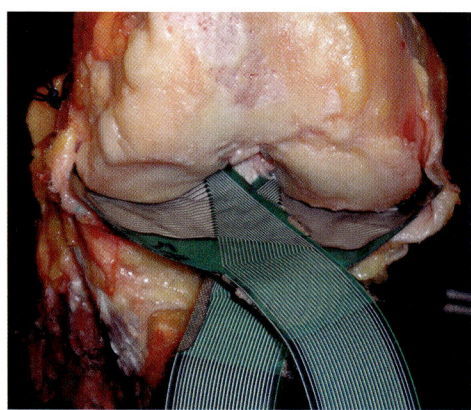

Fig 10-6   AP view of a knee specimen with pressure measurement sensors in the medial and lateral tibiofemoral compartment (K-Scan 4000, Tekscan).

In each set-up measurement was performed using pressure-sensitive films (K-Scan 4000, Tekscan, Boston, USA). Contact force (N), contact area (mm²), and contact pressure (MPa) as well as the topographic pressure distribution between the medial and lateral tibiofemoral joint were continuously recorded during the loading cycle (Fig 10-6).

■ **Experimental design for cartilage pressure measurements**
Custom-made fixture with seven cadaveric human knee joints.
Standardized loading protocol for 1000 N:
1. Pressure measurement with Tekscan sensors in the medial and lateral joint compartments
2. Testing of different weight-bearing axes (varus, neutral, valgus) prior to osteotomy
3. Open-wedge tibial head valgization osteotomy
4. Measurement at the Fujisawa point (62%) with intact and stepwise dissected medial collateral ligament

3.2   Results

Contact pressure distribution between the medial and lateral joint compartment was shown to be clearly dependent on the different load axes. For varus deformity (0%, ie, intersection of the loading axis with the joint line at the medial cortex), about 65% of the total pressure was measured in the medial compartment and 35% in the lateral compartment. The more the load axis was shifted laterally, the lower the contact pressure recorded medially and the higher in the lateral compartment (Fig 10-7, Fig 10-8, Fig 10-9). Surprisingly, after medial open-wedge osteotomy with intact medial collateral ligament under a loading of 1000 N, the percentage of contact force on the medial side was considerably higher than in the lateral compartment (71.4% versus 28.6%), although the load axis was slightly valgus positioned at the 62% point. Measurement with the same mechanical loading axis (62%) without osteotomy had produced a reverse pattern of contact pressure

distribution, ie, medial contact pressure was clearly lower than lateral contact pressure. Instead of decompressing the cartilage in the medial joint by shifting the weight-bearing axis into the valgus (62%); contact pressure was even slightly increased when the tibial osteotomy was performed without any ligament (Fig 10-10). Even without axial loading, some contact pressure was detected in the medial compartment. Only after stepwise dissection of the superficial distal portion of the medial collateral ligament medial decompression was achieved. Medial contact pressure was reduced and the lateral contact pressure increased reaching values that were previously recorded in the 62% position without osteotomy.

3.3   Analysis of the results

The results demonstrate that the topographical distribution of contact pressure between the medial and lateral compartment significantly depends on the direction of the loading axis in relation to the knee joint line. However, this varies to a relatively large extent within the specimens because difference in cadaveric specimen sizes, ligament tension, and individual structure of the joint cartilage affect cartilage contact pressure. The highly significant increase in pressure in the medial compartment after open-wedge HTO for all specimens proves that the applied intraligamentous osteotomy technique was associated with increased tension in the superficial layer of the medial collateral ligament bridging the osteotomy gap. This resulted in a considerable increase in medial contact pressure, which superimposed the effect of valgization and abolished it completely.

The results also indicate that intraarticular pressure is influenced by the amount of tension in the collateral ligaments and suggest that geometric correction of the axes without consideration of ligamentous tension may have an unexpected, paradoxical effect on cartilage pressure. The surgical technique presented in this study, which is also recommended by the Knee Expert Group of the AO (KNEG) and currently applied in the authors' clinic, is based on an intraligamentous technique, ie, an osteotomy performed within the medial collateral ligament (see chapter 9 "High-tibial open-wedge valgization osteotomy with plate fixator"). The opening of the osteotomy distracts the proximal and distal insertion of the ligament, which causes ligamentous tension that leads to a corresponding increase in contact pressure in the medial compartment that can only be decreased by a complete release of the superficial portion of the medial collateral ligament.

■ **Results of cartilage pressure measurement**
Testing prior to osteotomy:
- For varus alignment: medial 65%, lateral 35% of the total contact pressure.
- For neutral alignment: medial 40%, lateral 60% of the total contact pressure.
- For valgus alignment (Fujisawa point, 62%): medial 35%, lateral 65% of the total contact pressure.

Testing after open-wedge osteotomy:
- Despite valgus alignment (Fujisawa point), significant increase in medial contact pressure with intact medial collateral ligament (71% medial versus 29% lateral).
- Medial decompression was only achieved after dissection of the superficial medial collateral ligament (36% medial versus 64% lateral).

3.4   Summary

Although the presented biomechanical testing system is associated with certain simplifications as every experimental model in comparison to the in vivo situation, the results of these studies present a foundation regarding the amount of correction and the surgical technique of medial open-wedge valgization tibial osteotomy as a treatment of varus osteoarthritis.

The aim of correction osteotomy is redistribution of contact pressure from the medial to the lateral tibiofemoral compartment by shifting the mechanical axis laterally. Sufficient medial decompression is achieved by slight valgus overcorrection to the 62% Fujisawa point. However, the mechanical axis should not be corrected without addressing ligament tension. Applying valgization tibial osteotomy in open-wedge technique will lead to even greater mechanical loading in the medial compartment than in the original varus deformity due to excessive over-tensioning of the medial collateral ligament. Therefore, in this type of osteotomy a complete release of the distal superficial medial collateral ligament is mandatory to accomplish sufficient decompression of the medial joint compartment.

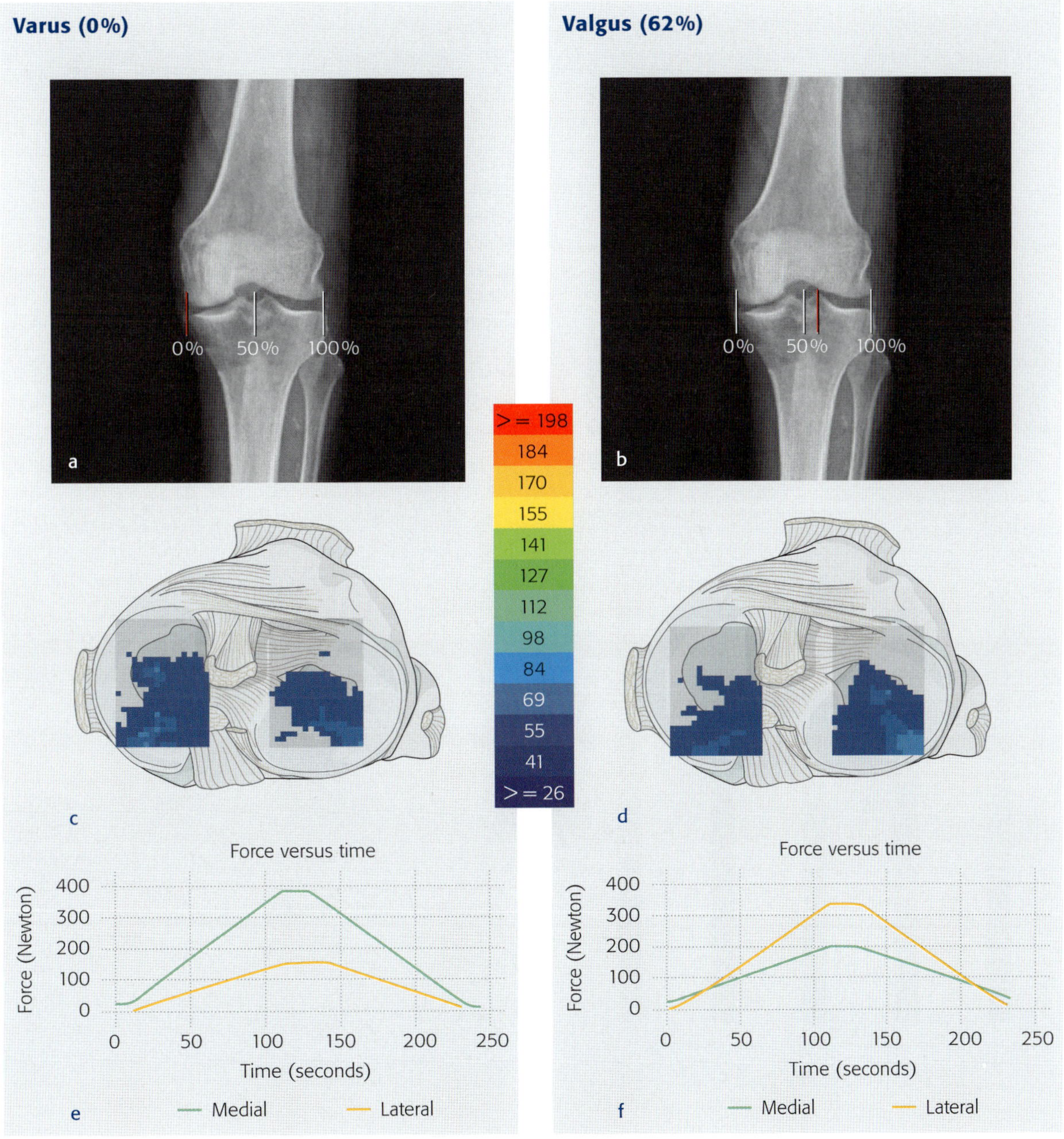

Varus (0%)

Valgus (62%)

Fig 10-7a–f   Contact pressure distribution between the medial and lateral compartment of the knee joint.
For a varus axis (0%) and 1,000 N applied axial force (plateau phase is shown in the lower panel), more load is transferred through the medial than through the lateral compartment. For a valgus axis (62%), this relationship is reversed. In both cases the loaded areas are located in the posterior aspect of the tibial plateau.

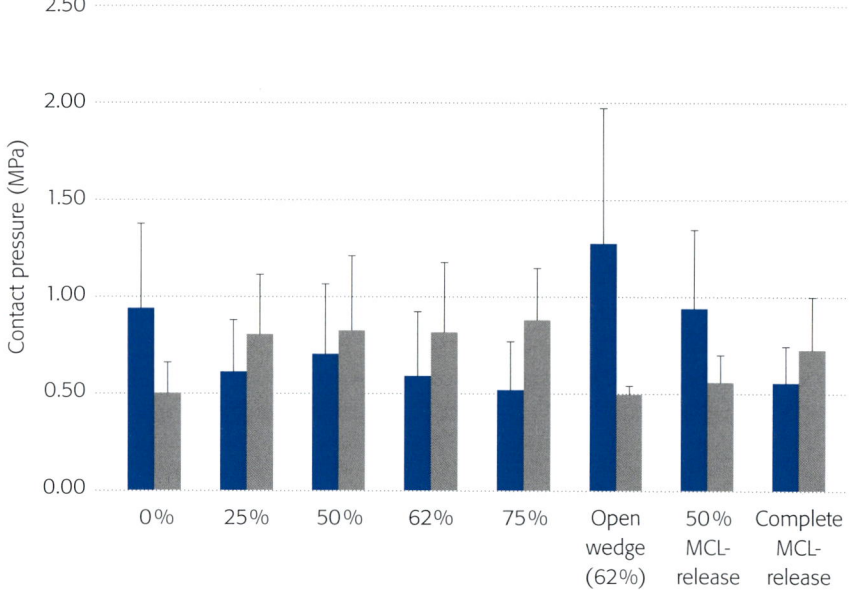
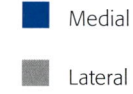

Fig 10-8 Contact pressure distribution (MPa) in the medial and lateral joint compartment in relation to the mechanical axis and following open-wedge high-tibial osteotomy. Significant increase in medial pressure with opened osteotomy gap and intact medial collateral ligament (MCL) despite valgus axis; reduction of medial pressure after release of the superficial medial collateral ligament.

■ Medial

■ Lateral

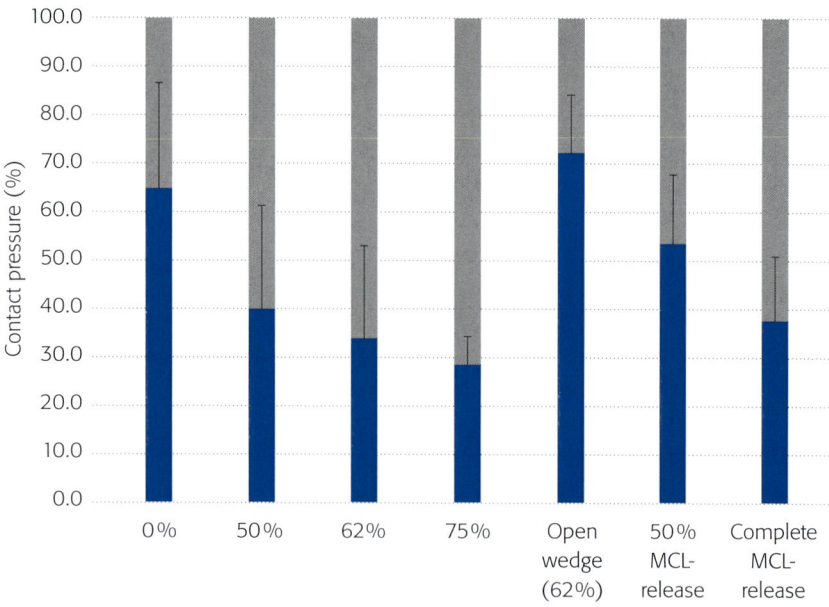
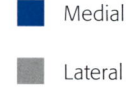

Fig 10-9 Contact pressure distribution (in %) between the medial and lateral tibiofemoral joint compartments under different mechanical set-ups.

■ Medial

■ Lateral

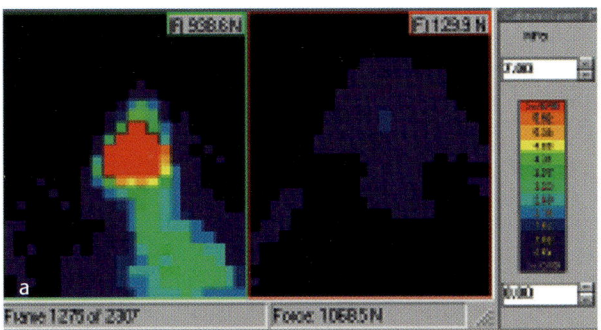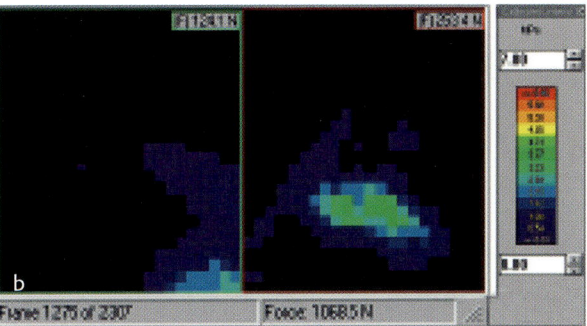

Fig 10-10a–b   Pressure distribution after open-wedge osteotomy (left field: medial compartment; right field: lateral compartment).

a   For open-wedge osteotomy and intact medial collateral ligament despite valgus axis (62%). Significant mechanical loading in the medial compartment with contact pressure peak in the middle of the tibial plateau.

b   After complete release of the superficial medial collateral ligament (see Fig 10-5c). Substantial reduction of contact pressure medially with simultaneous contact pressure increased laterally.

4   Acknowledgement

The study presented in this chapter was performed in collaboration with the Institute for Biomechanics and Biomaterials, Orthopedic Hospital of the Medical University Hanover (Director: PD Dr Christof Hurschler).

5   Bibliography

[1]   **Coventry MB** (1979) Upper tibial osteotomy for gonarthrosis. The evolution of the operation in the last 18 years and long term results. *Orthop Clin North Am;* 10:191–210.

[2]   **Coventry MB, Ilstrup DM, Wallrichs SL** (1993) Proximal tibial osteotomy. A critical long-term study of eighty-seven cases. *J Bone Joint Surg Am;* 75(2):196–201.

[3]   **Hassenpflug J, von Haugwitz A, Hahne HJ** (1998) [Long-term results of tibial head osteotomy.] *Z Orthop Ihre Grenzgeb;* 136(2):154–161. German.

[4]   **Insall JN, Joseph DM, Msika C** (1984) High tibial osteotomy for varus gonarthrosis. A long-term follow-up study. *J Bone Joint Surg Am;* 66(7):1040–1048.

[5]   **Ivarsson I, Myrnerts R, Gillquist J** (1990) High tibial osteotomy for medial osteoarthritis of the knee. A 5 to 7 and 11 year follow-up. *J Bone Joint Surg Br;* 72(2):238–244.

[6]   **Lootvoet L, Massinon A, Rossillon R, et al** (1993) [Upper tibial osteotomy for gonarthrosis in genu varum. Apropos of a series of 193 cases reviewed 6 to 10 years later.] *Rev Chir Orthop Réparatrice Appar Mot;* 79(5):375–384. French.

[7]   **Odenbring S, Egund N, Knutson K, et al** (1990) Revision after osteotomy for gonarthrosis. A 10-19-year follow-up of 314 cases. *Acta Orthop Scand;* 61(2):128–130.

[8] **Yasuda K, Majima T, Tsuchida T, et al** (1992) A ten- to 15-year follow-up observation of high tibial osteotomy in medial compartment osteoarthrosis. *Clin Orthop Relat Res;* 282:186–195.

[9] **Pape D, Adam F, Rupp S, et al** (2004) [Stability, bone healing and loss of correction after valgus realignment of the tibial head. A roentgen stereometry analysis.] *Orthopäde;* 33(2):208–217. German.

[10] **Hernigou P, Medevielle D, Debeyre J, et al** (1987) Proximal tibial osteotomy for osteoarthritis with varus deformity. A ten to thirteen-year follow-up study. *J Bone Joint Surg Am;* 69(3):332–354.

[11] **Coventry MB** (1984) Upper tibial osteotomy. *Clin Orthop Relat Res;* 182:46–52.

[12] **Engel GM, Lippert FG III** (1981) Valgus tibial osteotomy: avoiding the pitfalls. *Clin Orthop;* 160:137–143.

[13] **Kettelkamp DB, Wenger DR, Chao EY, et al** (1976) Results of proximal tibial osteotomy. The effects of tibiofemoral angle, stance-phase flexion-extension, and medial-plateau force. *J Bone Joint Surg Am;* 58(7):952–960.

[14] **Koshino T, Morii T, Wada J, et al** (1989) High tibial osteotomy with fixation by a blade plate for medial compartment osteoarthritis of the knee. *Orthop Clin North Am;* 20(2):227–243.

[15] **Myrnerts R** (1980) Knee instability before and after high tibial osteotomy. *Acta Orthop Scand;* 51(3):565–567.

[16] **Fujisawa Y, Masuhara K, Shiomi S** (1979) The effect of high tibial osteotomy on osteoarthritis of the knee. An arthroscopic study of 54 knee joints. *Orthop Clin North Am;* 10(3):585–608.

[17] **Dugdale TW, Noyes FR, Styer D** (1992) Preoperative planning for high tibial osteotomy. The effect of lateral tibiofemoral separation and tibiofemoral length. *Clin Orthop Relat Res;* 274:248–264.

[18] **Miniaci A, Ballmer FT, Ballmer PM, et al** (1989) Proximal tibial osteotomy. A new fixation device. *Clin Orthop Relat Res;* 246:250–259.

[19] **Noyes FR, Barber SD, Simon R** (1993) High tibial osteotomy and ligament reconstruction in varus angulated, anterior cruciate ligament-deficient knees. A two- to seven-year follow- up study. *Am J Sports Med;* 21(1):2–12.

[20] **Harrington IJ** (1983) Static and dynamic loading patterns in knee joints with deformities. *J Bone Joint Surg Am;* 65(2):247–259.

[21] **Hsu RW, Himeno S, Coventry MB, et al** (1990) Normal axial alignment of the lower extremity and load-bearing distribution at the knee. *Clin Orthop Relat Res;* 255:215–227.

[22] **Kettelkamp DB, Chao EY** (1972) A method for quantitative analysis of medial and lateral compression forces at the knee during standing. *Clin Orthop Relat Res;* 83:202–213.

[23] **Inaba HI, Arai MA, Watanabe WW** (1990) Influence of the varus-valgus instability on the contact of the femoro-tibial joint. *Proc Inst Mech Eng;* 204(1):61–64.

[24] **Izadpanah M, Keönch-Fraknóy J** (1977) [The effect of correction of the varus or valgus deformity of the knee.] *Z Orthop Ihre Grenzgeb;* 115(1):100–105. German.

[25] **McKellop HA, Sigholm G, Redfern FC, et al** (1991) The effect of simulated fracture-angulations of the tibia on cartilage pressures in the knee joint. *J Bone Joint Surg Am;* 73(9):1382–1391.

[26] **Riegger-Krugh C, Gerhart TN, Powers WR, et al** (1998) Tibiofemoral contact pressures in degenerative joint disease. *Clin Orthop Relat Res;* 348:233–245.

[27] **Agneskirchner JD, Hurschler C, Stukenborg-Colsman C, et al** (2004) Effect of high tibial flexion osteotomy on cartilage pressure and joint kinematics: a biomechanical study in human cadaveric knees. *Arch Orthop Trauma Surg;* 124(9):575–584.

[28] **Bai B, Kummer FJ, Sala DA, et al** (2001) Effect of articular step-off and meniscectomy on joint alignment and contact pressures for fractures of the lateral tibial plateau. *J Orthop Trauma;* 15(2):101–106.

[29] **Morris BA, D'Lima DD, Slamin J, et al** (2001) e-Knee: evolution of the electronic knee prosthesis. Telemetry technology development. *J Bone Joint Surg Am;* 83-A Suppl 2(Pt 1):62–66.

[30] **Anderson IA, MacDiarmid AA, Lance Harris M, et al** (2003) A novel method for measuring medial compartment pressures within the knee joint in-vivo. *J Biomech;* 36(9):1391–1395.

11   Osteotomy and ligament instability: tibial slope corrections and combined procedures around the knee joint

1   Introduction

High-tibial osteotomy (HTO) has become an established method for treatment of medial unicompartmental osteoarthritis of the knee by correction of varus alignment in the frontal plane. Transferring the mechanical axis from the degenerated medial joint compartment to the lateral compartment results in medial decompression, thus reducing pain and also delaying the progression of osteoarthritis.

Another indication for valgization HTO is treatment of patients with varus deformity and simultaneous chronic knee instability. Posterolateral instability with varus deformity results in lateral joint subluxation during weigth-bearing (known as varus thrust). In these patients, valgization osteotomy leads indirectly to joint stabilization since the shift of the mechanical axis to the lateral compartment eliminates posterolateral hyperdistraction.

As described in chapter 9 "High-tibial open-wedge valgization osteotomy with plate fixator", HTO for varus joint degeneration only aims for correction in the frontal plane (varus/valgus), whereas the sagittal plane (flexion/extension) remains unconsidered. Anatomically, the tibial plateau is not perpendicular to the tibial shaft axis, but the plateau declines caudally (tibial slope) at an angle of about 9–11° medially and 6–8° laterally with a large range of variation. It seems reasonable to assume that changes of the tibial slope will substantially affect knee biomechanics. In veterinary medicine it has been shown that anterior subluxation of the tibia in canine caused by a rupture of the anterior cruciate ligament can be treated by extension osteotomy (decreasing the tibial slope).

However, these anatomical and biomechanical conditions completely differ from human beings. Experimental studies investigating the exact relationships between tibial slope, sagittal translation of the tibia, ligament stability, and range of motion are currently lacking.

- **Tibial slope**
  Physiological: the slope of the tibial plateau is caudally inclined in relation to the horizontal plane.
  The slope is measured on the lateral x-ray with a long view of the tibial shaft. The tangent is marked at the medial and lateral tibial plateau.
  Definition of slope: angle between the tangents at the tibial plateau and the anatomical tibial axis minus 90° (see **Fig 11-11**).

The technique of medial open-wedge tibial osteotomy allows for alteration of the sagittal inclination of the tibial head by eccentric distraction of the osteotomy gap. If the osteotomy is opened anteriorly more than posteriorly, the tibial slope increases (flexion osteotomy); if it is opened posteriorly more than anteriorly, the slope decreases (extension osteotomy).

This chapter illustrates the effect of changes of the tibial slope on the biomechanics of the knee joint based on a biomechanical study conducted by the authors.

2 Biomechanical study with human cadaver knees

High-tibial flexion osteotomy cranial of the tibial tuberosity was performed on seven human cadaveric knee joint specimens without osteoarthritis or previous operations and with intact ligaments. The osteotomy was performed anteriorly in open-wedge technique, calibrated plastic wedges were inserted into the osteotomy gap from ventral in order to achieve standardized opening. The tibial slope was gradually raised from its original status (10° ± 4°) to 20° in steps of 5°. The osteotomy was stabilized with an external fixator (Fig 11-1).

A special computer-assisted test system (knee kinemator) was used to simulate physiological knee joint movements (Fig 11-1, Fig 11-2). An isokinetic extension movement between 120° flexion and full extension was achieved by tensioning the quadriceps tendon and applying an antagonistic force to the tibial shaft. Special suspension attachment of the tibia allowed for an unconstraint motion of the tibia on the femoral condyles,

ie, the proximal tibia was flexible in all planes (extension/flexion, varus/valgus, rotation, sagittal translation) and only restricted by the bony anatomy and the ligaments.

Joint kinematics were recorded using a specially designed three-dimensional ultrasound tracking system (Zebris), whereby parameters such as sagittal translation and rotation of the tibia in relation to the femur were analyzed with special software to an accuracy of 0.1 mm and 0.1°. A measuring sensor was inserted into the anteromedial bundle of the anterior cruciate ligament (ACL) to record any changes of its tension allowing for a continuously monitoring of ligament tension during the extension movement. Tibiofemoral cartilage pressure in the medial compartment was also evaluated (Tekscan sensors, also see chapter 10 "Effect of osteotomies on cartilage pressure in the knee").

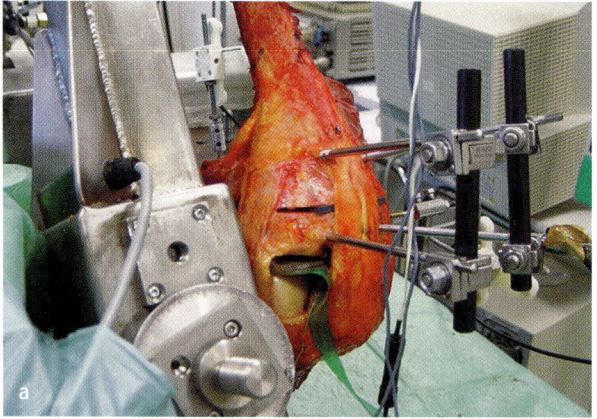 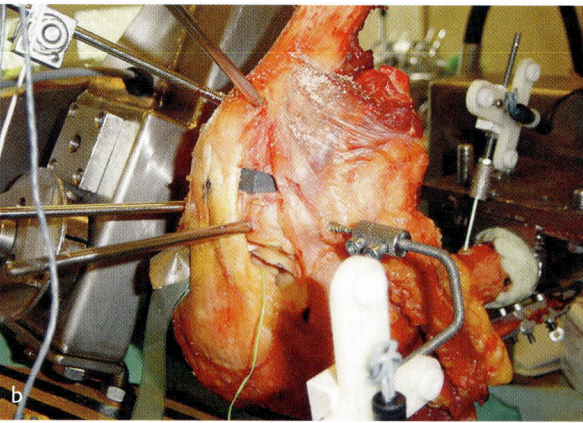

Fig 11-1a–b Experimental set-up. For biomechanical testing, the osteotomy was performed anterior cranial to the tibial tuberosity. Standardized plastic wedges were inserted into the osteotomy gap. To record knee kinematics, ultrasound sensors were inserted at defined points on the femoral and tibial joint surface.

The experiments were performed with intact ligaments and after transection of the posterior cruciate ligament (PCL) to simulate knee instability.

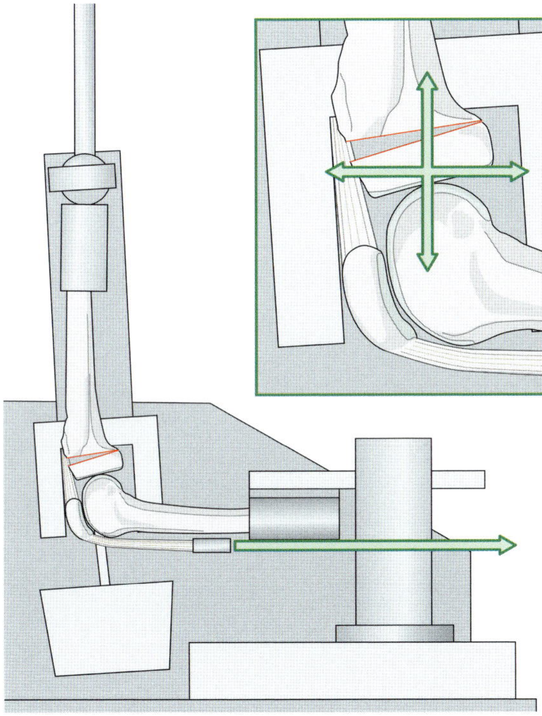

2.1   Results of the biomechanical studies

Between full extension and 60° knee flexion sagittal translation of the tibia (drawer phenomenon) was found to be highly significantly dependent on the degree of inclination of the tibia plateau (tibial slope). In comparison to the data obtained with the physiological slope, flexion osteotomy resulted in an anterior translation of the tibial head of up to 7 mm. The posterior drawer that occurred after transection of the posterior cruciate ligament was completely reduced by an elevation of the tibial slope of 5° and was even inverted into an anterior drawer (**Fig 11-3**).

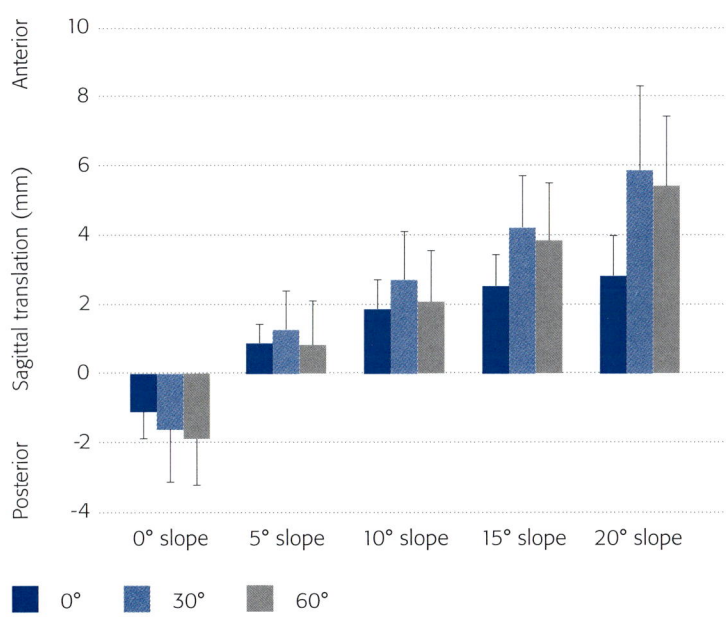

Fig 11-2   Schematic drawing of the knee kinemator. The femur was mounted horizontally with the patella facing downwards. Defined isokinetic extension movement via quadriceps tendon tensioning with antagonistic force at the tibia was applied by the computer, whereby the tibia was flexible in all planes. The kinematics of the tibial head were analyzed three-dimensionally.

Fig 11-3   AP translation of the proximal tibia after transection of the posterior cruciate ligament (PCL). The posterior translation (negative values) was already neutralized at an increase of the tibial slope of 5° and was even inverted into anterior translation with further slope inclination.

No significant changes after slope alteration were identified for tibial rotation, especially the final rotation movement of the tibia (external rotation of the tibia at the end of the extension movement) remained unaffected (Fig 11-4) as well as movements in the varus-valgus plane.

It would seem reasonable to assume that an increased anterior translation of the tibial head after slope elevation would lead to increased tension of the ACL. In this study the tension of the anterior cruciate ligament remained relatively constant during slope elevation to 10°. Minor increase occurred at slope elevations of 15° or 20° (Fig 11-5).

This fact can be explained by the surgical technique since the described opening procedure raises the proximal tibia in the region of the tibial insertion of ACL and thus relaxes the ligament.

Analysis of cartilage pressure showed that an increase of the tibial slope shifted the tibiofemoral contact area anteriorly (Fig 11-6, Fig 11-7), which is due to an earlier contact of the tibial plateau on the femoral condyle after slope elevation. The medial femoral condyle is moved anteriorly during tibial slope elevation leading to decompression of the posterior cartilaginous areas of the plateau and posterior horn of the medial meniscus (Fig 11-8).

■ Summary and conclusions based on biomechanical results

Alteration of the inclination of the tibial head (tibial slope) in open-wedge osteotomy affects the kinematics of the knee joint. Therefore, the tibial slope should not be increased or decreased during osteotomy in the frontal plane (valgus or varus correction) in patients with stable ligaments and normal range of motion.

Increase of the tibial slope shifts the tibial head anteriorly in relation to the femoral condyle. For example, in PCL insufficiency the tibial head can be reduced from the posterior drawer by increasing of the tibial slope. Alternatively, osteotomy with decrease of the tibial inclination can be applied in patients with anterior instability to reduce anterior subluxation of the tibia.

Increase of ACL tension during flexion osteotomy only occurs at slope elevation of more than 10°.

Increase of the tibial slope leads to anterior shift of the contact area between the femur and the tibia in extension. The greater the slope, the higher the load on the cartilage of the anterior half of the tibial plateau with simultaneous unloading of the posterior half. If there is cartilage damage of the posteromedial tibial plateau, eg, after partial resection of the posterior horn of the medial meniscus, osteotomy with slope elevation may selectively unload those damaged cartilaginous areas.

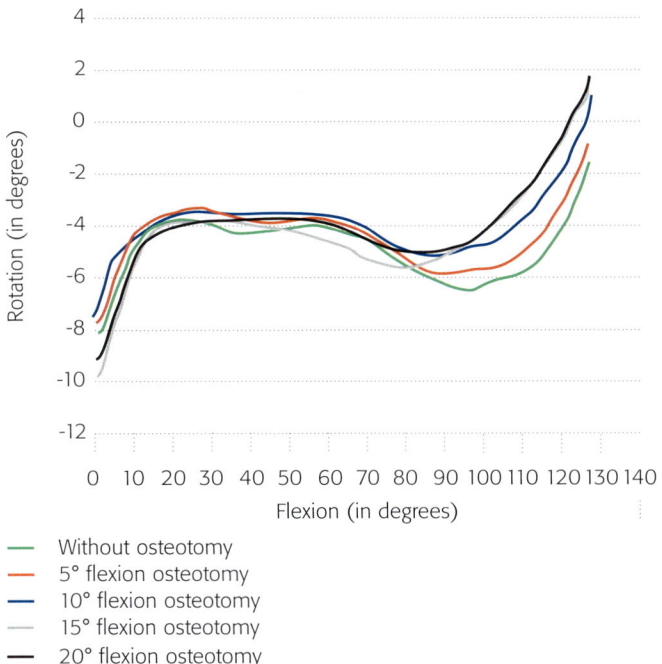

Without osteotomy
5° flexion osteotomy
10° flexion osteotomy
15° flexion osteotomy
20° flexion osteotomy

Fig 11-4   Rotation of the tibia in relation to the femoral axis depending on knee flexion and the inclination of the tibial slope. No significant effects of slope inclination on rotation.

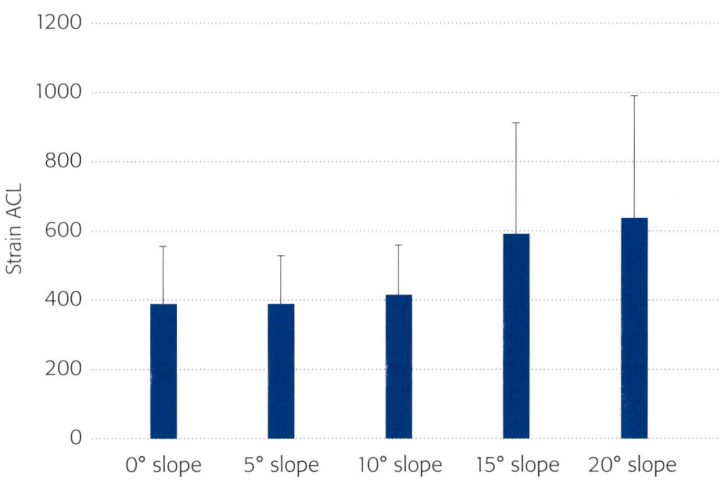

Fig 11-5   Tension of the ACL (measuring sensor in the anteromedial bundle) in relation to the tibial slope. A measurable increase in tension was only recorded at a slope increase of more than 10°.

In full extension

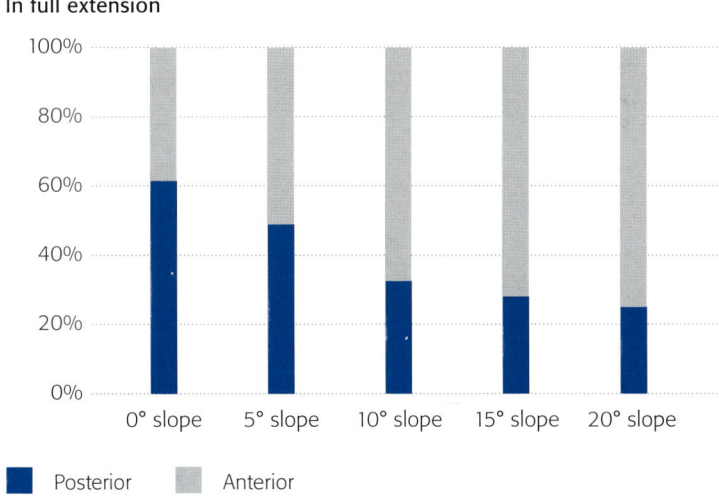

Posterior   Anterior

Fig 11-6   Topographical distribution of the tibiofemoral contact pressure on cartilage in the medial compartment. Slope increase resulted in a shift of the contact area from the posterior to the anterior half.

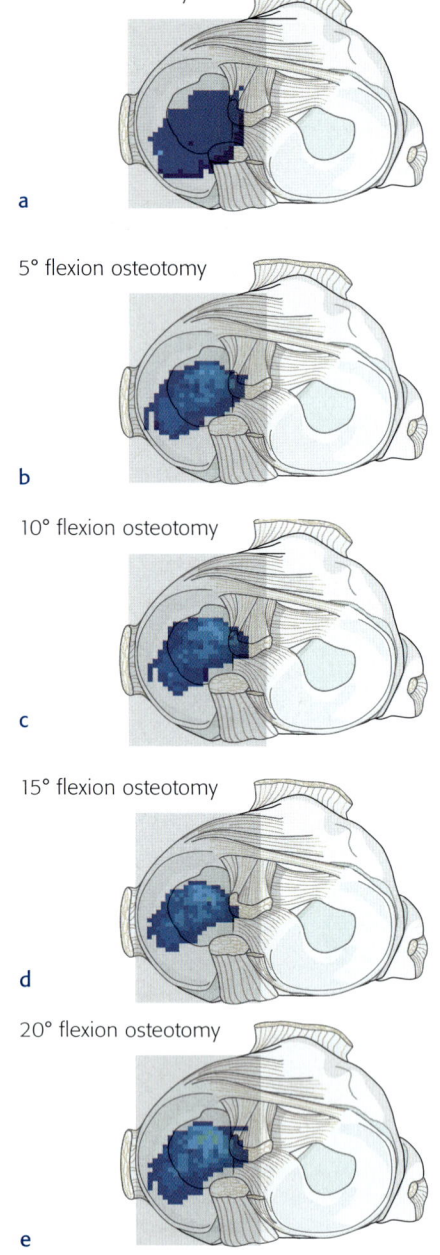

Without osteotomy

a

5° flexion osteotomy

b

10° flexion osteotomy

c

15° flexion osteotomy

d

20° flexion osteotomy

e

>= 198
184
170
155
141
127
112
98
84
69
55
41
>= 26

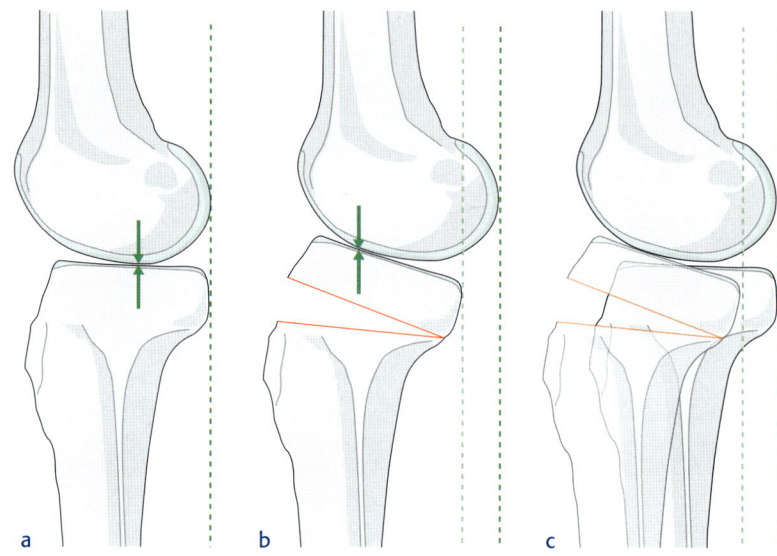

a   b   c

Fig 11-8a–c Schematic drawing of the knee joint to illustrate the effects of slope elevation on tibial translation and tibiofemoral contact in extension. Flexion osteotomy leads to anterior and superior translation of the proximal tibia (b–c). The sagittal translation leads to an anterior shift of the contact area between the femur and the tibia resulting in relative decompression of the posterior cartilaginous areas.

Fig 11-7a–e Example of the distribution of the tibiofemoral cartilage pressure in the medial compartment: the contact area between the medial femoral condyle and the tibial plateau is gradually shifted anteriorly as the slope is increased.

3   Technique of slope correction in open-wedge osteotomy of the tibial head

The technique of open-wedge tibial head osteotomy allows for continuous opening of the osteotomy intraoperatively. In closed-wedge technique size and shape of the excised bone wedge determine the amount correction and can hardly be changed intraoperatively once the wedge has been excised. In contrast, in open-wedge technique the horizontal gap can be adjusted by further spreading or closing. Under fluoroscopic control, axial correction can be precisely verified and altered as necessary prior to internal fixation. In particular, in cases of axis deviation with additional ligament instability preoperative planning on the x-rays is sometimes difficult due to the ligamentous component of the malalignment. In these cases, the possibility of intraoperative adjustment offered by open-wedge technique is advantageous and minimizes the risk of over- or undercorrection.

Furthermore, open-wedge technique allows excellent control and manipulation of the tibial slope, ie, in addition to valgus correction an extension or flexion correction can be achieved.

In literature, open-wedge osteotomy is often described as being associated with accidental elevation of the tibial slope, whereas closed-wedge osteotomy is assumed to lead to slope reduction. The authors' experience gained by the analysis of more than 900 tibial open-wedge osteotomies with measurement of the tibial slope on the postoperative lateral x-rays does not confirm these statements. The sagittal slope, like the extent of valgus correction, is a parameter that can be deliberately influenced depending on the specific characteristics of the operation technique. By strict adherence to surgical procedure as described in chapter 9" High-tibial open-wedge valgization osteotomy with plate fixator", especially with regard to the L-shaped ascending cut behind the tuberosity, any alteration of the preexisting anatomical slope will become apparent during the distraction of the osteotomy gap because of the incongruency of the anterior ascending osteotomy surfaces. A change in the slope will be indicated by a tilt of the ascending osteotomy surfaces: a decrease of the slope (extension) is indicated by bone contact in the cranial part of the anterior cut. By contrast, increase of the slope (flexion) is seen as bone contact in the caudal part of the anterior osteotomy cut (see also chapter 9 "High-tibial open-wedge valgization osteotomy with plate fixator", Fig 9-13).

Another key aspect for slope control is the medial collateral ligament (MCL). The osteotomy technique described here requires a release of the distal superficial fibers of the MCL, which covers the posterior part of the proximal tibia. The release of the superficial MCL fibers is not only necessary for decompression of the medial joint compartment (see chapter 10 "Effect of osteotomies on cartilage pressure in the knee"), but also in order to perform the transverse osteotomy in the posterior aspect. If the osteotomy is performed with the MCL left intact, the spreading of the osteotomy gap will lead to an eccentric opening osteotomy in the sagittal plane. The osteotomy opens anteriorly more than posteriorly since the MCL prevents the osteotomy segments from separating.

Considering all anatomical and technical features of tibial open wedge osteotomy as described in chapter 9" High-tibial open-wedge valgization osteotomy with plate fixator", this procedure can achieve valgus correction for treatment of medial osteoarthritis of the knee without altering the tibial slope.

Increase of the tibial slope (flexion osteotomy) can be obtained by eccentric opening of the osteotomy, whereby the opening is greater anteriorly than posteriorly. The application of two osteotomy spreaders, one anterior and one posterior in the osteotomy gap, is recommended for this purpose. A difference of about 4–5 mm between the anterior and the posterior opening of the osteotomy gap (eg, anterior 12 mm, posterior 7 mm) can realistically be achieved in the technique with the L-shaped osteotomy and can be performed with simultaneous valgus correction. The osteotomy gap should be spreaded with the knee in flexed position in order to counteract the long lever arms of the lower leg. With the spreaders in situ, the sagittal stability (drawer test) can be examined intraoperatively, and reduction/elimination of hyperextension can be assessed. Attention must be paid to avoid an exceeding offset in the frontal ascending osteotomy, which might compromise the stability as well as the healing process.

Decreasing the slope by extension osteotomy can be achieved by eccentric opening of the osteotomy posteriorly, whereby spreading of the osteotomy gap should be performed with the knee in extension. In this case it is sufficient to place only one osteotomy spreader in the posterior part of the horizontal osteotomy since that area is subject to the highest restoring forces. The anterior part of the osteotomy limits the extent to which the slope can be decreased since the tuberosity blocks the tilting of the tibial head segment when the horizontal gap is opened posteriorly. The described technique allows a slope reduction up to 5°. If more slope correction is required, a small slice of bone must be resected from the tibial head in the region of the anterior cut of the osteotomy, which then permits a greater degree of extensile tilting.

It is recommended that the sagittal inclination of the tibial slope be measured intraoperatively under fluoroscopy. The intraoperative slope should be compared with the preoperative lateral view.

- **Increasing tibial slope in open-wedge valgization osteotomy:**
  - Eccentric opening of the osteotomy gap: anteriorly more than posteriorly.
  - Opening of the osteotomy with the knee in flexion.
  - Application of two osteotomy spreaders in the horizontal gap.
  - Attention to bone surface contact in the anterior ascending cut of the osteotomy.
  - Intraoperative assessment of posterior translation (drawer test) and knee extension.

Decreasing tibial slope in open-wedge valgization osteotomy:
  - Eccentric opening of the osteotomy gap: posteriorly more than anteriorly.
  - Opening of the osteotomy with the knee in extension.
  - Application of one osteotomy spreader in the posterior part of the horizontal cut.
  - If indicated, minimal bone resection in the anterior cut of the osteotomy.
  - Intraoperative assessment of anterior translation (drawer test) and knee extension.

4   Clinical application

In addition to treatment of varus arthrosis of the knee high-tibial osteotomy can be indicated in patients with additional knee ligament instability.

4.1   Valgization osteotomy for medial joint degeneration, varus deformity, and increased lateral joint space (double varus)

Primary varus deformity is defined as an axial deviation exclusively caused by bony deformity of the tibiofemoral anatomy. If there is narrowing of the medial joint space in addition to the bone deformity, usually increased lateral joint distraction and decoadaptation between the lateral femoral condyle and the tibia is present (double varus) (**Fig 11-9**). The concomitance of varus deviation and lateral or posterolateral ligament insufficiency due to trauma or hyperextension leads to subluxation in the lateral joint segment, which causes a feeling of instability during weight bearing (varus thrust phenomenon). Lateral ligament reconstruction is contraindicated in these cases because of the bone deformity. In these patients, valgus correction osteotomy in the frontal plane achieves both decompression of the medial joint compartment and neutralization of the lateral distraction forces with elimination of varus thrust by shifting the mechanical axis laterally.

- Osteotomy for varus deformity and lateral joint distraction (double varus):
  Axial correction without alteration of the tibial slope.
  Valgus correction eliminates medial overload and lateral joint distraction (varus thrust).

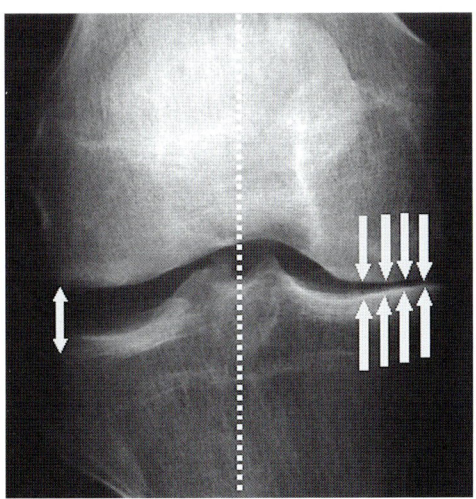

Fig 11-9   Double varus. Medial joint-space narrowing with compression, lateral joint-space opening with distraction and decoadaptation of the lateral femoral condyle and the tibia (lateral condylar lift off).

4.2 Valgization and flexion (slope increase) osteotomy in patients with varus deformity and complex posterior/posterolateral instability and hyperextension (triple varus)

The combination of varus deformity and lateral distraction with increased external rotation of the tibia due to posterolateral instability (triple varus) leads to a complex pathology of the bone and the ligaments (Fig 11-10). These patients often suffer from a posterior knee instability and hyperextension subsequent to PCL rupture. In cases of triple varus deformity complex ligament surgery with PCL replacement and lateral or posterolateral stabilization will remain unsuccessful. There is a risk of recurrent rapid insufficiency of the ligament graft due to the remaining osseous deformity. Valgization osteotomy restores the osseous anatomy in these patients and prevents varus thrust. The posterior instability can be treated simultaneously by elevation of the tibial slope to eliminate the posterior drawer under weight bearing (Fig 11-11). The increase of the slope and the concomitant flexion of the tibial head simultaneously reduces hyperextension of the knee. In cases of persistent, symptomatic instability, PCL, and/or posterolateral ligament reconstruction can be performed during a second operation; however, this is rarely preformed and only necessary in younger and very active patients.

- **Osteotomy in varus deformity and posterolateral and posterior ligament instability and hyperextension (triple varus).**
  Valgus correction:
  Elimination of medial overload.
  Reducation of lateral joint distraction (varus thrust)
  Increase of the tibial slope (flexion):
  Reduction of the posterior subluxation of the tibia.
  Elimination of hyperextension.

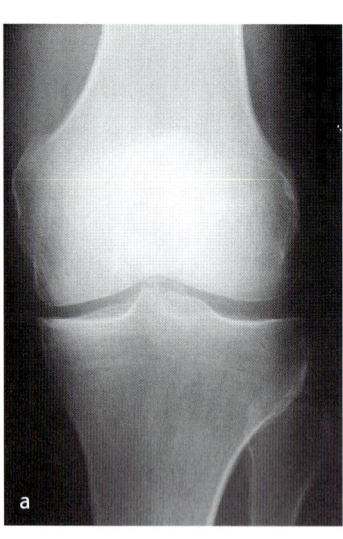
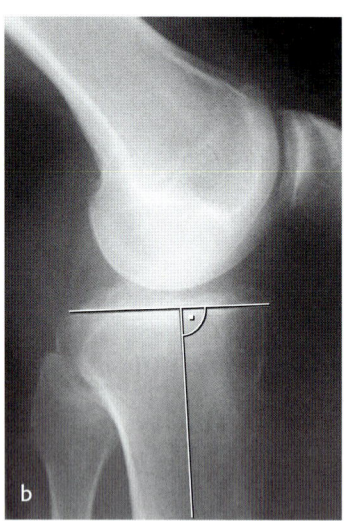
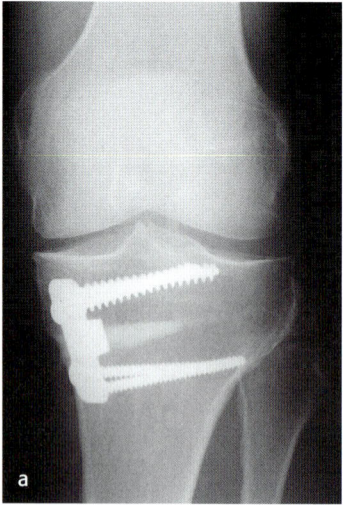
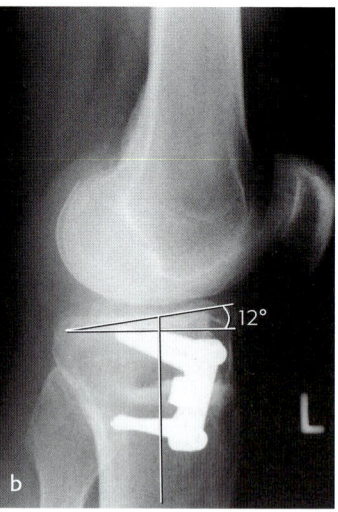

Fig 11-10a–b Patient with posterior and posterolateral ligament instability, hyperextension, and varus deformity (triple varus), preoperative tibial slope of 0°.

Fig 11-11a–b Open-wedge valgization and flexion osteotomy (tibial slope postoperative: 12°), posterior drawer eliminated in extension despite lacking PCL.

4.3   Valgization and extension (slope decrease) osteotomy in patients with varus deformity, medial osteoarthritis of the knee, and chronic anterior instability

Some patients suffer from symptomatic medial osteoarthritis due to varus deformity and chronic ACL insufficiency. Others present with chronic anterior knee instability without primary varus deformity. As a result of chronic knee instability, secondary joint destruction with medial joint-space narrowing develops due to loss of cartilage and meniscus, lateral joint distraction and, possibly, a varus thrust phenomena (double varus). If medial joint destruction progresses, symptoms of instability will be superimposed by symptoms of medial osteoarthritis. In these patients, valgization and extension HTO in open-wedge technique leads to decompression of the medial compartment with reduction of osteoarthritic pain. Decrease of the slope improves sagittal stability, ie, anterior translation of the tibia is reduced. Since the osteoarthritis in these patients is often associated with an extension deficit of the knee, slope reduction with extension of the tibia often has an additional positive effect. These patients seldomly require second surgery for ACL reconstruction after the combined osteotomy is performed. Nevertheless, arthroscopically-assisted ACL reconstruction with hamstring tendons or patellar tendon can easily be performed simultaneously (see below) or during second surgery.

4.4   Combination of valgization/extension osteotomy and ACL reconstruction in young, active patients with varus deformity, beginning medial osteoarthritis, and anterior instability

Symptomatic giving way and medial joint pain under weight bearing can especially be found in younger (<30 years) and active patients with severe anterior knee instability and primary varus deformity (Fig 11-12). Neither isolated high-tibial osteotomy nor isolated ACL reconstruction will result in a satisfactory outcome under these circumstances. Isolated osteotomy does not eliminate instability, isolated ligament reconstruction does not correct varus deformity. A single-stage procedure combining open-wedge valgization HTO with ACL reconstruction addresses both pathologies. Furthermore, the hamstring tendons can easily be harvested through the same incision at the anteromedial tibial head.

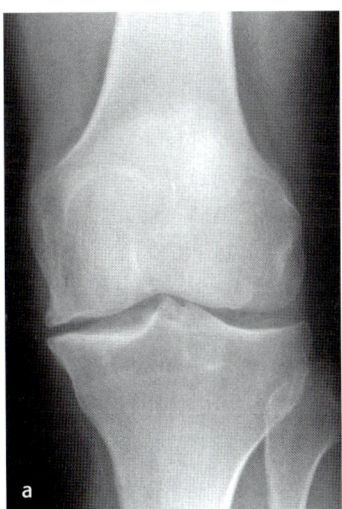 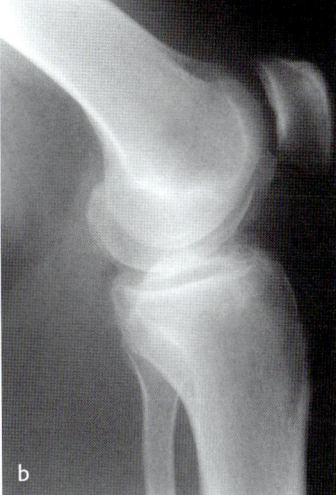

Fig 11-12a–b   Preoperative x-rays of a patient with varus osteoarthritis and symptomatic anterior knee instability.

Performing this combined procedure, the hamstring tendons must be harvested first, then the osteotomy can be performed, followed by ACL replacement (Fig 11-13). If ligament reconstruction was performed prior to the osteotomy, the ACL graft might be transected during sawing and the ligament tensioning might change after spreading of the osteotomy due to alteration of the tibial insertion (see subchapter 2.2 "Results of the biomechanical studies"). ACL reconstruction can be performed after osteotomy in standard arthroscopic technique, whereby the bolt in the anterior superior plate hole (hole A) may interfere with drilling of the tibial canal, when a TomoFix plate fixator is used. Therefore, in these cases, this bolt must be removed (Fig 11-14). Having drilled the tibial canal, the arthroscope can be introduced distally into the tibial canal and the bolt can either be replaced by a shorter bolt that does not penetrate into the tibial canal or be left away (Fig 11-13).

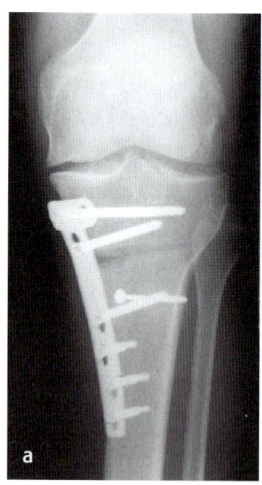 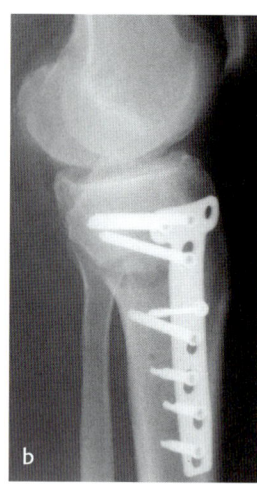 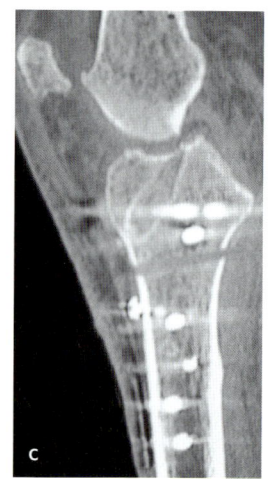 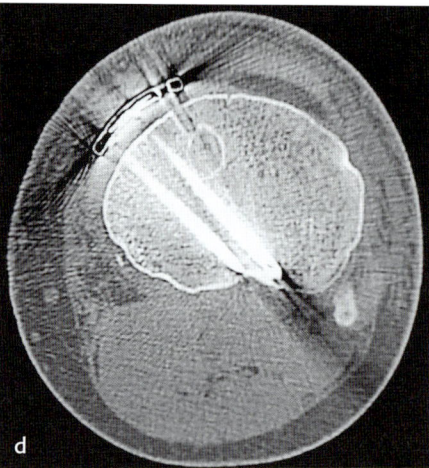

Fig 11-13a–d   Postoperative x-rays and CT scan after tibial open-wedge valgization and slight extension osteotomy and simultaneous ACL replacement (same patient as in Fig 11-12).
No bolt has been inserted into hole A of the TomoFix plate fixator as it would interfere with the tibial canal.

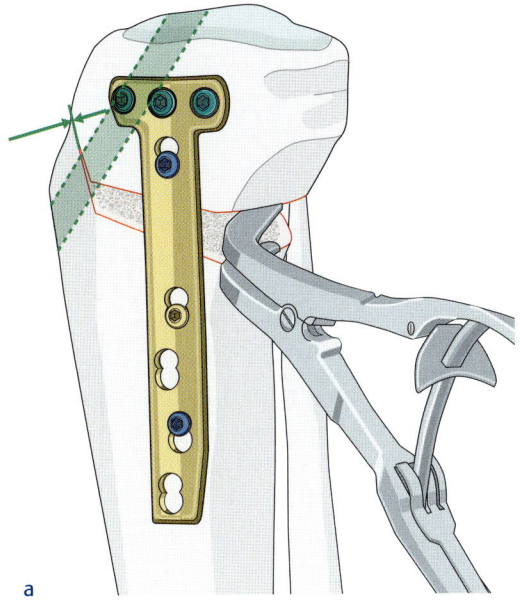

a

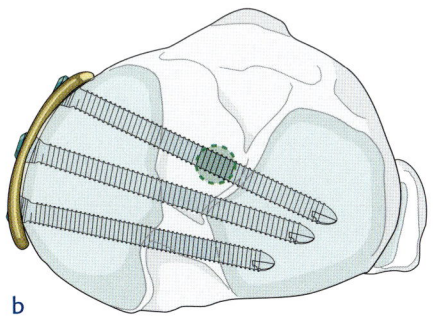

b

■ Osteotomy in varus osteoarthritis of the knee and anterior ligament instability

1. Valgization correction to treat medial osteoarthritis.
2. Decrease of the tibial slope (extension osteotomy) improves both sagittal stability by reducing anterior translation of the tibia and range of motion in knee extension deficit.

Combination of osteotomy and ACL replacement in young active patients with osteoarthritic pain and giving way symptoms is possible. The hamstring tendons must be harvested prior to the osteotomy. After stabilization of the osteotomy the arthroscopic ACL reconstruction is performed.

■ Conclusion

Valgization high-tibial osteotomy is an established procedure for treatment of complex pathologies of combined osseous deformity and ligament instability. The open-wedge technique facilitates excellent control of the amount of correction eeded for realignment in the frontal plane and ligament stability, which can be assessed intra-operatively. Biplanar correction with alteration of the tibial slope can be achieved by eccentric distraction of the medial osteotomy gap.

Fig 11-14a–b   Sagittal and transverse view of the relationship between the tibial canal and the TomoFix plate fixator in combined medial open-wedge osteotomy and ACL reconstruction.

5   Acknowledgement

The study presented in this chapter was performed in collaboration with the Institute for Biomechanics and Biomaterials, Orthopedic Hospital of the Medical University Hanover (Director: PD Dr Christof Hurschler).

6   Suggestions for further reading

Agneskirchner JD, Burkart A, Imhoff AB (2002) [Axis deviation, cartilage damage and cruciate ligament rupture—concomitant interventions in replacement of the anterior cruciate ligament.] *Unfallchirurg;* 105(3):237–245. German.

Agneskirchner JD, Hurschler C, Stukenborg-Colsman C, et al (2004) Effect of high tibial flexion osteotomy on cartilage pressure and joint kinematics: a biomechanical study in human cadaveric knees. Winner of the AGA-DonJoy Award 2004. *Arch Orthop Trauma Surg;* 124(9):575–584.

Bai B, Baez J, Testa N, et al (2000) Effect of posterior cut angle on tibial component loading. *J Arthroplasty;* 15(7):916–920.

Brazier J, Migaud H, Gougeon F, et al (1996) [Evaluation of methods for radiographic measurement of the tibial slope. A study of 83 healthy knees.] *Rev Chir Orthop Réparatrice Appar Mot;* 82(3):195–200. French.

Chiu KY, Zhang SD, Zhang GH (2000) Posterior slope of tibial plateau in Chinese. *J Arthroplasty;* 15(2):224–227.

Dejour H, Bonnin M (1994) Tibial translation after anterior cruciate ligament rupture. Two radiological tests compared. *J Bone Joint Surg Br;* 76(5):745–749.

Genin P, Weill G, Julliard R (1993) [The tibial slope. Proposal for a measurement method.] *J Radiol;* 74(1):27–33. French.

Giffin JR, Vogrin TM, Zantop T, et al (2004) Effects of increasing tibial slope on the biomechanics of the knee. *Am J Sports Med;* 32(2):376–382.

Imhoff AB, Linke RD, Agneskirchner J (2004) [Corrective osteotomy in primary varus, double varus and triple varus knee instability with cruciate ligament replacement.] *Orthopäde;* 33(2):201–207. German.

Jenny JY, Rapp E, Kehr P (1997) [Proximal tibial meniscal slope: a comparison with the bone slope.] *Rev Chir Orthop Réparatrice Appar Mot;* 84(5):435–438. French.

Jiang CC, Yip KM, Liu TK (1994) Posterior slope angle of the medial tibial plateau. *J Formos Med Assoc;* 93(6):509–512.

Julliard R, Genin P, Weil G, et al (1993) [The median functional slope of the tibia. Principle. Technique of measurement. Value. Interest.] *Rev Chir Orthop Réparatrice Appar Mot;* 79(8):625–634. French.

Lobenhoffer P, Agneskirchner JD (2003) Improvements in surgical technique of valgus high tibial osteotomy. *Knee Surg Sports Traumatol Arthrosc;* 11(3):132–138.

Lobenhoffer P, Lattermann C, Krettek C, et al (1996) [Rupture of the posterior cruciate ligament: status of current treatment.] *Unfallchirurg;* 99(6):382–399. German.

Matsuda S, Miura H, Nagamine R, et al (1999) Posterior tibial slope in the normal and varus knee. *Am J Knee Surg;* 12(3):165–168.

Meister K, Talley MC, Horodyski MB, et al (1998) Caudal slope of the tibia and its relationship to noncontact injuries to the ACL. *Am J Knee Surg;* 11(4):217–219.

Noyes FR, Goebel SX, West J (2005) Opening wedge tibial osteotomy: the 3-triangle method to correct axial alignment and tibial slope. *Am J Sports Med;* 33(3):378–387.

Slocum B, Devine T (1983) Cranial tibial thrust: a primary force in the canine stifle. *J Am Vet Med Assoc;* 183(4):456–459.

Slocum B, Slocum TD (1993) Tibial plateau leveling osteotomy for repair of cranial cruciate ligament rupture in the canine. *Vet Clin North Am Small Anim Pract;* 23(4):777–795.

12   Radiological examination of bone healing after open-wedge tibial osteotomy

1   Introduction

The general principles of fracture consolidation apply equally to the healing process of osteotomies. Osteotomies can be regarded as iatrogenic and targeted fractures, which are placed under optimal conditions and circumstances in order to reduce and stabilize the resultant bone fragments in the corrected position. The type of the deformity and its localization, the exact amount of correction, and the direction of correction must be considered when planning an osteotomy. Stabilization is performed according to the principles of internal fracture fixation.

Both adequate stability and good vascularity of the bone and soft tissues are premise for good bone healing and, consequently, for the good long-term results of open-wedge valgization osteotomy of the proximal tibia.

In addition to clinical aspects, radiological parameters and histological examination provide data to quantify bone healing. Regarding bone healing after open-wedge tibial osteotomy, the question often arises as to whether the interposition of solid material or osteoconductive/osteoinductive substances into the osteotomy gap is beneficial. The author has performed over 500 open-wedge osteotomies with the TomoFix implant without filling the osteotomy gap.

2   Bone healing

The pattern of consolidation after bone injury depends on the size of the defect and biomechanical stability of the internal fixation. There is a basic differentiation between primary bone healing (contact healing) and secondary bone healing (gap healing). Primary bone bridging under stable conditions is possible to a threshold of 0.5 mm [1].

In primary healing (contact healing) every osteon passes through a regeneration cycle divided into three phases: activation, resorption, and formation (ARF sequence) [2, 3]. A basic cellular unit consisting of osteoclasts, an axial blood vessel, and osteoblasts performs the remodeling sequence. The osteoclasts extend the resorption canal in an axial direction, whereas the osteoblasts are responsible for centripetal apposition of new bone lamellae that gradually narrow the resorption canal concentrically until the definitive dimension of the Haversian canal is reached. The apposition rate is about 1 µm per day. The lamellar osteoid matrix mineralizes after about 8–10 days. This process of restructuring is referred to as remodeling of the Haversian system [1].

In secondary healing or gap healing bone regeneration occurs directly without preceding osteoclastic resorption or intermediate cartilaginous phases. It is a two-stage consolidation process. During the first phase a trabecular scaffold of fibrous bone forms within 1–2 weeks and its meshes are later filled out with lamellar bone [1]. This structure is replaced in subsequent weeks by osteons running perpendicular to the fracture gap. Secondary bone healing takes place where micromotion between the fragments occurs. In plate osteosynthesis, callus always forms at the contralateral cortex. In internal and external fracture fixation or metadiaphyseal osteotomy primary and secondary instabilities at the contralateral cortex cause biomechanical stress on the fixation system.

3   Revascularization and bone remodeling after fractures and osteotomies

Both biomechanical stability and adequate blood supply are vital to fracture healing [4–11]. The earlier the traumatic and iatrogenic vascular damage, eg, due to heat necrosis during sawing, is resolved by restoration of cortical blood supply, the more rapidly the bone heals [5, 6, 9]. The revascularization process begins within the compacta and is attended by intracortical remodeling in the zone between the well vascularized and the poorly vascularized bone. Necrotic material is resorbed and replaced by regenerated bone [12]. The first basic cellular unit consists of osteoclasts and osteoblasts with a central blood vessel. These reach the medullary cavity after 4 weeks. Bone remodeling is a relatively slow process [13–15], whereby the process depends on cortical thickness. Experimental studies have shown that remodeling in the rabbit with its relatively thin cortex takes 4 weeks, but will take 12 weeks in specimens with thicker cortices, eg, sheep or dogs. Duration of more than 12 weeks is assumed in human individuals [5, 6, 13].

4   Open-wedge tibial osteotomy with autogenous and heterogeneous interposition material

Open-wedge osteotomy of the proximal tibia creates a highly unstable situation, but it also allows for correction and stabilization in various degrees of freedom (Fig 12-1). Whether open-wedge valgization osteotomy of the tibia should be performed with or without interposition material is currently under discussion. Several reports in literature describe the interposition of autogenous materials (generally one or more bicortical iliac crest grafts) or insertion of homogenous and heterogeneous bone substitutes in medial open-wedge tibial osteotomy [16–25]. As for synthetic materials, hydroxylapatite (HA) is generally preferred and can be inserted into the osteotomy gap in the form of compressed wedges to supplement plate fixation. Koshino et al [21] investigated these substances histologically and found a bone integration rate of 72% in the HA pores. Plain x-rays did not show any alteration of radiological density of the osteotomy gap when filled with the HA wedge. The planned mechanical axial alignment of 3–6° valgus was achieved in 75% of patients in this study. The author reports an average axial correction of 10.3°. No loss of

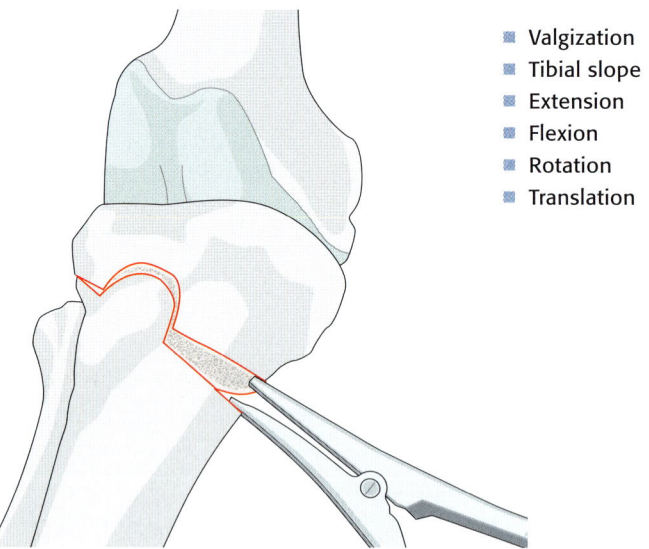

- Valgization
- Tibial slope
- Extension
- Flexion
- Rotation
- Translation

Fig 12-1   Correction in different directions can be achieved by open-wedge tibial osteotomy. Combined corrections can be useful in cases of complex deformities.

correction in the subsequent course, however, two cases of delayed healing and one case of pseudarthrosis were recorded.

Hernigou and Ma [19] investigated 245 patients after medial open-wedge HTO stabilized by application of conventional plates and insertion of acrylic bone cement into the osteotomy gap. They present this procedure as an efficient method of preventing secondary loss of correction but do not specify the contribution of the cement to stability.

5   Open-wedge tibial osteotomy without interposition material

The principles of angular stable internal fixation with the TomoFix implant have been presented in detail in chapter 7 "Principles of angular stable fixators" and chapter 9 "High-tibial open-wedge valgization osteotomy with plate fixator". Currently, surgeons who apply this implant to stabilize the tibia after open-wedge osteotomy are not definitively agreed on the maximum gap width beyond which autogeneous or heterogeneous graft is indicated. Galla and Lobenhoffer (see chapter 9 "High-tibial open-wedge valgization osteotomy with plate fixator") recommend filling the gap from a vertical width of 13 mm and more, but in the author's own procedures and those of other working groups the gap is either not filled or only filled from a vertical width of 20 mm or more [18, 26].

With regard to consolidation after open-wedge osteotomy without interposition material, two basic questions remain:
1. How does new bone regenerate in the osteotomy gap?
2. Does the regenerated bone correspond to normal bone in terms of biomechanical stability and stability under load?

5.1   Evaluation of x-rays

Preoperative imaging for correction osteotomies are described in chapter 2 "Clinical and radiological evaluation". The postoperative evaluation requires an AP radiographic view of the knee joint, lateral view in 90° flexion, and a full-length weight-bearing view immediately postoperatively and after 6, 12, 24, and 52 weeks. It is important to ensure neutral rotation and complete extension of the knee joint to obtain images suitable for evaluation.

Bone healing

The author's experience indicates that bone healing in the osteotomy gap progresses from lateral to medial [27]. A lateral bone bridge is left intact intraoperatively, ie, the so-called hinge, which is defined at about 10% of the bone width (see Fig 12-2a). This hinge is not cut during osteotomy and yields to plastic deformation when the osteotomy gap is opened (see chapter 9 "High-tibial open-wedge valgization osteotomy with plate fixator"). The author finds a distance of 5–10 mm to the lateral cortex to be optimal.

An early sign of bone regeneration is an increase in bone density at the osteotomy surfaces. Band-shaped zones of new bone form at the osteotomy surfaces as part of the healing process (Fig 12-2). In this way, the osteotomy gap is successively consolidated from lateral to medial. Awfter 6 weeks bone contact is seen along almost one-third of the osteotomy surface at the interface between the tibial head and the tibial shaft. The author observed very rapid bone consolidation at the ascending anterior osteotomy (often already after 3 weeks). This area acts as a stabilizing column during the healing process. The anterior osteotomy accounts for about 5% of the total bone contact surface.

Table 12-1 and Table 12-2 show the series of patients and the progress of bone consolidation in the osteotomy gap for our study of 53 patients.

Initial bone resorption is seen in 55% of all patients 3–4 weeks postoperatively (see Fig 12-3, Fig 12-7). This leads to slight temporary instability with increased load on the implant. This phenomenon was seen more frequently in smokers and after secondary fracture of the lateral hinge. In 10% of all cases the latter caused displacement of the lateral cortex by more than 5 mm. This occurred in the first phase of the learning curve immediately after implant development (Fig 12-4). It was noticeable that the fissures extending distally were much more unstable than transverse fissures extending laterally or slightly ascending fissures. In severe deformity requiring more extensive correction with a larger osteotomy gap, a lateral hinge fracture is unavoidable, especially if full extension needs to be reached through the osteotomy (Fig 12-6). Nevertheless, temporary

	Average age in years	Number of male patients	Average width of the osteotomy gap in mm
Patients (n = 53)	50 (18–71)	39	10 (5–20)

Table 12-1   Basic data.

Postoperative radiological follow-up (AP view)	Total bone-contact surface in %
Day 1	23 ± 15 (0–50)
3 weeks	25 ± 15 (10–60)
6 weeks	32 ± 20 (0–60)
3 months	57 ± 14 (30–80)
6 months	73 ± 14 (50–100)
9 months	80 ± 10 (70–90)
12 months	88 ± 10 (80–100)
At implant removal	90 ± 10 (80–100)
After implant removal	94 ± 6 (80–100)

Table 12-2   Progress of bone consolidation in the osteotomy gap at the postoperative AP radiological follow-ups.

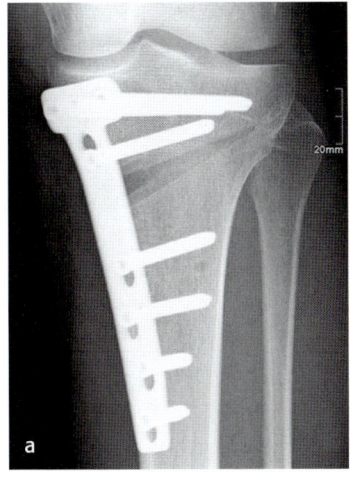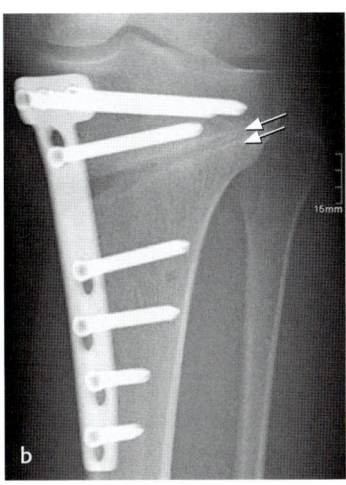

Fig 12-2a–b Early radiological sign of primary bone healing. Band-shaped radiopaque zones of new bone are noticeable at the osteotomized surfaces (arrows).

insertion of a compression screw into combination hole 1 will resolve this problem. The screw pretensions the plate and leads to secondary reduction and compression of the lateral hinge (see chapter 9 "High-tibial open-wedge valgization osteotomy with plate fixator"). The formation of callus at the posterolateral tibia during the course of consolidation is considered as a sign of temporary tilting instability (**Fig 12-3**, **Fig 12-7**), which is triggered by increasing pressure in flexion and which must be neutralized by the implant. However, there is no correlation between the extent of the cortical fracture and the intensity of callus formation.

■ Overall, we did not observe loosening or implant failure in our patient sample.

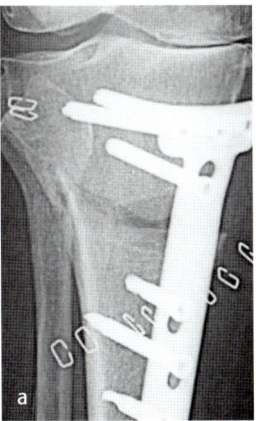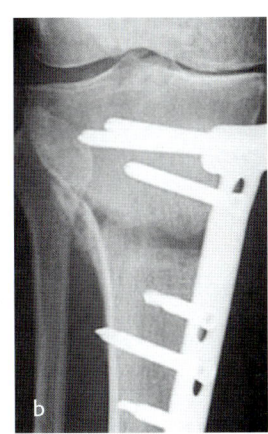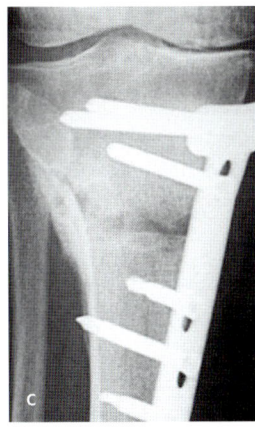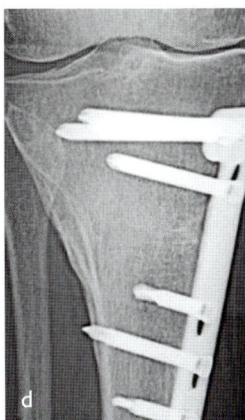

Fig 12-3a–d Progress of secondary bone healing for a relatively distal osteotomy (1st series) with initial bone resorption after the procedure (a) immediately postoperatively (resorption), (b) 3 weeks postoperatively, (c) 6 weeks postoperatively, and (d) remodeling after 18 months.

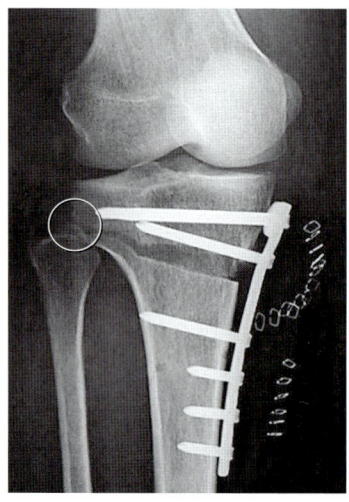
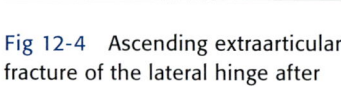
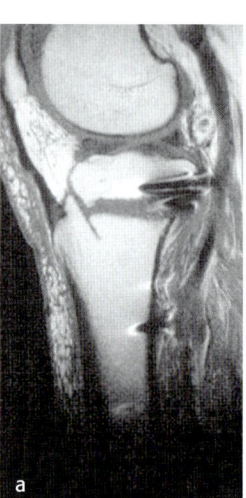
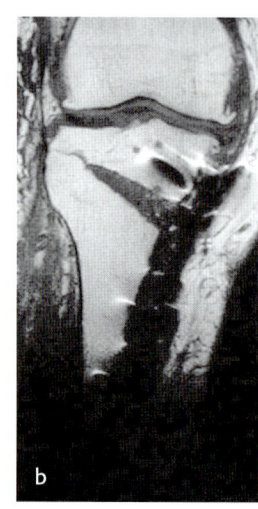
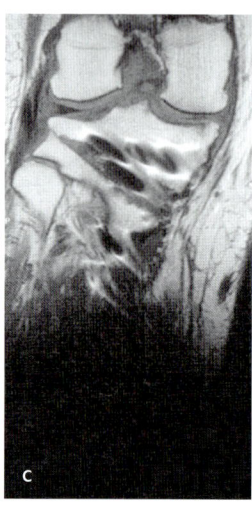
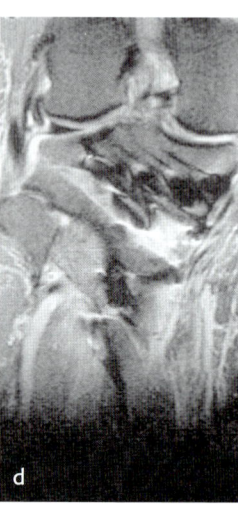

Fig 12-4   Ascending extraarticular fracture of the lateral hinge after open-wedge HTO (circle).

Fig 12-5a–d   Nondislocated fissures are only visible on magnetic resonance images (MRIs). These do not destabilize the lateral hinge.

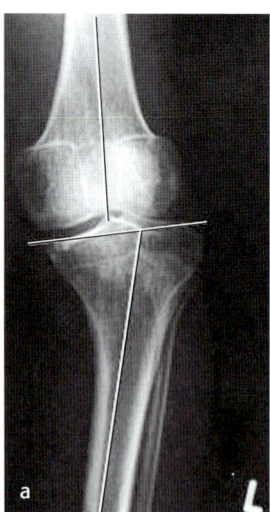
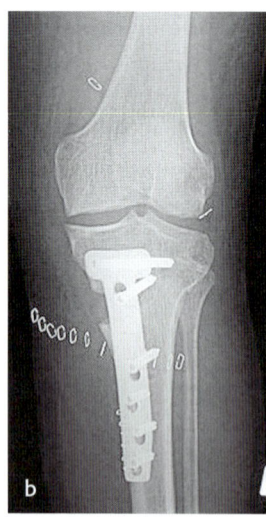
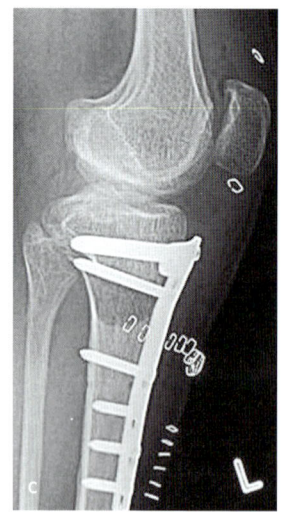

Fig 12-6a–c   Open-wedge HTO without interposition material in a 19-year-old patient with a deformity of the lower extremity due to epiphyseal dysplasia (15° correction at the proximal tibia).

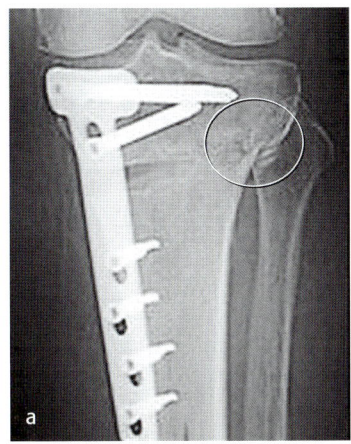
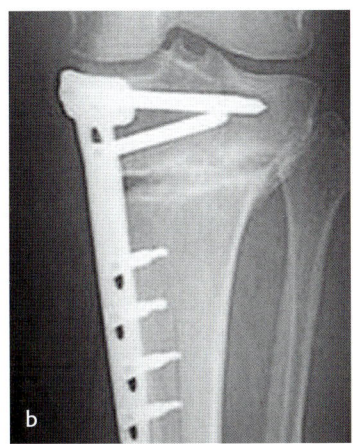
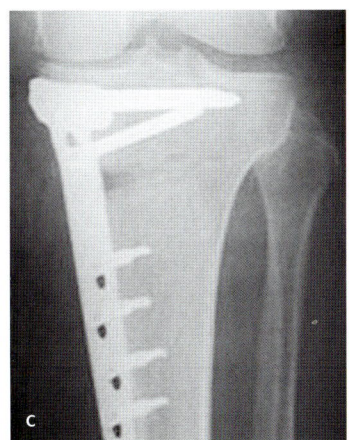
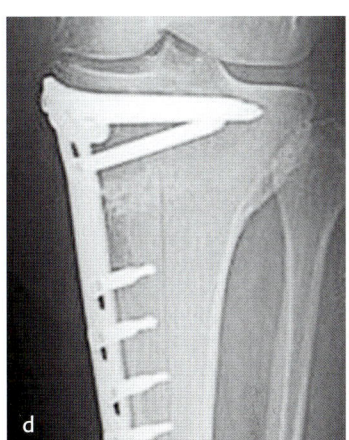

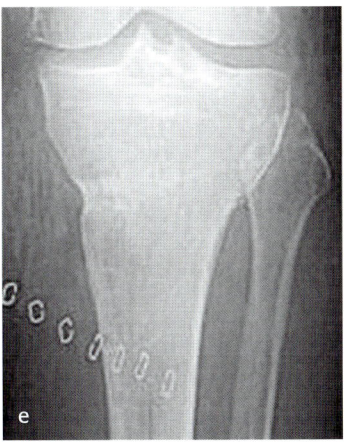
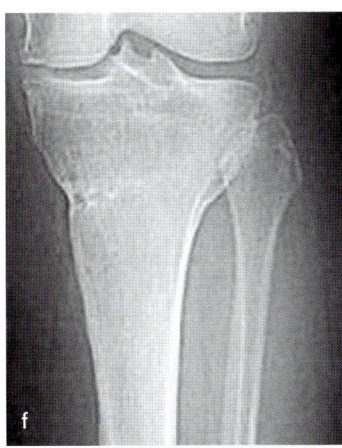

Fig 12-7a–f

a   Secondary bone healing with callus formation in the region of the posterolateral tibia as a sign of temporary tilting instability. This instability develops under increasing pressure during flexion and is neutralized by the implant.

b   Three months postoperatively.

c   Six months postoperatively.

d   One year postoperatively.

e   Eighteen months postoperatively.

f   Forty-two months postoperatively.

Secondary loss of correction with revarization

Loss of correction after implant removal was only observed in patients who had the implants removed less than 6 months postoperatively and in patients whose primary correction was insufficient (< 175° femorotibial axis).

Local infection without joint involvement became manifest in one patient with insulin-dependent diabetes mellitus after simultaneous HTO and ACL reconstruction and was treated by repeated debridement and early implant removal 2.5 months after the first operation. The osteotomy was consolidated with a correction loss of 3° and persistent medial pain during weight bearing. In another patient with osteopenia, the screws migrated through the cancellous bone of the proximal metaphysis. The authors conclude that the tibial metaphysis, especially in patients with osteopenic or osteoporotic bone stock, offers insufficient screw anchorage, particularly if the mechanical axis is undercorrected.

Based on this observation and in consideration of the fact that bone density diminishes exponentially with increasing distance from the tibial plateau, we recommend that the proximal screws A, B, and C are positioned below the tibial plateau in the subchondral bone. In order to achieve adequate stability, screws must be inserted into every plate hole. In one of our patients (66-year-old male) who underwent HTO on both knee joints within a 6-month period, the author observed secondary loss of correction after the second operation in the previously corrected contralateral extremity because the first osteotomy had not yet consolidated and was overloaded (Fig 12-8). The interval between first and second surgery of both knees should be at least 1–1.5 years for open-wedge correction procedures. Revision valgization osteotomy to salvage undercorrection or secondary loss of correction with persistent symptoms is possible and advisable with the TomoFix implant [22]. The author clearly advices against simultaneous bilateral open-wedge correction osteotomies.

- Bone healing in the osteotomy gap progresses from lateral to medial. The ascending anterior osteotomy consolidates very rapidly and consequently acts as a stabilizing column against tilting and rotational instabilities. A lateral bone hinge of 5–10 mm should be left laterally. The occurrence of fissures within this lateral hinge depends on the width of the osteotomy gap, but can be placed under compression by insertion of a temporary lag screw in combination hole 1. Screws A, B, and C should be placed subchondrally at the tibial plateau. To achieve good biomechanical stability, screws must be inserted into every plate hole. Simultaneous bilateral open-wedge correction osteotomies should not be performed. If bilateral corrections are indicated, the time between these two interventions should be at least 1–1.5 years.

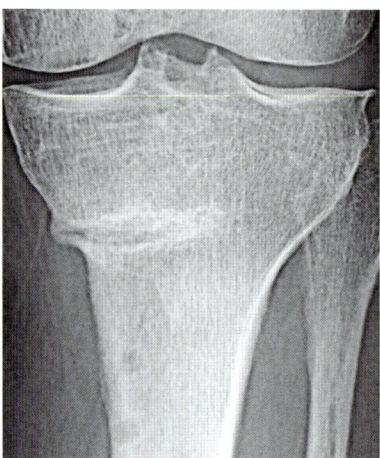

Fig 12-8 Small osteophyte at the medial aspect of the osteotomy indicating sintering with revarization as a result of early implant removal.

5.2   Evaluation of magnetic resonance imaging

In all patients postoperative magnetic resonance imaging (MRI) showed hematoma in the osteotomy gap on postoperative day 1 (Fig 12-9). In two patients examined on postoperative days 4 or 6, a 1 mm wide contrast enhanced band was already visible along the distal diaphyseal osteotomy surface. There was no evidence of bone marrow edema in any of the patients at this early stage.

Three weeks postoperatively, 1–5 mm wide band-shaped zones of regenerated tissue had formed at the osteotomy surfaces in all patients. The newly formed tissue filled the greater part of the gap volume (average 75%). Since the osteotomy gap is wedge-shaped and narrows laterally, the lateral portion was generally filled completely with tissue whereas a medial gap remained. Bone marrow edema was noticeable in the tibial head in all patients after 3–6 weeks (Fig 12-10). A fissure in the proximal tibial segment (epiphysis and metaphysis) was observed in 78% of patients.

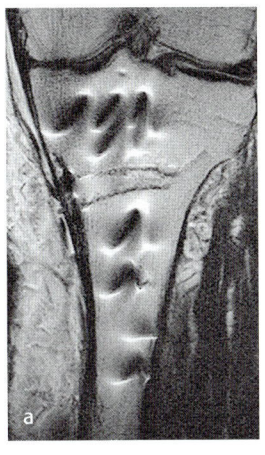 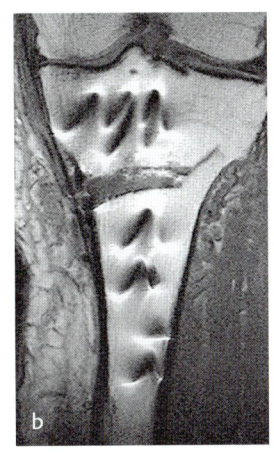 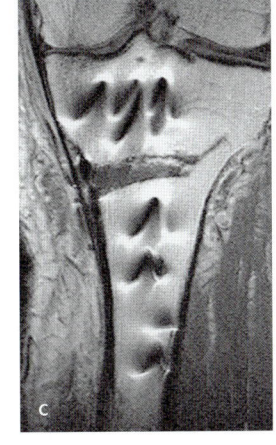

Fig 12-9a–c   MRIs on first postoperative day.
a   Hematoma in the osteotomy gap.
b   T2 sequence.
c   No enhancement after application of contrast media.

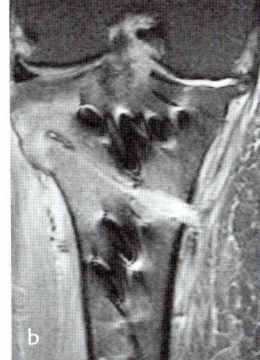 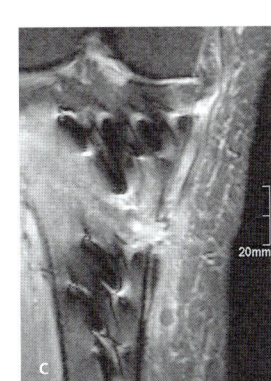

Fig 12-10a–c
a–b MRIs immediately postoperatively without bone marrow edema (a), and 3 weeks postoperatively showing bone marrow edema (b).
c   Increase in signal intensity 6 weeks postoperatively.

Six weeks after surgery the regenerated tissue filled almost the entire gap volume (average 93%) (Fig 12-11). Residual hematoma remained as a central defect of 1–2 mm thickness in half the patients. Evidence for bone marrow edema in the tibial head close to the osteotomy surfaces was found in 63% of all cases and fissure in 50% of the patients.

Three months after surgery, the osteotomy gap was filled out entirely by regenerated structures in palisade formation (Fig 12-12). In one patient a 1 mm wide structure with relatively high signal intensity on T1-weighted images was observed. This signal was interpreted as the beginning of tissue calcification or bone regeneration at the margin of the osteotomy since the intensified T1 signal can be attributed to dispersed calcium. The borders of the anterior oblique osteotomy and the lateral third of the osteotomy could no longer be identified in this patient due to complete consolidation. Bone marrow edema had receded completely and contrast enhancement in the tissue within the osteotomy gap was minimal, indicating a relatively weak perfusion. The tissue was interpreted as firm connective tissue.

After the sixth postoperative month, a 1–2 mm wide zone with moderate contrast enhancement at the surfaces of the osteotomy was already apparent in 57% of the patients examined. The osteotomy surfaces were seen as bands of low signal intensity (Fig 12-13).

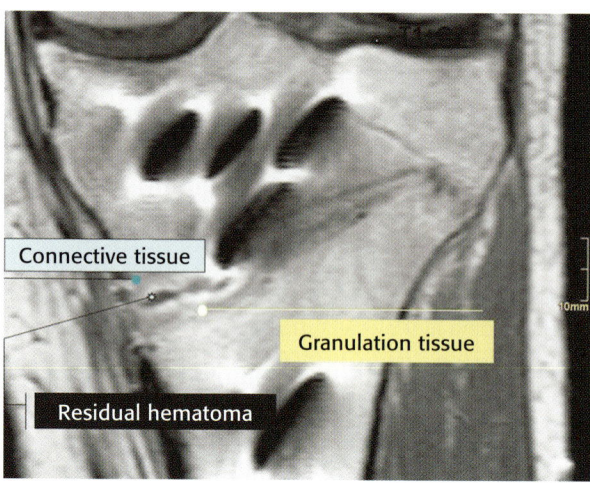

Fig 12-11   MRI showing regenerated tissue in the osteotomy gap 6 weeks postoperatively. (Residual hematoma = dark grey; connective tissue = light grey; granulation tissue = white.)

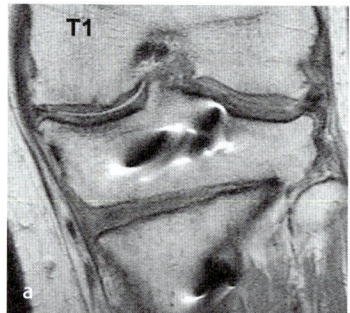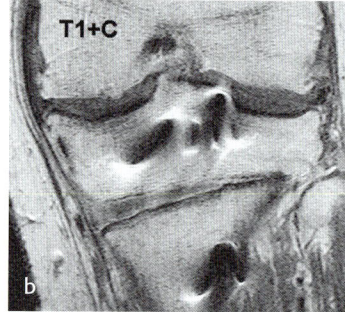

Fig 12-12a–b   Palisade-formed structures with minimal contrast enhancement (T1+C) at the surface of the osteotomy gap 3 months postoperatively. The lateral hinge is entirely consolidated.

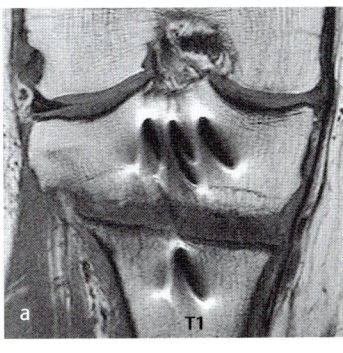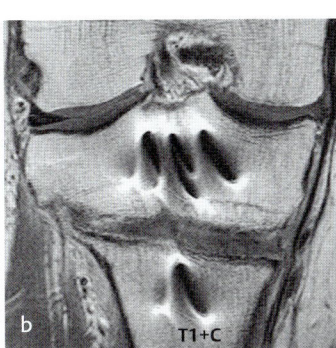

Fig 12-13a–b Six months postoperatively, 1–2 mm band-shaped contrast enhancement at the osteotomy surfaces. The surfaces themselves are visible as well defined narrow, band-shaped structures with low-signal strength.

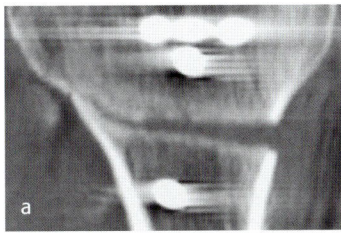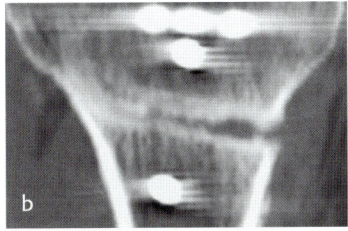

Fig 12-14a–b CT scan. Bone consolidation of the osteotomy gap progressing from lateral to medial, originating from the osteotomy surfaces.
a   Bone consolidation 6 weeks after open-wedge tibial osteotomy.
b   Bone consolidation 6 months after open-wedge tibial osteotomy.

5.3   Evaluation of computer tomography

The mineralization process of the regenerated bone in the osteotomy gap was also studied by computer tomography (CT).

From the third month after surgery bone regenerate was identified at the osteotomy surfaces of every patient. As already apparent on the magnetic resonance images, small bone structures in palisade formation developed, originating perpendicularly from the osteotomy surfaces. The palisades were 1–3 mm wide. Bridging, stabilizing callus formation at the posterolateral osteotomy surface, and the posterolateral border of the tibia was seen in 50% of patients.

Six months after open-wedge tibial osteotomy, the palisade-shaped bone regeneration at the osteotomy surfaces had reached a width of 2–4 mm in 86% of patients. The new bone layers from the proximal and from the distal osteotomy surfaces had contact in half the patients. The gap began to fill up from lateral to medial (Fig 12-14). In one patient, the osteotomy gap had already filled completely with bone at that time.

6   Evaluation of the postoperative anatomical femorotibial axis

The femorotibial axis can only be correctly evaluated by means of a weight-bearing view of the entire lower extremity with the knee joint in full extension. The anatomical femorotibial axis was corrected on average by 9–2° ± 3.4° in our patients. All patients were examined as outpatients until bone consolidation of the osteotomy had been confirmed and documented. In all patients with postoperatively correctly aligned mechanical axis and who did not require early implant removal, the postoperative femorotibial axis was maintained without loss of correction.

7   Accidental alteration of the tibial slope

The tibial slope shows a tendency to increase during opening of the osteotomy because the posteromedial capsuloligamentous complex and the pes anserinus counteract distraction of the osteotomy in the posterior portion. To avoid flexion deformity of the tibial plateau, multistage, subperiosteal, subligamentous release of the superficial fibers of the medial collateral ligament is essential (see chapter 10 "Effect of osteotomies on cartilage pressure in the knee", chapter 9 "High-tibial open-wedge valgization osteotomy with plate fixator", and chapter 11 "Osteotomy and ligament instability: tibial slope corrections and combined procedures around the knee joint"). During the consolidation phase the tibial slope showed no further statistically significant alterations.

8   Primary undercorrection and secondary loss of correction

Good clinical long-term results can only be achieved in correct surgical technique after precise planning of axial correction. The best outcomes have been described when the primarily planned correction is accomplished and the femorotibial axis remains within the range of 173–176° during consolidation without loss of correction [18]. There is a clear tendency towards undercorrection of the deformity [18, 22, 28]. This is a technical problem related to planning and surgical technique that can be avoided by working with a navigation system.

In our series of patients, accidental undercorrection was the most common cause of poor clinical outcome with subsequent revision osteotomy in two patients and secondary total knee replacement in seven patients.

Undercorrection combined with poor bone stock, eg, in older patients, may lead to postoperative loss of correction, particularly if the implant is removed too early. On the basis of our experience we recommend that an open-wedge osteotomy should no longer be performed in cases with severe osteoporosis.

9   Comparison of imaging procedures: x-ray, MRI, and CT

The purpose of the retrospective study conducted by Treumann and Staubli [27] was to evaluate the efficacy of three imaging techniques, x-ray, MRI, and CT, in the assessment of tissue regeneration and bone healing after medial open-wedge HTO without interposition material. The aim was to determine adequate methods for evaluation of the postoperative consolidation process.

Conventional radiological findings indicate that healing of the osteotomy gap progresses from lateral to medial, and that about 75% of the entire tibial width has already filled 6 months after surgery. By contrast, CT images after 6 months show narrow, vertical bone structures in palisade formation at the osteotomy surfaces without complete osseous consolidation. It can be concluded that radiographic images provoke an overestimation of the amount of gap filled. CT studies show that the bone healing process takes longer than has been assumed from the evaluation of plain x-rays. The reason for this discrepancy is the fact that the x-ray beam in conventional technique does not lie in the osteotomy plane but at an oblique angle to it. The osteotomy gap is partially superposed by parts of the tibial head. Therefore, x-rays in their current application do not represent an absolutely reliable method of assessing osteotomy healing. For precise evaluation the x-ray tube has to be tilted into the plane of the osteotomy gap.

MRI is an eligible diagnostic method to visualize early mineralization processes in the osteotomy gap.

Parameters defining sufficient consolidation and stability of the tibial head under loading to permit implant removal are not yet available. The author's observations indicate that loss of correction does not occur if the plate is removed after 12–18 months. The point at which bone remodeling is definitively completed has not been clarified to date.

10   Additional radiological findings

The persistent medial defect under the plate that the author observed in 20% of cases after plate removal seems to be of no clinical relevance and has no effect on stability since the intact cortical frame of the tibia and extensive bone regeneration in the osteotomy gap ensure sufficient mechanical stability. The defect is located where the horizontal saw cut is performed (Fig 12-15). Possible reasons why this small area is not bridged might be:

- Reduced distribution of forces at the medial aspect of tibia after valgization correction and stress protection under the plate
- Intraoperative interposition of partially detached soft tissues
- Necrosis that inhibits the regeneration of tissue

In a few cases minimal residual notching is visible at the posteromedial cortex of the tibia, which likewise has no influence on stability.

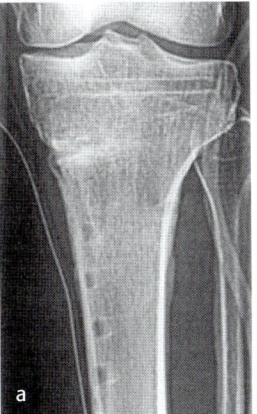 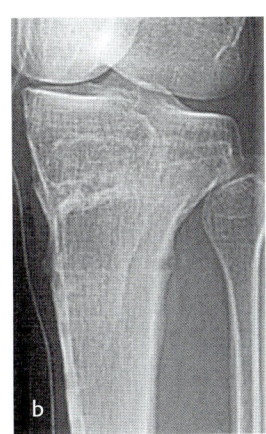 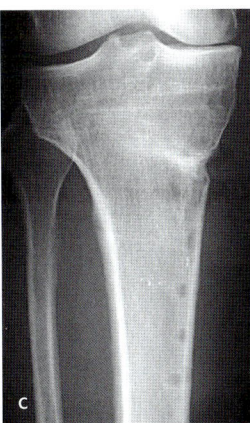

Fig 12-15a–c Persistent medial defect at the proximal tibia at the level of the osteotomy visible on the AP x-rays after implant removal.

11   Nicotine abuse

Nicotine abuse significantly delays bone healing. This is an established fact in fracture healing and is also valid for open-wedge tibial osteotomy as shown by prospective studies with open-wedge hemicallotasis HTO [29–31]. The author observed this matter of fact in his patients (Fig 12-16) and drew the conclusion that the significantly higher complication rate must be pointed out to the patient. In patients with chronic nicotine abuse and lack of compliance, we only perform this kind of osteotomy in selected cases [32, 33].

■ Secondary loss of correction after open-wedge HTO is seen after primary undercorrection of the mechanical axis and after early implant removal. The consolidation process and the quality of the regenerated bone depend on the quality of individual bone stock (eg, osteoporosis) and patient compliance (eg, nicotine abuse). In most patients it takes at least 1 year for mechanically stable bone to form in the osteotomy gap. The option of inserting heterogeneous materials into the gap to accelerate bone regeneration is currently still under discussion. The advantages of these materials must first be proven in prospective, randomized studies. Our experience indicates that the osteotomy gap will heal uneventfully without the application of interposition materials.

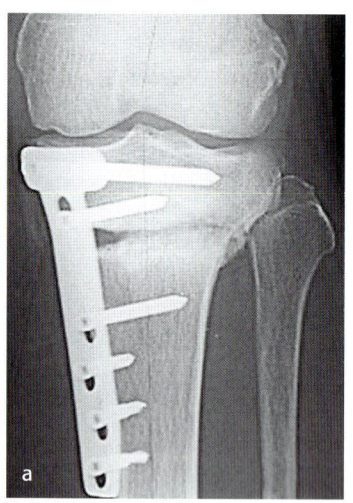
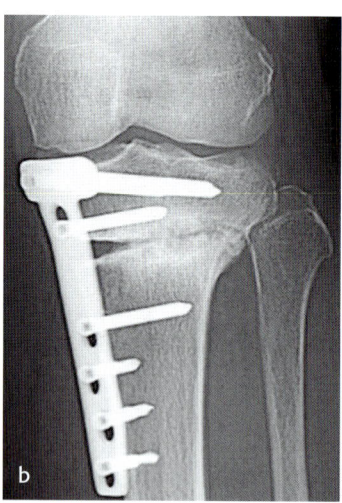
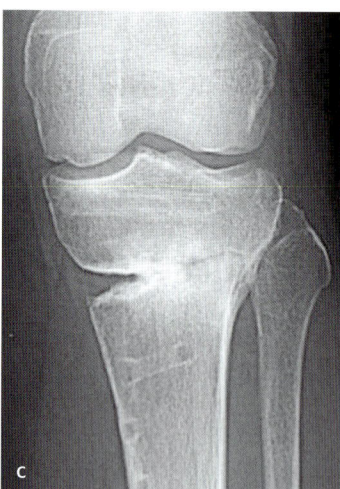

Fig 12-16a–c   Radiological follow-up after tibial open-wedge valgization correction in a patient with extreme nicotine abuse. Delayed bone healing is clearly apparent after more than 1 year.
a   Seven months postoperatively.
b   Thirteen months postoperatively.
c   Fifteen months postoperatively.

12   Bibliography

[1] **Schenk RK, Willenegger HR** (1977) [Histology of primary bone healing: modifications and limits of recovery of gaps in relation to extent of the defect.] *Unfallheilkunde;* 80(5):155–160. German.

[2] **Bonetta M** (2006) [Influence of the drill cutting on the Development of the callus at defects of the tibia. A histomorphological analysis on tibia of sheet.] *Disertation.* Freiburg i.Br.: Albert-Ludwigs-Universität. German.

[3] **Schenk RK** (1978) [Histology of primary bone healing in light of new concepts of bone reconstruction.] *Unfallheilkunde;* 81(4):219–227. German.

[4] **Kelly PJ, Montgomery RJ, Bronk JT** (1990) Reaction of the circulatory system to injury and regeneration. *Clin Orthop Relat Res;* 254:275–288.

[5] **Kessler SB, Rahn BA, Schweiberer L, et al** (1983) [Revascularization of intermediary fragments following interlocking nailing.] *Hefte Unfallheilkunde;* 161:38–41. German.

[6] **Kessler SB, Rahn F, Eitel L, et al** (1983) [Revascularization of the corticalis of the bone after nailing. Comparing analyses on different animals in vivo.] Lausanne: *D-O-Ch Unfall;* 1–4. German.

[7] **Perren SM** (2002) Evolution of the internal fixation of long bone fractures. The scientific basis of biological internal fixation: choosing a new balance between stability and biology. *J Bone Joint Surg Br;* 84(8):1093–1110.

[8] **Pfister U, Rahn BA, Perren SM, et al** (1979 [Vascularization and bone reconstruction after nailing of long bones.] *Aktuel Traumatol;* 9:191–195. German.

[9] **Pfister U** (1982) [Vascularization and bone reconstruction after nailing in tibia of the sheet.] *Hefte Unfallheilkunde;* 158:51–52.

[10] **Smith SR, Bronk JT, Kelly PJ** (1990) Effect of fracture fixation on cortical bone blood flow. *J Orthop Res;* 8(4):471–478.

[11] **Trueta J** (1963) The role of the vessels in osteogenesis. *J Bone Joint Surg;* 45B:402–418.

[12] **Rahn BA** (1995) [Bone healing after nailing.] *Osteosynthese International;* 4:240–245. German.

[13] **Pfister U** (1988) [Biomechanical and histological analyses after nailing of the tibia.] *Aktuel Traumatol;* 18:40. German.

[14] **Pfister U** (1988) [Current status of intramedullary nailing osteosynthesis.] *Aktuelle Traumatol;* 18 Suppl 1:40–45. German.

[15] **Stürmer KM, Schuchardt W** (1980) [New aspects of closed intramedullary nailing and marrow cavity reaming in animal experiments. III. Bone-healing, revascularisation and remodelling.] *Unfallheilkunde;* 83(9):433–435. German.

[16] **Bonnevialle P, Abid A, Mansat P, et al** (2002) [Tibial valgus osteotomy using a tricalcium phosphate medial wedge: a minimally invasive technique.] *Rev Chir Orthop Réparatrice Appar Mot;* 88(5):486–492. French.

[17] **Bové JC** (2002) [Utilization of a porous alumina ceramic spacer in tibial valgus open-wedge osteotomy: fifty cases at 16 months mean follow-up.] *Rev Chir Orthop Réparatrice Appar Mot;* 88(5):480–485. French.

[18] **Hernigou P** (1996) [A 20-year follow-up study of internal gonarthrosis after tibial valgus osteotomy. Single versus repeated osteotomy.] *Rev Chir Orthop Réparatrice Appar Mot;* 82(3):241–250. French.

[19] **Hernigou P, Ma W** (2001) Open wedge tibial osteotomy with acrylic bone cement as bone substitute. *Knee;* 8(2):103–110.

[20] **Hinz P, Wolf E, Schwesinger G, et al** (2002): A new resorbable bone void filler in trauma: early clinical experience and histologic evaluation. *Orthopedics;* 25(5 Suppl):s597–s600.

[21] **Koshino T, Murase T, Saito T** (2003): Medial opening-wedge high tibial osteotomy with use of porous hydroxyapatite to treat medial compartment osteoarthritis of the knee. *J Bone Joint Surg Am;* 85(1):78–85.

[22] **Müller W** (2001) High Tibial Osteotomy. *European Instructional Course Lectures EFORT;* Volume 5:194–206.

[23] **Puddu GC, Cerullo G, Cipolla M, et al** (1998) [Usage of a plate for open-wedge osteotomies of the tibia.] *Rodilly;* 6:33–37. Italian.

[24] **Seeherman H** (2001) The influence of delivery vehicles and their properties on the repair of segmental defects and fractures with osteogenic factors. *J Bone Joint Surg Am;* 83 Suppl 1(2):S79–S81.

[25] **Szpalski M, Gunzburg R** (2002) Applications of calcium phosphate-based cancellous bone void fillers in trauma surgery. *Orthopedics;* 25(5 Suppl):s601–s609-

[26] **Siguier M, Brumpt B, Siguier T, et al** (2001) [Original valgus tibial osteotomy by internal opening and without loss of bone contact. Technique and incidence of consolidation speed: a preliminary series of 33 cases.] *Rev Chir Orthop Réparatrice Appar Mot;* 87(2):183–188. French.

[27] **Treumann T, Staubli AE** (2008) Osteotomy gap healing after open-wedge high tibial osteotomy determining the best method of assessment (unpublished data).

[28] **Lobenhoffer P, Agneskirchner JD** (2003) Improvements in surgical technique of valgus high tibial osteotomy. *Knee Surg Sports Traumatol Arthrosc;* 11(3):132–138.

[29] **Brown CW, Orme TJ, Richardson HD** (1986) The rate of pseudarthrosis (surgical nonunion) in patients who are smokers and patients who are nonsmokers: a comparison study. *Spine;* 11(9):942–943.

[30] **Dahl, W.** (2004): Cigarette smoking delays bone healing: a prospective study of 200 patients operated on by the hemicallotasis method. *Acta Orthop Scand* 75, 347–351.

[31] **Heppenstall RB, Goodwin CW, Brighton CT** (1976) Fracture healing in the presence of chronic hypoxia. *J Bone Joint Surg Am;* 58(8):1153–1156.

[32] **Lobenhoffer P, De Simoni C, Staubli AE** (2002): Open wedge high-tibial osteotomy with rigid plate fixation. *Techniques in Knee Surgery;* 1:93–105.

[33] **Staubli AE, De Simoni C, Babst R, et al** (2003) TomoFix: a new LCP-concept for open wedge osteotomy of the medial proximal tibia—early results in 92 cases. *Injury;* 34 Suppl 2: B55–B62.

13 Supracondylar varization osteotomy of the femur with plate fixation

1 Introduction

The aim of varization osteotomy of the distal femur is to relieve lateral single-compartment degeneration at the knee by shifting the mechanical axis medially. Degeneration of the lateral knee with valgus deformity is a frequent consequence of subtotal or total lateral meniscectomy. Valgus deformities that are posttraumatic or subsequent to growth disorders or partial epiphyseodesis also require surgical correction.

Varization osteotomy of the distal femur can be performed by a medial closed-wedge or lateral open-wedge technique. Less frequently used dome osteotomies can also be performed in the supracondylar region of the femur. Supracondylar varization osteotomy of the femur today is generally performed as a medial closed-wedge osteotomy. Stabilization of the osteotomy is achieved by application of conventional blade plates, angular-stable plates, or insertion of a distal femoral nail [1].

In recent years incomplete open-wedge osteotomy through a lateral approach has gained increasing acceptance due to the development of spacer plates [2]. The authors have, however, observed that this technique may result in disturbed bone healing and symptoms at the lateral aspect of the femur due to friction as the iliotibial tract moves over the plate. In this chapter an improved technique for medial closed-wedge osteotomy is described that involves an incomplete osteotomy and application of a special internal plate fixator.

2 Principles of medial closed-wedge femoral osteotomy

Stable osteosynthesis is of great importance in a supracondylar osteotomy of the femur as it permits undisturbed bone healing and functional rehabilitation. In addition to the angled blade plate [3–11], the curved semitubular plate [12, 13] and a more recently developed plate fixator [14] can be considered for osteotomy stabilization. In biomechanical investigations substantial differences have been found in the primary stability of different fixation methods, and these differences must be respected when planning postoperative rehabilitation [15].

Apart from the fixation technique, the type of osteotomy, its orientation and localization also play an important role in primary stability. An incomplete, medial closed-wedge osteotomy with an intact lateral bone bridge is far more stable than a complete osteotomy that cuts through the lateral cortex. In terms of closed-wedge osteotomies of the distal femur, an oblique, proximal to distal, descending osteotomy will yield greater primary stability than a transverse osteotomy since the osteotomy surfaces are more congruent and the medial cortical support is more secure [12, 15]. Primary stability is also markedly increased by compression of the osteotomy surfaces, whereby optimal cortical contact is essential for effective compression to avoid risk of overcorrection due to subsidence of the distal fragment into the proximal fragment. Compression also accelerates bone healing and prevents delayed union and nonunion.

■ Type, direction, and localization of the osteotomy as well as the fixation technique are very important for the primary stability of the osteotomy. An incomplete medial closed-wedge osteotomy with an intact lateral cortical bridge is far more stable than an osteotomy that cuts through the bone bridge. Oblique, proximal to distal descending osteotomies are more stable than transverse osteotomies.

3 Design of the fixed-angle plate fixator TomoFix MDF

The specific plate fixator TomoFix MDF was developed in collaboration with the Knee Expert Group (KNEG) of the AO. It is a special "spoon-shaped" locking compression plate (LCP) that has four threaded holes in the distal part and four combination holes in the proximal shaft (Fig 13-1). Alignment and angulation of the distal threaded holes are designed to fit the anatomy of the supracondylar zone of the distal femur. Left and right versions facilitate correct positioning of the plate in the anteromedial segment of the distal femur and secure anchorage of the locking head screws in the condylar block. Utilization of an LCP guide sleeve to predrill the screw holes ensures correct alignment of the distal locking head screws. The screws are inserted with the torque screwdriver and locked at a fixed angle in the conical threaded hole. Self-tapping locking head screws are inserted in the distal part and self-tapping/self-drilling locking head screws combined with self-tapping screws with predrilling in the proximal part. The proximal locking head screws can be anchored mono- or bicortically (Fig 13-2). Secondary correction loss during screw tightening is avoided since the fixed-angle locking head screws do not develop a lag screw effect. This feature permits stable fixation of the TomoFix plate fixator even in osteoporotic bone. Temporary insertion of a 3 mm spacer in the most proximal plate hole preserves the periosteal blood flow.

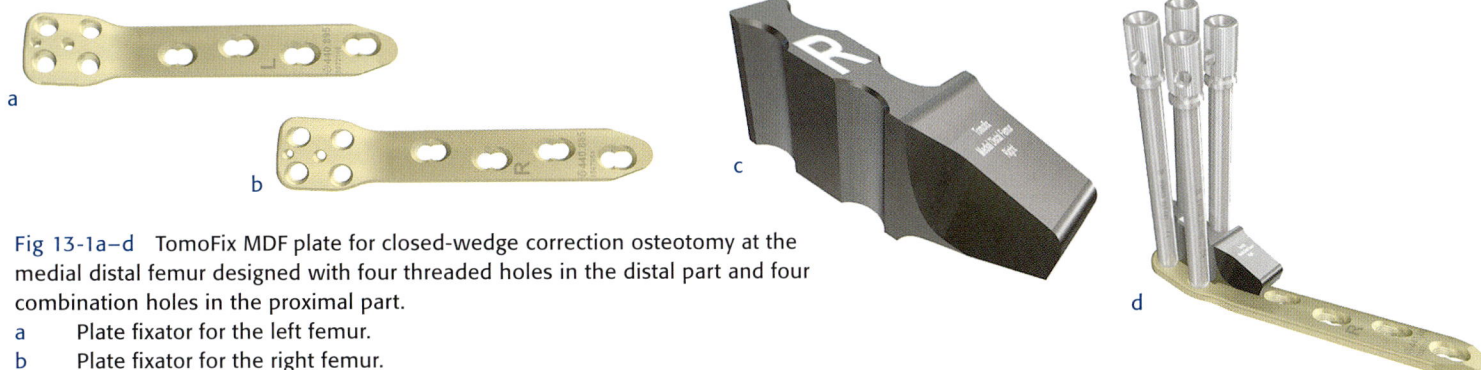

Fig 13-1a–d   TomoFix MDF plate for closed-wedge correction osteotomy at the medial distal femur designed with four threaded holes in the distal part and four combination holes in the proximal part.
a   Plate fixator for the left femur.
b   Plate fixator for the right femur.
c–d   The drill sleeves are attached to the plate by application of the positioning device (black).

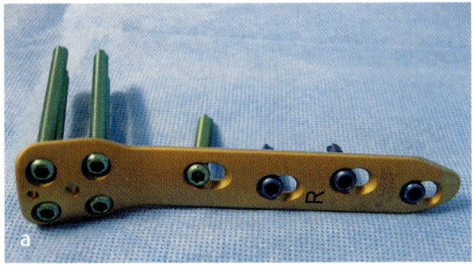
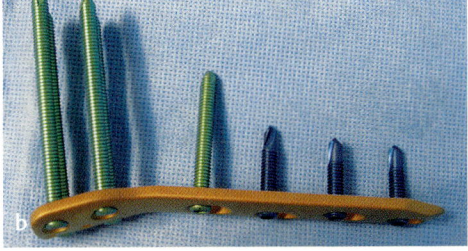
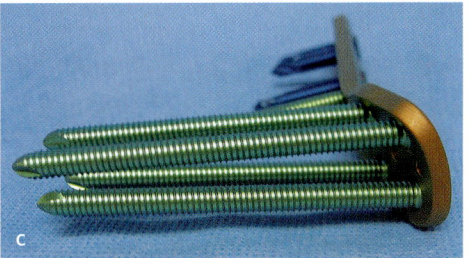

Fig 13-2a–d   TomoFix MDF plate with the bicortical (green) and monocortical (blue) locking head screws inserted.
a   Medial view.
b   Frontal view.
c   Caudal view.
d   Angulation of the locking head screws in the transverse plane in a bone model.

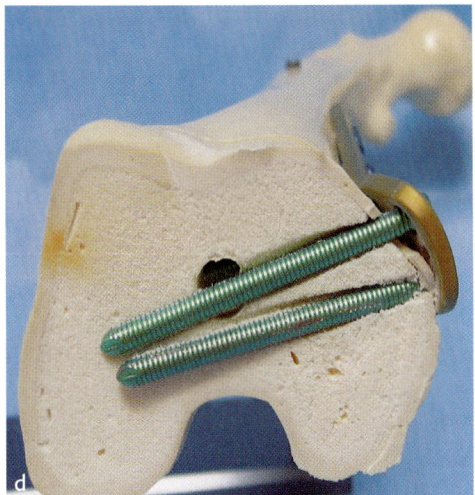

4 Indications and contraindications

The indication for varization osteotomy of the distal femur and plate fixation is lateral single-compartment degeneration at the knee with valgus deformity of the lower extremity. The patient should have a desire to be active and should not be older than 55 (female) to 60 (male) years of age. The procedure can be combined with other reconstructive measures in the lateral compartment, eg, osteochondral autogenous transplantation (OATS), autogenous chondrocyte transplantation (ACT), and matrix-induced autogenous chondrocyte implantation (MACI).

Relevant symptomatic valgus deformities due to growth disorders or as the result of trauma should likewise be corrected prior to the development of manifest arthrosis. Planning must always respect the need for the surface of the knee joint to be as horizontal as possible after correction. If there is a deformity at the proximal tibia in addition to the femoral deformity, a double osteotomy must be considered since isolated varization of the femur may lead to excessive deviation of the knee base-line from the horizontal, leading to long-term symptoms (see chapter 14 "Double osteotomies of the femur and the tibia").

The preoperative range of motion at the knee should be at least extension/flexion 0-0-90°. Extension and flexion deficits can be corrected to some extent by the osteotomy involving additional wedge extraction in the sagittal plane. This requires a complete femoral osteotomy.

Contraindications include obesity, loss of the inner meniscus, arthrosis, or third degree cartilage damage of the medial compartment as classified by Outerbridge [16], or restricted movement at the knee, especially an extension deficit greater than 15–20°. The operation should not be performed if the soft-tissue situation at the distal femur is inadequate or if there is acute or chronic infection. In addition there should be no nicotine abuse.

- Indications: Single-compartment lateral joint degeneration with valgus deformity, patients aged 55–60 years.
  Contraindications: Obesity, extension deficit of >20°, loss of the inner meniscus, third degree cartilage injury of the medial compartment, or manifest arthrosis, insufficient soft-tissue situation, and nicotine abuse.

5 Preoperative work-up

Correction of axial deformity by osteotomy of the distal femur requires thorough preoperative planning. Full explanation of the possible complications and risks must be given to the patient. This does not just include information on general risks such as vessel and nerve injuries, thrombosis, embolism, disturbed wound healing, early and late infections, but also the possibility of delayed bone healing. Hematoma at the distal thigh, protracted swelling, and lymph edema are often to be expected postoperatively. Despite the submuscular approach, recovery of full flexion may require a long rehabilitation period.

5.1 Preoperative diagnostics

Clinical examination includes assessment of the range of motion and the laxity of the knee ligaments. The skin and soft-tissue situation should be normal. Radiological diagnosis requires views of the knee in three planes and an x-ray of the whole leg under loading. Additional information about the extent of damage of the knee can be derived from a weight-bearing view in 45° flexion, known as the Rosenberg view, and MRI, but these procedures are not essential. Stress views may be valuable if there is also ligament laxity. It is essential to take soft-tissue and ligament laxity with asymmetrical opening of the joint into account during preoperative planning of the overall correction angle (see chapter 4 "Basic principles of osteotomies around the knee").

Until the indication is certain, preoperative prescription of a varus brace (lateral unloader brace) may be helpful. Application of this brace should lead to a substantial decrease of symptoms. Prior to the correction or at the same operation, arthroscopy may be performed to assess the joint surfaces. The cartilage surfaces and inner meniscus should be more or less intact medially. Lateral cartilage damage is recorded in detail and frayed body or cartilaginous tissue is cut away. Sometimes microfracturing is useful for localized defects.

5.2   Radiology: preoperative planning

Currently, there is a lack of agreement on the desired realignment of the mechanical axis of the leg. One group recommends restoration of the mechanical axis to normal values (mechanical femorotibial axis 0°) [2], whereas other groups advocate a realignment of the mechanical axis more or less into the medial compartment. Mechanical femorotibial angles of between 1° and 3° are proposed [3, 5, 7, 8] or anatomical angles of 6–10° [4, 9–11]. The authors correct the mechanical axis to the normal position or beyond so that it lies slightly medially. In valgus deformities involving an intact lateral joint compartment, the mechanical axis of the contralateral side can be used as a reference. In patients with an oblique knee joint line, planning aims to achieve a horizontal knee baseline and normal mechanical axis after correction.

Radiological planning of a supracondylar closed-wedge femoral osteotomy is shown in **Fig 13-3**. The same principles apply as for the preoperative planning of proximal tibial head osteotomy. The correction angle for the osteotomy is calculated on the basis of the preoperative x-rays and is reproduced intraoperatively with the help of an appropriate saw guide and a calibrated goniometer. In addition, the height of the osteotomy wedge base can be determined by radiological planning (taking into account the magnification factor); these measurements can be checked intraoperatively with a ruler or depth gauge.

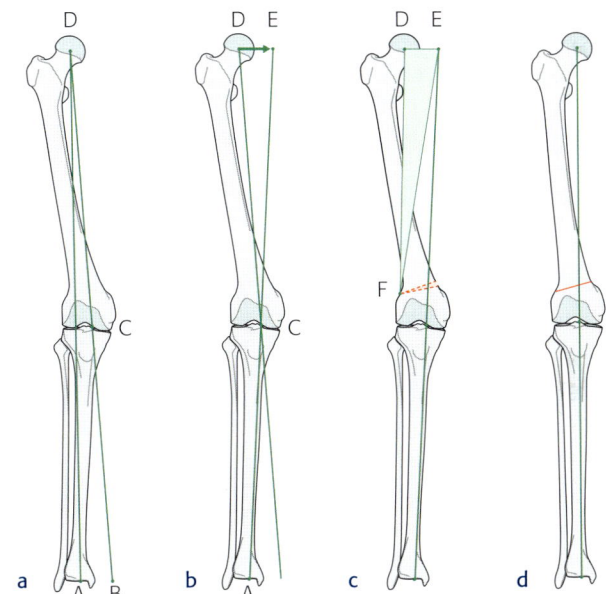

Fig 13-3a–d Planning a varization osteotomy of the distal femur. The postoperative mechanical axis should be somewhat medial of the medial intercondylar eminence (C). Position E is at the level of the center of the femoral head (D) on a connecting line between C and the center of the upper ankle joint (A). Position F is the hinge point of the closed-wedge osteotomy. The angle between the lines DF and EF correspond to the correction angle at the distal femur. This angle is projected at the distal femur. Osteotomy width and level of the wedge base can then be measured taking into account the magnification factor.

5.3 Positioning, implants, and instruments

Closed-wedge medial femoral osteotomy is performed with the patient in the supine position and under general anesthesia, local anesthesia close to the spinal cord, or single-leg anesthesia. The patient is positioned so that hip, knee, and ankle joints can be assessed. Draping leaves the entire leg and iliac crest free so that the leg axis can be assessed intraoperatively. A sterile tourniquet is not generally necessary but, if required, it should be placed as far proximal as possible to leave sufficient room for the surgical approach. Systemic antibiotic prophylaxis is given preoperatively as a single-shot. The image intensifier for intraoperative screening is positioned on the side of the leg to be operated on, the surgeon stands on the contralateral side.

In addition to the standard instrument set for bone surgery, the following are required:

- TomoFix MDF plate fixator with bicortical and monocortical locking head screws
- Oscillating saw with 90 mm long, wide saw blade
- Special saw guide or K-wires to mark the osteotomy
- Image intensifier
- Sterile metal rod to evaluate leg axis
- Sterile ruler or standard depth gauge to determine the height of the osteotomy wedge base

6 Surgical technique

Arthroscopy is performed first to assess the cartilage situation and to carry out arthroscopic surgery if indicated.

Surgery begins with the knee in extension. The anatomical landmarks are drawn on the skin. The longitudinal skin incision starts a hand's width above the patella and extends to the upper one third of the patella (Fig 13-4a). This anterior longitudinal incision is chosen so that wound healing problems are avoided if subsequent operations are required (eg, total knee replacement). After division of the subcutaneous tissue, the muscle fascia is incised (Fig 13-4b). The vastus medialis is stripped from the intermuscular septum by partially sharp and partially blunt dissection, and retracted cranially. A blunt Hohmann retractor is passed over the femur to expose the anteromedial aspect of the supracondylar area of the femur (Fig 13-4c). The intermuscular septum in the metaphyseal area of the femur is carefully incised longitudinally close to the bone. The vessels beneath are preserved. The posterior side of the femur is approached subperiosteally with a rasp, and a blunt Hohmann retractor is

positioned after that to avoid damage to the neurovascular structures. To enhance exposure distally, part of the medial patellofemoral ligament and the distal insertion of vastus medialis are incised to expose the medial femoral condyle (Fig 13-4d). Proximally, the shaft is exposed sufficiently for the plate to be positioned by dissection of the vastus medialis from the septum. The periosteum should not be violated.

The oblique osteotomy begins in the medial supracondylar area and ends within the lateral femoral condyle. The distal osteotomy should run laterally about 10 mm above the intercondylar groove. The upper margin of the intercondylar groove can be palpated from the medial aspect via a small arthrotomy, alternatively, the margin of the intercondylar groove can be located with the image intensifier. The starting point for the distal osteotomy at the medial femur is best defined by temporary application of the plate fixator. The distal osteotomy should be placed within the solid portion of the plate. The level of the osteotomy can be marked on the bone with the electrocautery.

The authors use a precise saw guide (Balansys, the Mathys company) (Fig 13-5) for closed-wedge osteotomy of the distal femur. A new special saw guide for this type of osteotomy has been developed by the Knee Expert Group of the AO and should soon be available on the market. The planned wedge for extraction can also be marked by insertion of K-wires under image intensification, whereby these wires also serve to guide the saw. The saw cuts should be made under constant irrigation for cooling (Fig 13-6). At the posterior aspect, attention must be paid to proper retraction of the soft tissues, particularly the vessels.

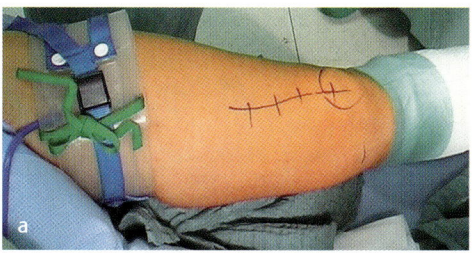

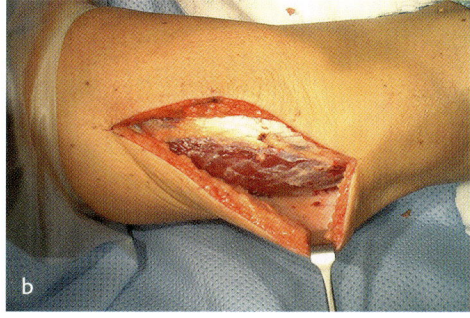

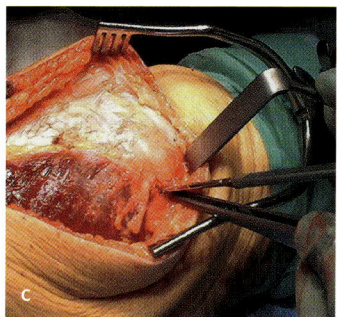

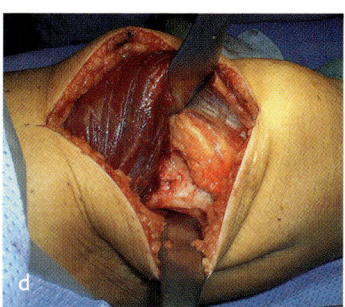

Fig 13-4a–d   Surgical approach for closed-wedge correction osteotomy at the medial distal femur.
a   The anterior skin incision begins a hand's width above the patella and extends to the upper one third of the patella.
b   The fascia of vastus medialis is incised and the muscle is stripped from the medial intermuscular septum and retracted cranially.
c   The medial patellofemoral ligament is partly incised to enhance distal exposure.
d   The intermuscular septum is incised and a Hohmann retractor passed posterior to the femur.

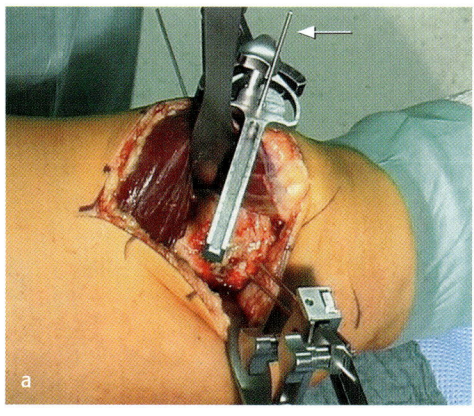

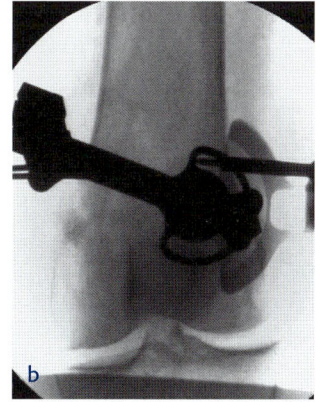

Fig 13-5a–b   Positioning of the saw guide. The hinge point of the osteotomy is located 10 mm medial to the lateral cortex in the upper portion of the lateral femoral condyle. The hinge point is marked by anteroposterior insertion of a K-wire (arrow). The saw cuts stop at the K-wire and the posterior vessels are carefully protected by the Hohmann retractor.
a   Operative site.
b   Image intensification.

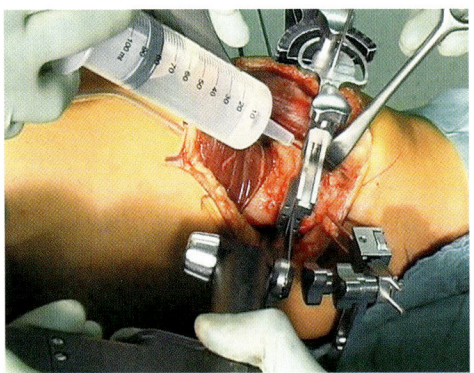

Fig 13-6 Both osteotomies are conducted using the saw guide with thorough cooling of the saw blade.

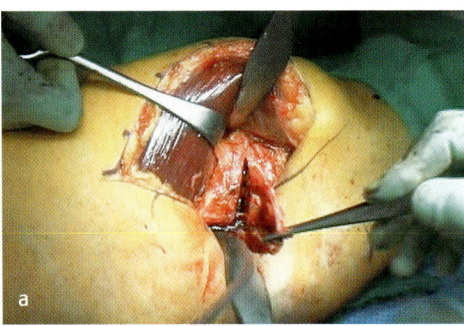

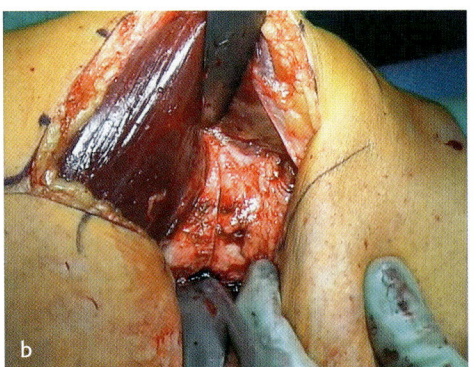

Fig 13-7a–b Wedge extraction. After completion of both saw cuts, the bone wedge is extracted. The size of the osteotomy gap can now be compared with the preoperative radiological plan (a). After cleaning the osteotomy surfaces, possibly weakening the lateral cortex by drill holes, and making the rotation marks, the osteotomy is slowly closed by application of controlled axial pressure on the foot (b).

The cuts for the osteotomy stop 10 mm before reaching the lateral cortex so that a wedge with a medial base can be created. The wedge is extracted and wedge height can be checked using a sterile ruler. It is especially important that wedge extraction should be complete and that no fragments of cortical bone persist in the posterior part of the osteotomy (Fig 13-7a). Now two longitudinal lines are marked on the medial shaft with the cautery in order to assess rotational alignment. Alternatively, a K-wire can be inserted proximal and distal to the osteotomy. After wedge extraction, the lateral aspect of the osteotomy is thoroughly inspected. Residual bone fragments have to be carefully removed; the wedge height should be compared again with the preoperative plan. If the extracted wedge is too small, the osteotomy surface can be cut again. If the medial defect is larger than planned, the osteotomy gap must only be partially closed to avoid over-correction. The osteotomy is now carefully closed by applying consistent pressure on the lateral lower leg with simultaneous stabilization of the joint region (Fig 13-7b). It may take several minutes to achieve complete closure of the osteotomy by plastic deformation of the lateral cortex. The rotation markers are examined to check rotational alignment. Step-off at the anterior cortex is assessed by palpation. Bearing the intended plate position in mind, the osteotomy can now be stabilized with two crossed K-wires.

However, after closing the wedge leaving the inge intact, a stable situation is present and crossed K-wires are not necessary.

The alignment of the mechanical axis of the leg is now evaluated (Fig 13-8) by placing a long metal rod between the radiologically determined center of the femoral head and the center of the ankle (see chapter 9 "High-tibial open-wedge valgization osteotomy with plate fixator", subchapter 5 "Surgical technique"). At the center of the knee joint or slightly medial to it, the axis should pass through the medial compartment as planned preoperatively.

The osteotomy is stabilized with the TomoFix MDF plate fixator. The implant is prepared by mounting the drill sleeves in the four distal threaded holes. The positioning device should be used to ensure precise insertion of the drill sleeves into the plate holes (see Fig 13-1c–d). The distal plate holes have been designed with a laterally ascending angle of 20° to prevent posterior perforation of the locking head screws at the distal femur. Therefore, right and left versions of the plate are available. The plate with the mounted sleeves is now slid under the vastus medialis and the distal part of the plate is positioned anteromedially on the distal femur. The solid part of the plate should lie over the osteotomy (Fig 13-9a–b). The plate shaft is aligned parallel to the femoral shaft and the plate is temporarily stabilized in the distal part with a 2 mm thick K-wire (Fig 13-9c–e). This is guided by inserting a guide sleeve into one of the preassembled drill sleeves. Plate position and orientation of the wire in relation to the osteotomy and the intercondylar space of the distal femur are monitored under image intensification. The internal fixator has been designed so that form-fit seating of the implant at the distal femur is not necessary. However, it is very important that the distal holes are correctly aligned in the femoral condylar block so that the optimal (longest) length of locking head screw can be later achieved. If the condyles are deformed, the plate can be positioned more anteriorly or rotated to alter the angulation of the locking head screws so that posterior penetration of the femoral condyles is prevented.

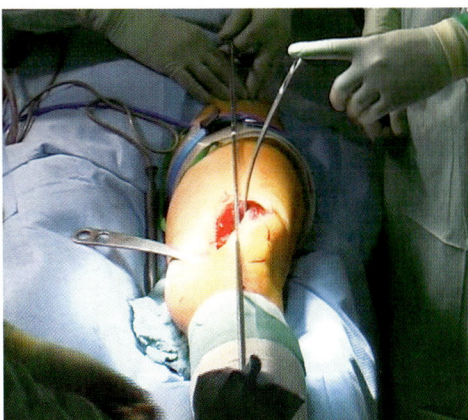

Fig 13-8   The alignment of the corrected mechanical axis is now evaluated and adjusted with the help of a long metal rod that is positioned under image intensification from the center of the femoral head to the center of the upper ankle joint. The osteotomy is either held closed manually or stabilized temporarily by crossed wires.

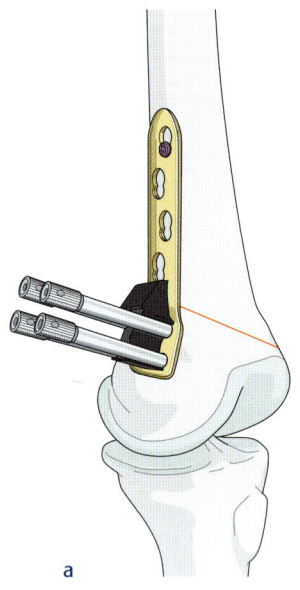

a

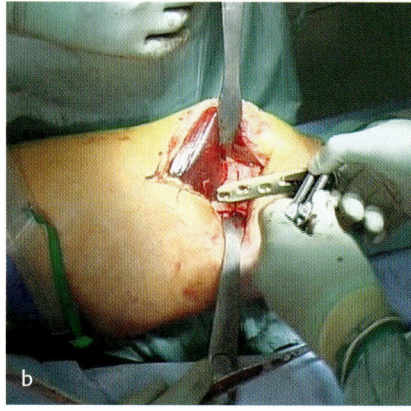

b

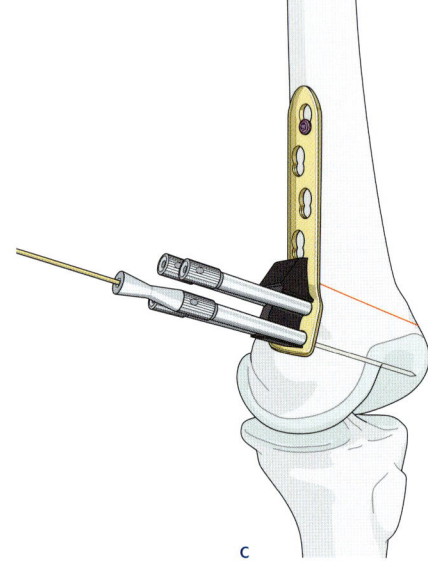

c

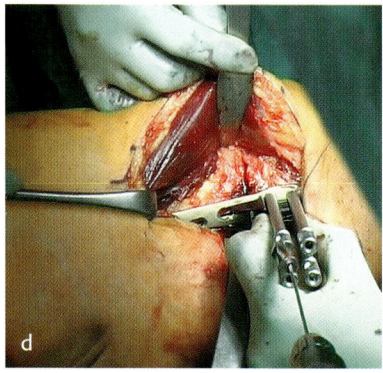

d

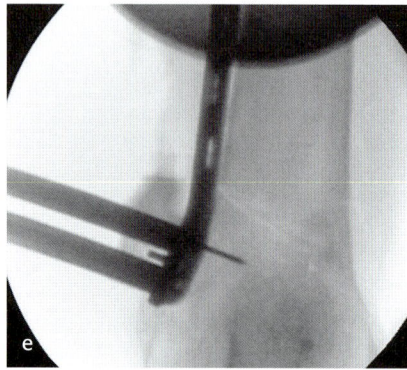

e

Fig 13-9a–e   Position of the TomoFix MDF plate on the distal femur.

a–b   The distal drill sleeves are mounted in their exact positions with the help of the positioning device (black) before submuscular slide insertion of the plate fixator. The solid part of the plate should rest at the level of the osteotomy.

c–e   The plate is temporarily stabilized with a 2 mm K-wire in a guide sleeve at its distal part. The position of the locking head screws and their angulation can be tested, if necessary, by insertion of one or more wires through the drill sleeves under image intensification prior to drilling.

The holes for the self-tapping 5.0 mm locking head screws are now drilled through the drill sleeves with a calibrated 4.3 mm drill. The length of the locking head screws can be read from the scale on the drill, whereby lateral protrusion of the screw tips should be avoided. Alternatively, the drill sleeves can be removed and locking head screws length can be determined using the depth gauge for screws. The depth gauge can also be used to examine the integrity of the bone posteriorly before the locking head screws are inserted. The locking head screws are locked manually with the torque screwdriver or with the 4.0 Nm torque limiter for the Compact Airdrive. A click must be heard clearly during locking. Finally, K-wire and guide sleeve are removed and replaced by locking head screws.

The osteotomy is compressed manually at this stage. Additional compression can now be applied by eccentric positioning of a 4.5 mm self-tapping cortex screw in the dynamic part of the combination hole directly above the osteotomy. A 3.2 mm spiral drill is used in combination with the 4.5 mm/5.0 mm drill sleeve or the LCP drill sleeve in compression mode. If even greater compression is desired, a tensioning device can be inserted into the dynamic part of the last combination hole, however, this requires proximal extension of the approach. If it is the lateral osteotomy hinge that needs to be placed under compression (especially in the case of intraoperative fracture of the lateral hinge), an additional compression mode can be used. In this mode the self-tapping cortex screw in the combination hole directly proximal to the osteotomy is not inserted at right angles to the shaft but at an ascending angle from proximal to lateral instead as for the proximal tibial osteotomy, (see chapter 9 "High-tibial open-wedge valgization osteotomy with plate fixator"). Gradual tightening of the screw produces a caudally oriented compression vector acting on the lateral femur. The screw should be tightened carefully under image intensification until any lateral gaping has been eliminated. Screws are inserted into the residual holes in the plate shaft from distal to proximal. The authors work with monocortical, self-drilling, and self-tapping locking head screws, whereby the medial femoral cortex is only punchmarked with the short 4.3 mm spiral drill. In general, 26–30 mm self-drilling, self-tapping locking head screws are used for monocortical fixation: power-driven insertion of the locking head screws until just before locking, then tightening with the torque screwdriver. The spacer in the most proximal plate hole is removed and replaced by a monocortical locking head screw. Finally, the cortical lag screw is replaced by a bicortical self-tapping 5.0 mm locking head screw (**Fig 13-10**). It must be emphasized again that all locking head screws are only to be locked manually using the torque screwdriver or power-driven with the 4.0 mm torque limiter for the Compact Airdrive or other power-driven devices.

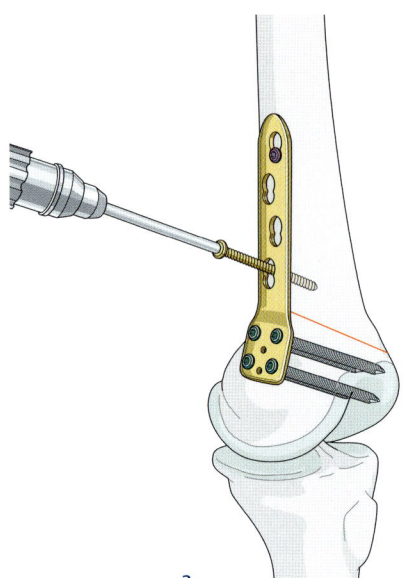
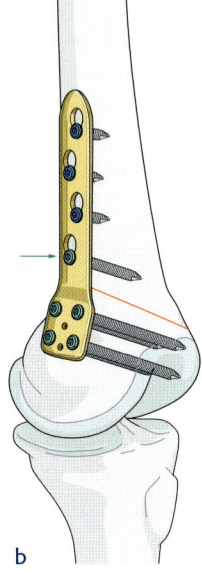
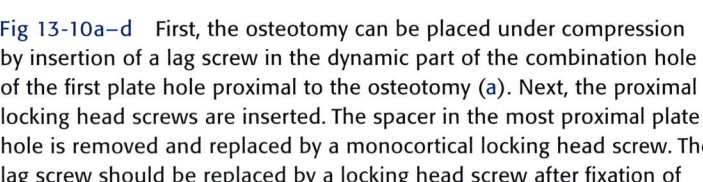

a

b

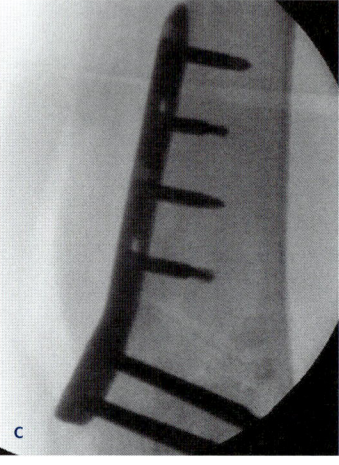
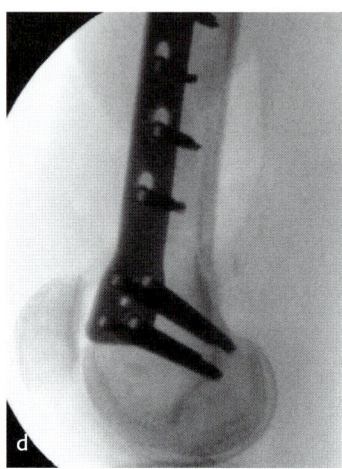

c

d

Fig 13-10a–d First, the osteotomy can be placed under compression by insertion of a lag screw in the dynamic part of the combination hole of the first plate hole proximal to the osteotomy (a). Next, the proximal locking head screws are inserted. The spacer in the most proximal plate hole is removed and replaced by a monocortical locking head screw. The lag screw should be replaced by a locking head screw after fixation of the plate. A self-tapping locking head screw is inserted bicortically (see arrow) in the fixed-angle part of the combination hole after drilling through a drill sleeve (b). Alternatively, a self-tapping and self-drilling locking head screw can be inserted if the lateral bone bridge has remained intact after closure of the osteotomy (c–d).

Next, the stability of the osteotomy and the position and length of the locking head screws are assessed by image intensification. The anterior arthrotomy is continuously closed. The partially incised patellofemoral ligament and the partially released distal insertion of vastus medialis at the patella are carefully reconstructed. A suction drain are placed beneath the vastus medialis and brought out distally in order to reduce hematoma formation beneath the muscle, to prevent development of compartment syndrome, and to monitor postoperative blood loss. The fascia over the vastus medialis is closed, followed by subcutaneous and skin suture. An elastic compression bandage is applied and postoperative x-rays in two planes are obtained.

A clinical example is shown in **Fig 13-11**, **Fig 13-12**, and **Fig 13-13**.

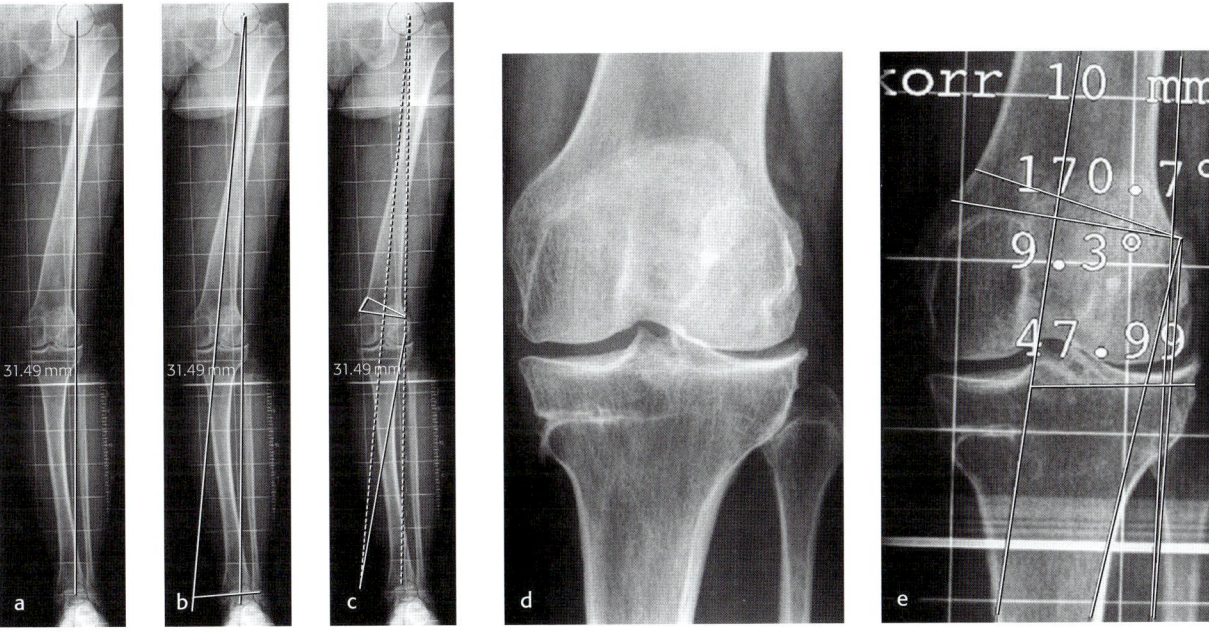

Fig 13-11a–e   46-year-old female with posttraumatic valgus degeneration at the knee after metaphyseal tibial fracture as a child. Valgus deformity of 10°. Osteotomy planning. Detailed view of the knee joint showing the planned bone wedge for extraction.

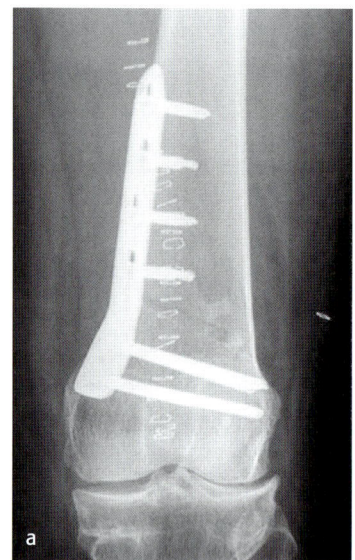
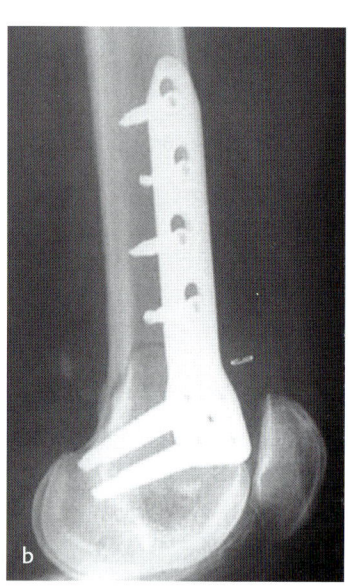

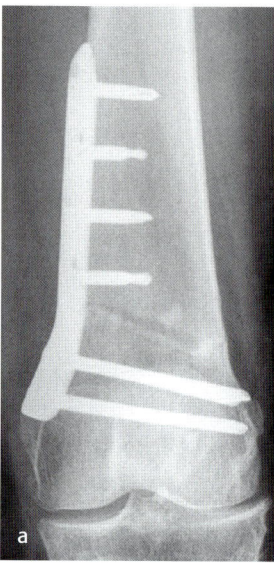
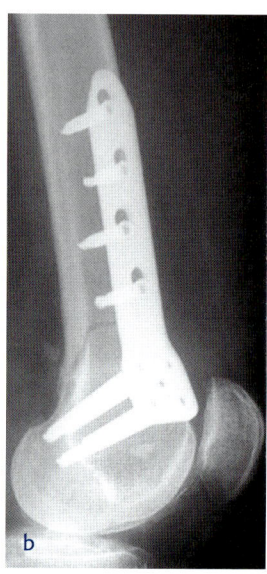

Fig 13-13a–b Radiographic views in two planes 6 weeks postoperatively. Free range of motion and transition to full weight bearing without walking aids is allowed.

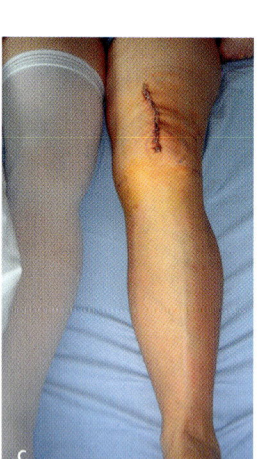
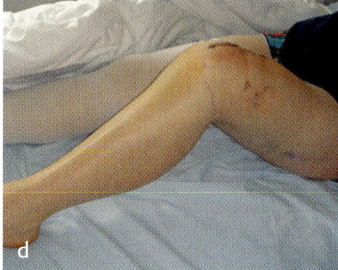
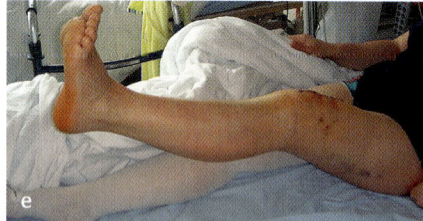

Fig 13-12a–e Postoperative course after medial closed-wedge femoral osteotomy for a 10° correction with the TomoFix MDF.
a–b Radiographic views in both planes after mobilization.
c–e Clinical axis and clinical function on postoperative day 5.

7   Postoperative management

On the day of surgery, gentle movements can already be performed with the compression bandage in place. Swelling can be reduced by cryotherapy and application of an intermittent vein pump. The bandage is changed on postoperative day 1 and the soft-tissue situation evaluated. Mobilization starts on postoperative day 1 with underarm crutches and partial loading up to 15–20 kg bodyweight (monitored with a scale). Partial loading should be performed for 6 weeks, range of motion is unrestricted, and a splint is not generally necessary. In week 7 after surgery, loading is increased up to the pain threshold, whereby the loading depends on the extent of osseous consolidation as confirmed by the postoperative x-rays at 6 weeks. If the osteotomy is not fully closed or fixation stability is not optimal, loading should be increased step-by-step over 2–4 weeks. Full weight bearing can be permitted if radiological assessment shows the osteotomy to be fully consolidated.

During the rehabilitation period, the patient should not apply torsional loading to the leg since the authors' biomechanical study has shown that this implant, like all implants available for supracondylar femoral osteotomy, is particularly sensitive to torsional weight bearing. Until full loading is possible, medication for thromboembolism prophylaxis should be continued in the form of low-molecular heparin with regular checks of the thrombocyte count. The physical therapy program includes active and passive exercises. Daily manual lymph drainage is recommended due to the frequent occurrence of postoperative lymph edema. Electrotherapy for muscle stimulation (EMS device) is recommended, especially for the vastus medialis.

Sutures are removed on postoperative days 10–12. Radiological assessment of the osteotomy should take place immediately postoperatively, after mobilization of the patient, and at 6 weeks and 3 months postoperatively.

8   Possible pitfalls and complications

Application of the TomoFix plate fixator requires an in-depth knowledge of the implant and its specific locking technique. Fixed-angle locking has to be performed precisely and requires absolute respect for the orientation of the locking head screws as dictated by plate-hole design. Special attention must also be paid to correct positioning of the TomoFix implant. The plate shaft is aligned parallel to the longitudinal axis of the femur and the distal plate head is placed anteromedially onto the medial femoral condyle. Implant contouring is not necessary and is also undesirable since the principle of the plate fixator does not require form-fit seating of the plate on the bone. Special attention should be paid to the angulation of the locking head screws in

the frontal plane so that the screws do not protrude posteriorly from the condylar block.

To prevent over- or undercorrection of the physiological axis, thorough preoperative planning is absolutely essential. Intraoperative assessment of the corrected axis is also highly recommended prior to stabilization so that any planning errors can be identified and dealt with. With regard to the soft tissues, it is especially important to reconstruct the incised medial patellofemoral ligament and distal insertion of the vastus medialis, otherwise patellar instability with lateral subluxation may occur.

Osteotomy of the posterior femoral cortex is associated with a significant risk of injury to the femoral artery and vein. The sciatic nerve and vascular bundle are also situated near the bone at the posterior aspect and can be injured. For this reason, the posterior femoral cortex should only be cut if the soft tissues beyond it are safely protected by a blunt bone retractor or anatomically shaped spatula. In addition, the genicular arteries and veins are situated directly posterior to the intermuscular septum and are susceptible to bleeding if the septum is divided. Therefore, the septum should only be incised with extreme care directly at its bony insertion. Hemorrhage must be coagulated immediately.

Accidental injury to large blood vessels during osteotomy results in heavy bleeding when the tourniquet is released. This requires revision by vascular surgery. An anteromedial or direct posterior approach can be chosen for this purpose.

Extensive postoperative soft-tissue swelling and lymph edema can be prevented to a large extent by early drug therapy and physical therapy. In addition to oral antiphlogistic treatment, we also recommend manual lymph drainage and use of an intermittent vein compression pump. The risk of crural thrombosis or lung embolism must be remembered and immediate clarification initiated at the first signs.

The medial subvastus approach rarely leads to compartment syndrome. However, a large postoperative hematoma may cause compartment syndrome even with this medial approach. The clinical signs are firm, elastic swelling of the extremity and disturbed sensation. This condition requires immediate surgical relief of the hematoma.

Early postoperative infection is treated by surgical revision with debridement, systemic antibiosis, and possible inlay of antibiotic carriers. The plate fixator does not need to be removed if the osteosynthesis is stable and the soft tissue cover intact, otherwise a change of management to an external fixator, eg, a ring fixator, is possible.

Delayed bone healing of the osteotomy is often expressed by persistent pain on loading. In these cases, a small amount of callus will be visible laterally on the x-rays. Treatment consists of secondary cancellous bone grafting, which the authors only perform if no sign of bone healing can be seen after more than three months. Otherwise, the period of partial weight bearing should be continued.

9   Biplanar osteotomy technique

At the end of 2006 an alternative to the closed-wedge technique described above was introduced by Dr Alex E Staubli. Based on the experience with the biplanar open-wedge HTO technique a biplanar distal femur osteotomy technique was developed. In this technique, the saw cuts for the closed-wedge part of the procedure are made at the posterior 2/3 of the distal femur after which the wedge is removed. Starting at the lower cut of the osteotomy cuts, an ascending bone cut is made parallel to the posterior side of the femur (Fig 13-14a). In normal femurs the ascending bone cut has an angle between 90–100° to the closed-wedge osteotomy cuts in the sagittal plane. Because of the antecurvation of the femur, the anterior cut will end a few centimeters proximally. After the anterior bone cut is completed the osteotomy cut can be closed and the plate fixator is applied (Fig 13-14b).

An advantage of the biplanar technique is that the fat pad between the suprapatellar bursa and the dorsal side of the quadriceps muscles and tendon on the one side and the anterior part of the distal femur on the other side remain intact (Fig 13-15a). This fat pad is an important structure facilitating sliding of soft tissues during flexion and extension of the knee. The fat pad is protected during surgery by retraction of the quadriceps muscle while performing the anterior saw cut with a thin saw blade under intense rinsing (Fig 13-15b–e). Additional advantages of the biplanar technique are increased postoperative stability against rotational instability and the ability to position the closed-wedge saw cuts more distal in the femur condyles as the trochlea does not limit the height of the closed-wedge cuts.

Observations in the first 40 patients treated with the biplanar osteotomy technique are very promising [17]: patients reach normal range of knee motion faster due to undisturbed fat pad and soft tissues sliding mechanism, and regain normal quadriceps muscle force also faster as compared to the conventional technique. Bone healing is faster as the anterior bone cut often heals within 6 weeks, time to full weight bearing is shorter as due to the very stable situation during functional aftertreatment, and bone healing is faster as compared to the conventional technique. This is anticipated that after additional biomechanical testing and clinical evaluation the biplanar osteotomy technique in combination with the TomoFix medial distal femur plate will become the standard surgical technique for medial closed-wedge corrections of the distal femur.

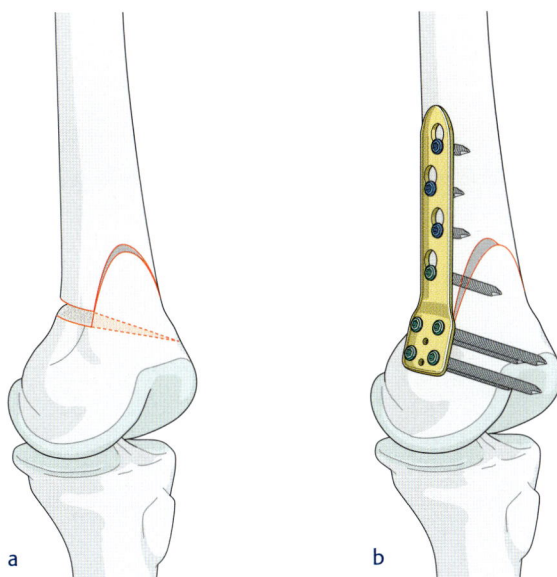

a   b

Fig 13-14a–b   Biplanar medial distal femur closed-wedge osteotomy technique. Bone cuts shown after wedge removal: oblique descending bone cuts and anterior ascending bone cut (a) after closing and fixation with TomoFix medial distal femur plate (b).

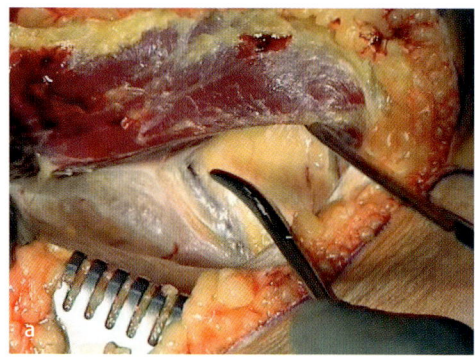
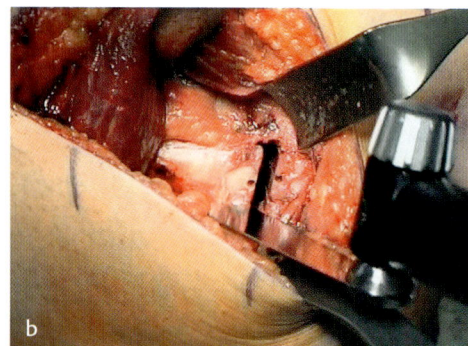
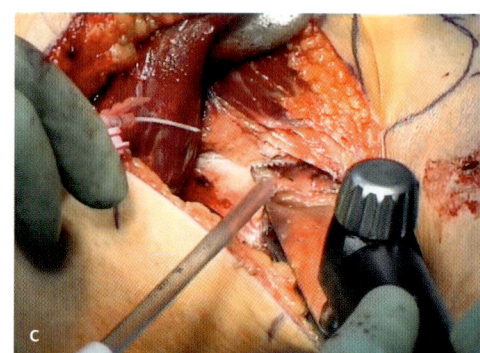

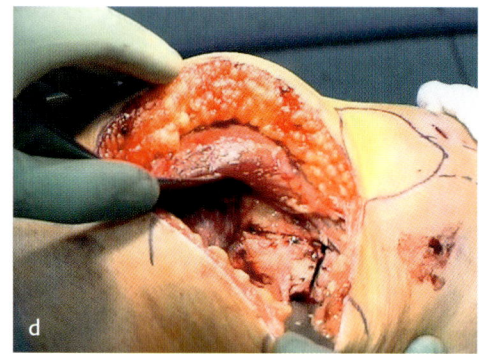
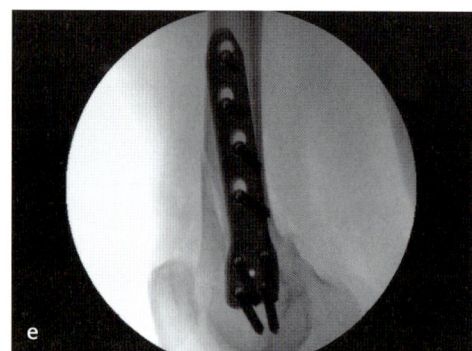

Fig 13-15a–e   Intraoperative views of biplanar osteotomy technique.

a   Fat pad on anterior side of the femur.
b   Introduction of thin saw blade after wedge removal out of posterior 2/3 of the femur.
c   Anterior ascending osteotomy cut under intense rinsing.
d   After closing of the gap the anterior fat pad is undisturbed.
e   Fluoroscopy view after fixation shows ascending bone cut.

10   Results

By the end of 2006, a total of 59 procedures had been performed in the authors' departments using the technique described [14]. The average wedge size was 7.3 mm (range 4–12 mm), and the mean age of the patients was 37.5 years (17–79 years). 57 osteotomies healed uneventfully, and two patients required secondary bone grafting and reosteosynthesis. There was one infection which healed after revision and one hematoma requiring evacuation.

Starting at the end of 2006 the biplanar technique was also used at the three departments and compared with the single plane technique. By 2008, more than 100 patients medial closed-wedge osteotomies have been stabilized with the TomoFix MDF plate without implant failures observed. More than 40 patients have been operated on using the biplanar technique.

11   Bibliography

[1]   **Paley D** (2000) Hardware and osteotomy considerations. *Paley, D (ed), Principles of deformity correction.* Berlin Heidelberg: Springer-Verlag, 291–410.

[2]   **Franco V, Cipolla M, Gerullo G, et al** (2004) [Open wedge osteotomy of the distal femur in the valgus knee.] *Orthopäde;* 33(2):185–192. German.

[3]   **Cameron HU, Botsford DJ, Park YS** (1997) Prognostic factors in the outcome of supracondylar femoral osteotomy for lateral compartment osteoarthritis of the knee. *Can J Surg;* 40(2):114–118.

[4]   **Finkelstein JA, Gross AE, Davis A** (1996) Varus osteotomy of the distal part of the femur. A survivorship analysis. *J Bone Joint Surg Am;* 78(9):1348–1352.

[5]   **Healy WL, Anglen JO, Wasilewski SA, et al** (1988) Distal femoral varus osteotomy. *J Bone Joint Surg Am;* 70(1):102–109.

[6]   **Learmonth ID** (1990) A simple technique for varus supracondylar osteotomy in genu valgum. *J Bone Joint Surg Br;* 72(2):235–237.

[7]   **Marti RK, Schröder J, Witteveen A** (2000) The closed wedge varus supracondylar osteotomy. *Op Tech Sports Med;* 8:8–55.

[8]   **Mathews J, Cobb AG, Richardson S, et al** (1998) Distal femoral osteotomy for lateral compartment osteoarthritis of the knee. *Orthopedics;* 21(4):437–440.

[9]   **McDermott AG, Finkelstein JA, Farine I, et al** (1988) Distal femoral varus osteotomy for valgus deformity of the knee. *J Bone Joint Surg Am;* 70(1):110–116.

[10]   **Miniaci A, Grossmann SP, Jakob RP** (1990) Supracondylar femoral varus osteotomy in the treatment of valgus knee deformity. *Am J Knee Surg;* 3:65–72.

[11]   **Miniaci A, Watson LW** (1994) Distal femoral osteotomy. *Fu FH, Harner CD, Vince KG (eds), Knee Surgery.* Philadelphia: Lippincott William & Wilkins,1173–1180.

[12]   **Stähelin T, Hardegger F, Ward JC** (2000) Supracondylar osteotomy of the femur with use of compression. Osteosynthesis with a malleable implant. *J Bone Joint Surg Am;* 82(5):712–722.

[13]   **Stähelin T, Hardegger F** (2004) [Incomplete, supracondylar femur osteotomy. A minimally invasive compression osteosynthesis with soft implant.] *Orthopäde;* 33(2):178–184.

[14]   **Van Heerwaarden R, Wymenga A, Freiling D, et al** (2007) Distal medial closed wedge varus femur osteotomy stabilized with the Tomofix plate fixator. *Operat techn Orthop;* 17(1):12–21.

[15] **Brinkman JM, Hurschler C, Agneskirchner JD, et al** (2008)
      Axial and torsional stability of supracondylar femur osteotomies:
      A biomechanical investigation of five different plate and
      osteotomy configurations. Clin Orthop submitted.

[16] **Outerbridge RE** (1961) The etiology of chondromalacia
      patellae. *J Bone Joint Surg Br;* 43:752–757.

[17] **Freiling D, Lobenhoffer P, Staubli A, et al** (2008) [Medial
      closed-wedge varus osteotomy of the distal femur.] *Arthroskopie;*
      21:6–14. German.

Authors   Ronald J van Heerwaarden, Frank Wagenaar, Siegfried Hofmann

14   Double osteotomies of the femur and the tibia

1   Introduction and definition

In addition to single osteotomies of the femur or tibia, their combination in form of a double osteotomy around the knee allows for treatment of complex deformities of the lower extremity. Double osteotomies can generally be performed in the frontal, sagittal, or transverse plane. In this chapter, the authors discuss one-stage corrections of the distal femur and proximal tibia. The overall correction of the weight-bearing line in the frontal plane is made by two simultaneous osteotomies at different levels. Precise planning and the surgical technique are the premises for achieving the desired correction [1, 2]. The same principles that apply to single osteotomies of the femur or tibia must also be applied to double osteotomies; however, a double osteotomy is a more extensive procedure. This explains why it is only indicated in well-selected cases. Originally, double osteotomy of the femur and tibia was performed to relieve pressure on a knee compartment in cases of joint degeneration [3]. However, in patients with rheumatoid arthritis, satisfactory outcomes were not achieved with this procedure [4, 5]. Due to more recent biomechanical findings the principles of double osteotomy have been redefined [1, 6].

2   Biomechanical principles

The biomechanical principles, on which planning and correction of deformities of the lower extremity are based, have already been presented in other chapters of this book. There are some additional biomechanical considerations that need to be taken into account when planning a double osteotomy. Five aspects should be considered to analyze bone deformities around the knee:

1. Frontal weight-bearing axis
2. Sagittal leg axis
3. Joint line
4. Patellofemoral joint
5. Rotational deformity of the leg

The physiological axes of the lower extremity are discussed in chapter 1 "Physiological axes of the lower limb". The pathology is most frequently localized in the frontal plane and in the sagittal plane.

In double osteotomies for axial correction of the knee, precise planning is mandatory. Imprecise planning may aggravate the existing deformity or even cause new symptomatic deformities. For example, a slight decrease of the tibial slope in a high-tibial osteotomy can lead to severe gait disturbance with hyperextension of the knee if a distal femoral osteotomy leads to simultaneous recurvatum deformity of the femur as well.

The relevance of the midjoint line as an important third plane has been given not enough consideration in the past [1, 7]. The midjoint line (MJL) is centered between the knee baseline of the femur and the baseline of the tibial plateau and forms femorolateral and mediotibial angles of 87 ± 3° with the mechanical axis (Mikulicz line) (Fig 14-1). Slight varus inclination of this knee baseline is physiological and is explained by the greater distance between the centers of the hip joints in relation to the centers of the ankle joints. During stance and gait the planes of the knee joint and ankle joint shift into a horizontal position [8], thus ensuring optimal biomechanical load distribution. Any correction in the frontal plane should take these patterns into consideration and should result in parallelism of the knee-joint line and the ankle-joint line as well as achieving correct loading of the joints [9]. Frontal plane correction can result in a pathological alteration of the joint line if the correction is not performed at the site of the bone deformity, therefore leading to subsequent loading on an incorrectly aligned plane (Fig 14-2). It has been possible to prove

that only 31% of patients with varus deviation of the leg have osseous deformity at the tibia only. In 59% the varus deformity is located at the femur and in 10% both femur and tibia are affected. The situation for valgus deformity of the leg is similar. In these cases the deformity is situated in the femur in only 22%. In 45% the valgus deformity is located at the tibia and in 33% it affects both femur and tibia [2]. The frequently quoted tenet for correction of varus malalignment at the tibia and valgus malalignment at the femur is, consequently, incorrect for about 50% of varus and valgus joint degeneration deformities.

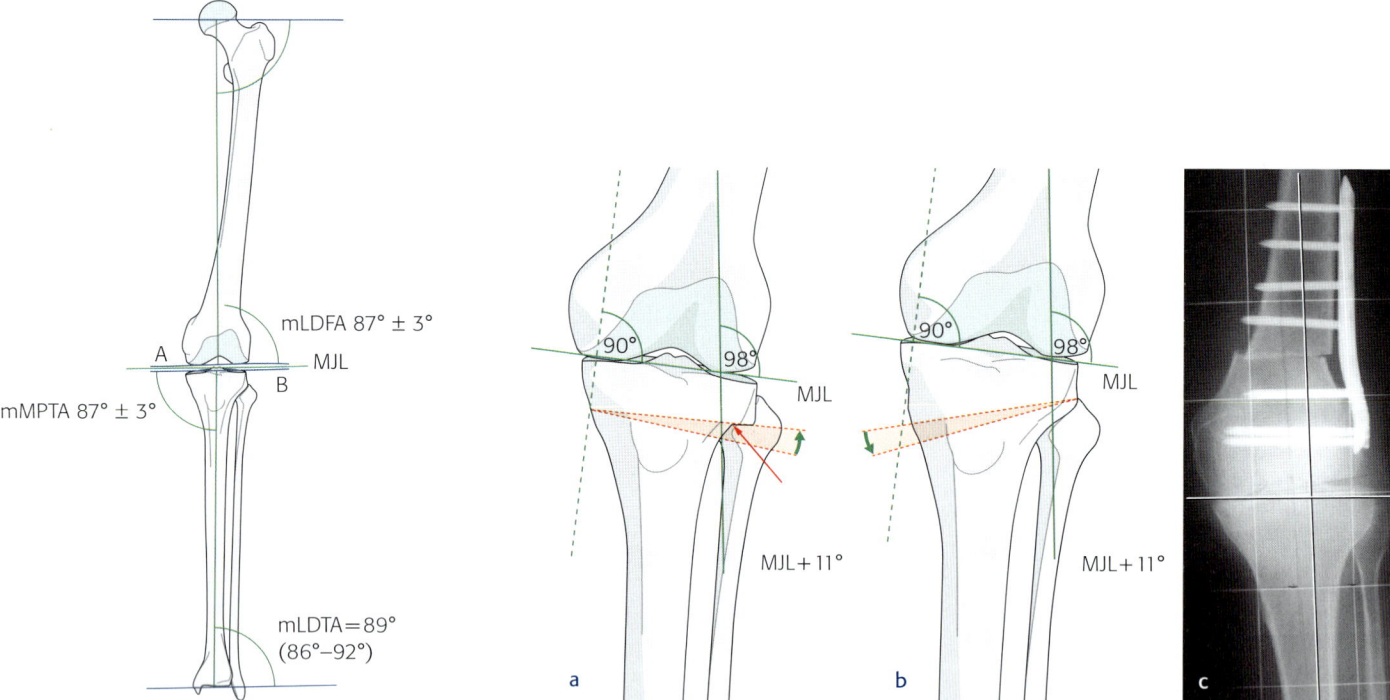

Fig 14-1 Mechanical axes and joint angles with standard values. The midjoint line (MJL) (green) is centered between the baselines of the femur (A) and the tibia (B). Mechanical lateral distal femoral angle (mLDFA) = 87° ± 3°, mechanical medial proximal tibial angle (mMPTA) = 87° ± 3°.

Fig 14-2a–c Example of preoperative planning in a patient with a varus deformity of 7°. Valgus correction by lateral closed-wedge osteotomy (a) or medial open-wedge osteotomy (b) of the proximal tibia results in a pathological joint line obliquity of 98° with 11° lateral inclination. Additionally, there is a marked step-off at the lateral cortex (red arrow) for the lateral osteotomy. Lateral closed-wedge distal femoral osteotomy results in axial correction with a normal joint-line orientation of 86° (c).

Cartilage can distribute mechanical loading very effectively due to the "cushion principle". This compensatory mechanism is, however, limited with regard to shear forces [10]. Chronic shear forces lead to overload and damage of the cartilage surface. In addition, the development of a pathological joint line (see above) may lead to overload of the capsuloligamentous structures [9]. After biomechanically correct adjustment of the axes in the frontal plane, alterations of the joint line and/or tibial slope that have been overlooked can cause persistent symptoms [11]. Based on his 1965 study, Coventry postulated that an inclination of the joint line in the frontal plane of up to 10° is acceptable after a correction osteotomy [12]. A more recent study from the Mayo Clinic, conducted with a computer-assisted biomechanical analysis programs (OASIS), has shown that the maximal inclination of the joint line should not exceed 4° [1]. As a result of precise observance of the joint line, the survival rate of 8 years after double osteotomy for this prospective study was 96%, which is comparable to the results achieved after minimally invasive implantation of a unicompartmental prosthesis. The clinical outcomes are also remarkable with a total of 85% very good and good scores for double osteotomy.

Several authors held the opinion that combined deformities of the femur and tibia had to be corrected at both levels, otherwise the pathology would partially remain or be aggravated [7–9, 11]. Correction at only one level (the femur alone or the tibia alone) may achieve correction of the overall leg axis in patients with combined tibial and femoral deformities, but may simultaneously result in an alteration of the joint line beyond the standard values. To achieve a biomechanically correct axial correction, on the one hand, and to maintain a correct joint line, on the other, requires combined femoral and tibial double osteotomy in about 10% of patients with axial deformities around the knee [1, 2].

The fourth aspect of preoperative analysis in a correction osteotomy is the patellofemoral joint. The role of the patella in indication for axial correction is still subject of discussion. In the past, no great importance was attributed to the patella with regard to correction osteotomies. By contrast, Schoettle states "any preoperative disorder of the patella" is a contraindication for correction osteotomy [13]. Biomechanically important parameters are the so-called Q-angle and patella contact pressure. Identification of the tibial tuberosity trochlear groove (TTTG) distance by easily reproducible CT scan diagnostics is, however, superior to measuring the Q-angle [14] (see chapter 15 "Rotational osteotomies of the femur and the tibia"). Correction of the leg axis, especially in rotational osteotomies can lead to a change in the TTTG distance. This must be taken into account during preoperative planning. An unphysiological gliding mechanism of the patella can be corrected by reorientation of the trochlea or by medial or lateral translation of the tibial tuberosity [15]. Furthermore, the height of the patella is altered in both closed- and open-wedge osteotomies of the proximal tibia. In cases of a preexisting patella infera, an anterior osteotomy of the tuberosity extending distally should be combined with medial open-wedge tibial osteotomy [16] in order to prevent further reduction of the distance between the tip of the patella and the tibial tuberosity when the osteotomy gap is opened.

Rotational deformities of the lower extremity are the fifth aspect of preoperative analysis of correction osteotomies around the knee, and must be taken into account in the clinical and radiological examination. Preoperative clinical and radiological diagnosis of rotation deformities is discussed in detail in chapter 15 "Rotational osteotomies of the femur and the tibia".

■ In a combined deformity of femur and tibia, both segments must be corrected; otherwise new bone deformities are created. Correction of only one segment (either tibia or femur) may result in a straight leg axis but may lead to a pathological alteration of the joint line.

3 Patient selection

The indication for a double osteotomy is a complex axial deformity of the leg such that correction at one level, femur or tibia, would lead to a significant deviation from the physiological orientation of the knee-joint line [17]. A further indication for double osteotomy is the combination of an existent pathological joint-line obliquity with only slight or no axial deformity of the leg. Typical causes are hereditary cartilaginous exostosis adjacent to the growth plates, status after epiphysiodesis, or previous correction osteotomy that straightened the leg at the cost of a highly pathological joint line. These patients complain primarily of knee instability and joint pain. Persistent shear stress on the joint can rapidly lead to slackening of the collateral ligaments, which increases instability and induces knee-joint degeneration.

The indications and contraindications for double osteotomy correspond to those defined in previous chapters for single osteotomy (see chapter 9 "High-tibial open-wedge valgization osteotomy with plate fixator" and chapter 13 "Supracondylar varization osteotomy of the femur with plate fixator"). Nevertheless, in these cases, the authors are particularly meticulous in their analysis of both the deformity and the correction (see chapter 13 "Supracondylar varization osteotomy of the femur with plate fixator"). It can generally be stated that a double osteotomy should be considered if single correction would shift the midjoint line orientation beyond 90 ± 4°.

3.1 Double osteotomies for deformities around the knee

As already described, the Mikulicz line, the mechanical lateral distal femoral angle (mLDFA), and the mechanical medial proximal tibial angle (mMPTA) represent the essential characteristics of a bone deformity around the knee (see chapter 1 "Physiological axes of the lower limb", **Fig 1-5**). The position of the midjoint line should always be measured in the weight-bearing views. The above-mentioned parameters allow correct classification of the deformity (**Table 14-1**).

Mechanical axis	Position of the midjoint line		
	Varus	**Neutral**	**Valgus**
Varus	mLDFA ↓ mMPTA ↓ MJL -	mLDFA ↑ mMPTA ↓ MJL =	mLDFA ↑ mMPTA ↑ MJL +
Neutral	mLDFA ↓ mMPTA ↓ MJL -		mLDFA ↑ mMPTA ↑ MJL +
Valgus	mLDFA ↓ mMPTA ↓ MJL -	mLDFA ↓ mMPTA ↑ MJL =	mLDFA ↑ mMPTA ↑ MJL +

Table 14-1   Classification of deformities around the knee.

mLDFA = mechanical lateral distal femoral angle
(normal: 87° ± 3°, ↑: > 90°, ↓: < 84°)
mMPTA = mechanical medial proximal tibial angle
(normal: 87° ± 3°, ↑: > 90°, ↓: < 84°)
MJL = midjoint line
(normal: 87–90°, -: varus < 86°, +: valgus > 94°)

3.2   Preoperative diagnostics

Clinical examination includes assessment of the range of motion and ligamentous laxity of the knee joint. Of special importance are the movement of the patella, the alignment of the extensor mechanism, and any instability of the patella. A rotation profile (examination protocol according to Staheli; see chapter 15 "Rotational osteotomies of the femur and the tibia") is always included in order to exclude additional rotational deformity. Skin and soft tissue should be in good condition.

Radiological diagnosis requires x-rays of the knee in three planes and a weight-bearing view of the entire leg. A weight-bearing view in 45° knee flexion, a so-called Rosenberg view, and/or MRI may offer additional information on the extent of damage to the knee, but are not mandatory. MRI can nevertheless reveal zones of subchondral bone marrow edema (BME) as a sign of overloading, thus facilitating the decision to operate. It has been shown that for patients with varus degeneration where MRI shows BME in the medial joint compartment, there is a 4.5 times greater risk that degeneration will progress than for patients without edema. BME in knee degeneration is however a nonspecific sign and must be differentiated from other forms of BME (eg, transient bone marrow edema) [2, 18].

Stress views may be valuable if there is additional ligament instability. It is absolutely essential to take ligament laxity with asymmetrical opening of the joint gap into account during preoperative planning of the overall correction angle.

Computed tomography to evaluate the TTTG distance is required if pathological alignment of the patella is evident or suspected (see chapter 15 "Rotational osteotomies of the femur and the tibia"). Measurement of the TTTG distance allows preoperative planning of an osteotomy of the tibial tuberosity. Additional transverse CT scans at the level of the femoral neck, the distal femoral condyles, tibial head, and ankle should be obtained if an additional rotational deformity of the extremity is suspected.

4   Planning

The planning procedure for a double osteotomy corresponds to that of a single osteotomy (see chapter 4 "Basic principles of osteotomies around the knee" and chapter 13 "Supracondylar varization osteotomy of the femur with plate fixator"). Assessment of the leg axis is also possible by measuring the femorotibial angle on the AP x-ray of the knee (angle between the anatomical tibial axis and the anatomical femoral axis: standard value 173–175° valgus). The femorotibial angle can however deviate substantially from the mechanical axis and therefore cannot be regarded as a substitute for the weight-bearing x-ray of the entire lower extremity [6].

The aim of axial correction in the frontal plane depends on the degree of joint degeneration. If a deformity around a nonarthrotic joint is corrected, planning should aim to restore physiological joint angles and normal alignment of the knee midjoint line [8]. The authors also prefer to restore normal anatomical axes even in patients with mild degenerative joint alteration (Fig 14-3). However, if there is already monocompartmental degeneration due to axial deformity in the frontal plane, the affected compartment should be unloaded by the correction. For medial joint degeneration the authors utilize the Fujisawa point (62% of the width of the tibial plateau as measured from

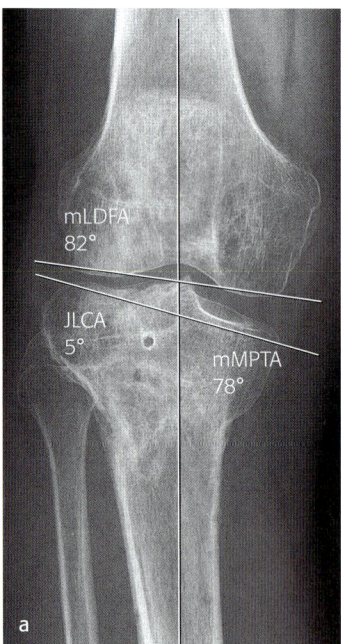

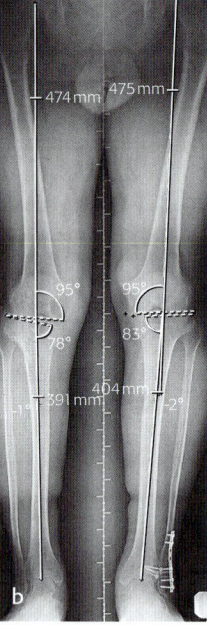

Fig 14-3a–b   Posttraumatic varus deformity of the proximal tibia (mMPTA = 78°) and preexisting valgus deformity of the distal femur (mLDFA = 82°). Medial instability causes medial joint opening under load (JLCA—joint line convergence angle = 5°). The position of the mechanical axis is normal, but the patient cannot walk without pain for more than 5 minutes because joint instability combined with pathological varus joint line obliquity (pathological MJL) causes lateral subluxation of the tibia.

its medial cortex) (see chapter 9 "High-tibial open-wedge valgization osteotomy with plate fixator") as the target for the postoperative weight-bearing line of the leg. In valgus degeneration, correction should aim for neutral or slight varus weight-bearing leg alignment depending on the degree of

degeneration (see chapter 13 "Supracondylar varization osteotomy of the femur with plate fixation"). Overcorrection in these cases will produce a slight deviation of the midjoint line from the physiological value, which is nevertheless acceptable as long as it does not exceed 4° [1] (Fig 14-4).

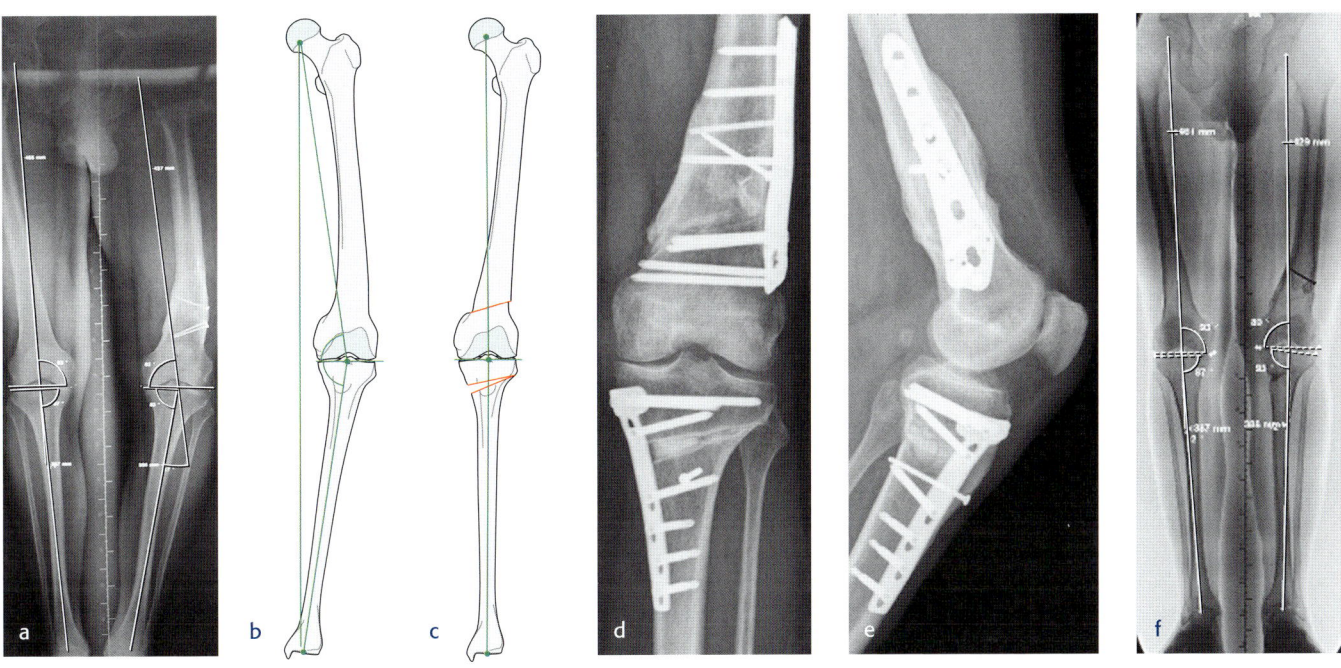

Fig 14-4a–f   Double osteotomy for a varus deformity with a neutral MJL orientation.

a   Frontal plane weight-bearing view. The tibiofemoral angle is 17° varus. There are posttraumatic deformities at the distal femur (mLDFA = 98°) and the proximal tibia (mMPTA = 83°). The MJL orientation is normal and the lateral joint opening (JLCA) is 2°.

b–c Planning a double osteotomy: The mechanical axis runs medial to the medial compartment; the MJL is in normal alignment. Vitallium screws from a previous osteosynthesis are located in the former fracture zone, which is the area of planned correction due to healing in malalignment. Correct positioning of the mechanical axis and joint line by 11° closed-wedge distal lateral femoral osteotomy and 6° open-wedge medial proximal tibial osteotomy.

d–e Radiographic views in the frontal and sagittal plane after double osteotomy with TomoFix implants (lateral distal femur, medial proximal tibia). The osteotomy gap at the tibia has been filled with bone substitute since the wedge extracted from the femur contained vitallium screws and therefore could not be used. The biplanar tibial osteotomy was performed with a tuberosity osteotomy extending distally in order to prevent a patella baja.

f   Frontal plane weight-bearing view after bone healing and implant removal. Normal tibiofemoral angle, mLDFA = 87°, mMPTA = 91° (slight overcorrection in valgus), MJL = 91°, lateral joint opening of 3°.

Table 14-2 shows the different combinations of femoral and tibial osteotomies for the treatment of the deformities listed in Table 14-1. Although various osteotomy combinations are possible, the authors' experience shows that the best option for correction of varus deformities is a closed-wedge lateral femoral osteotomy combined with an open-wedge medial tibial osteotomy (see Fig 14-4). For valgus deformities the most frequent procedure performed is a medial closed-wedge femoral osteotomy combined with a medial closed-wedge tibial osteotomy. If leg lengthening is also required, this can be achieved by a lateral open-wedge femoral osteotomy with bone grafting of the opened gap (Fig 14-5).

Mechanical axis	Position of the midjoint line		
	Varus	**Neutral**	**Valgus**
Varus	F: medial closed-wedge DFO* + T: medial open-wedge HTO* *Alternative: lateral open-wedge DFO	F: lateral closed-wedge DFO* + T: medial open-wedge HTO	F: lateral closed-wedge DFO + T: medial closed-wedge HTO* *Alternative: lateral open-wedge HTO
Neutral	F: medial closed-wedge DFO* + T: medial open-wedge HTO *Alternative: lateral open-wedge DFO		F: lateral closed-wedge DFO + T: medial closed-wedge HTO* *Alternative: lateral open-wedge HTO
Valgus	F: medial closed-wedge DFO* + T: medial open-wedge HTO *Alternative: lateral open-wedge DFO	F: medial closed-wedge DFO* + T: medial closed-wedge HTO** *Alternative: lateral open-wedge DFO **Alternative: lateral open-wedge HTO	F: lateral closed-wedge DFO + T: medial closed-wedge HTO* *Alternative: lateral open-wedge HTO

Table 14-2   Double osteotomies. Combination of femoral (F) and tibial (T) osteotomies for deformities around the knee (see Table 14-1).

DFO = distal femoral (supracondylar) osteotomy
HTO = high-tibial osteotomy

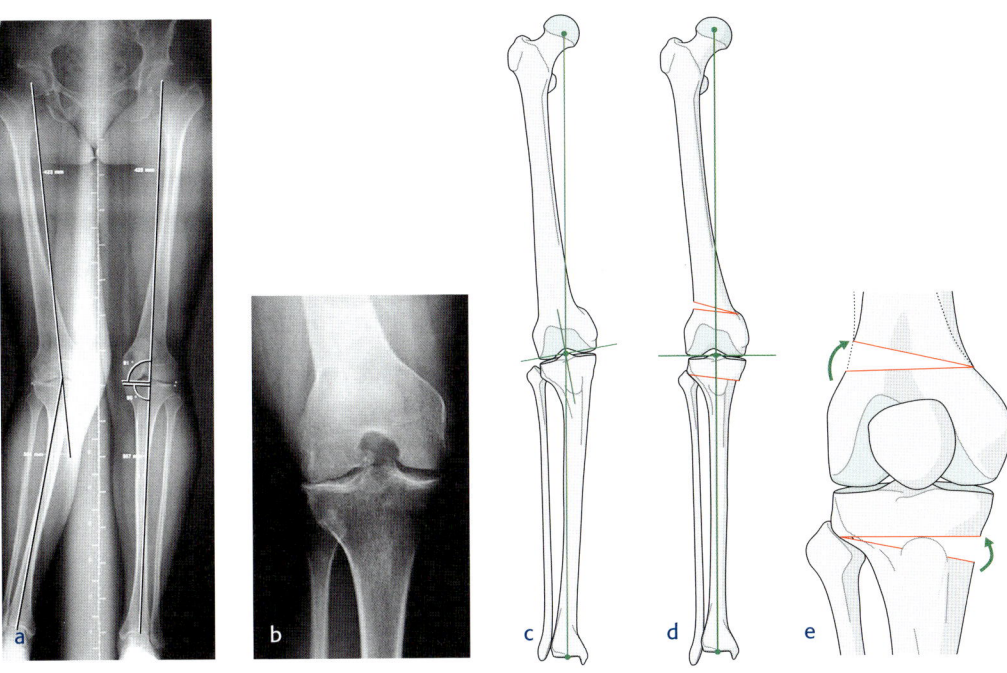

Fig 14-5a–l   37-year-old female patient with progressive joint degeneration and increasing valgus deformity with clinical symptoms. The range of motion was found to be reduced to E/F 0/15/90° due to contracted valgus deformity and osteophytic formations (excerpt from [19]).

a   Frontal plane weight-bearing view of the leg with lateral displacement of the mechanical axis. Tibiofemoral angle 16° valgus, 5° of the deformity are located within the femur, additional pathological mMPTA of 97°. The midjoint line is orientated in a normal, joint line convergence angle (JLCA) of 2°.

b   45° view (Rosenberg view) showing serious lateral joint degeneration and notch osteophytes. All other x-rays show normal patellar height and a normal TTTG distance.

c–d Planning of correction. A single, closed-wedge medial distal femoral osteotomy will produce a pathological orientation of the MJL with a new deformity of the distal femur (mLDFA) and a residual deformity of the proximal tibia (mMPTA = 97°). Combining a closed-wedge medial tibial osteotomy with an open-wedge lateral distal femoral osteotomy will restore normal anatomy (mLDFA and mMPTA are normal)

e   Planning the double osteotomy. A 10° closed-wedge medial tibial osteotomy, combined with a 5° open-wedge lateral distal femoral osteotomy produces a neutral respectively slight varus alignment of the mechanical axis and a neutral midjoint line (MJL) since the medial joint opening is eliminated. The osteophytes are excised to improve the range of motion.

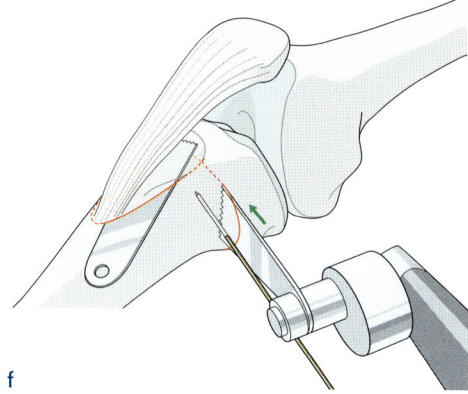

f

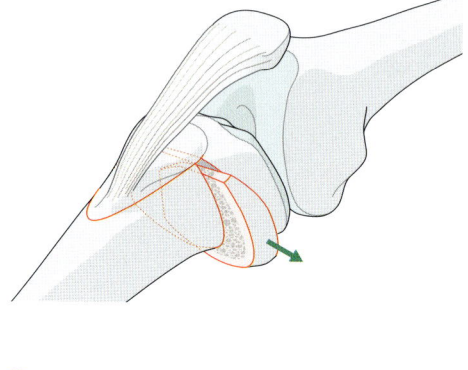

g

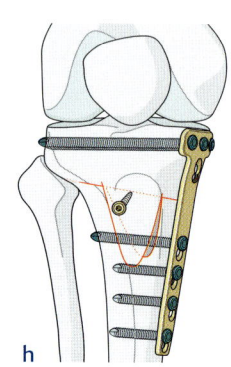

h

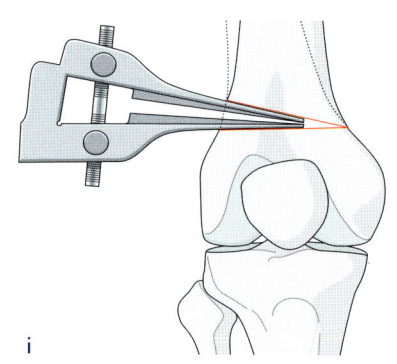

i

Fig 14-5a–l (cont)   37-year-old female with progressive joint degeneration and increasing valgus deformity with clinical symptoms. The range of motion was found to be reduced to E/F 0/15/90° due to contracted valgus deformity and osteophytic formations (excerpt from [19]).

f–g   Medial closed-wedge tibial osteotomy with distal tuberosity osteotomy. After the tuberosity osteotomy, a small saw blade is inserted to protect the tuberosity during the subsequent osteotomy of the tibia. The ascending transverse tibial osteotomy runs obliquely and ends 1 cm before the lateral cortex. The bone wedge is removed and the osteotomy closed.

h   Stabilization of the osteotomy with three bicortical locking head screws proximally and three monocortical locking head screws distally in the TomoFix implant. The tuberosity osteotomy is secured by insertion of a bicortical lag screw.

i   Lateral open-wedge osteotomy of the distal femur: Oblique descending osteotomy that ends just before the cortex of the medial femoral condyle. Distraction of the osteotomy with a calibrated spreader and correction until normal alignment of the mechanical axis is achieved. The wedge size can be measured with a ruler. The wedge extracted from the tibia is prepared and inserted into the gap in the distal femur.

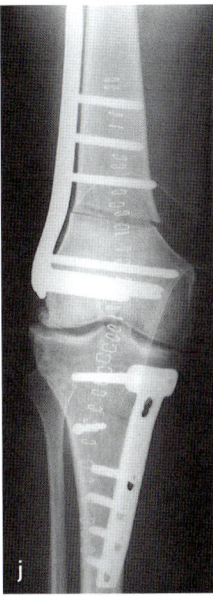

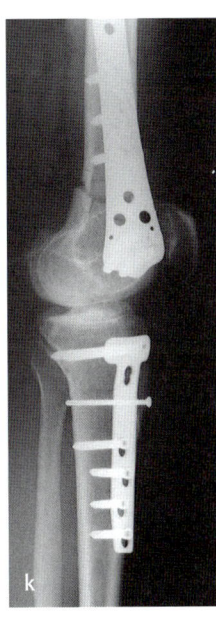

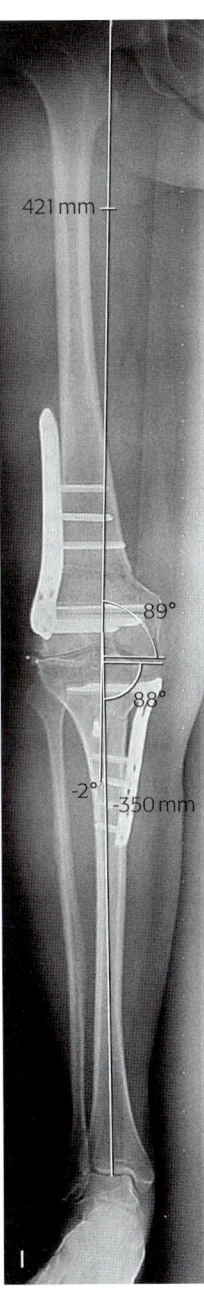

Fig 14-5a–l (cont)   37-year-old female with progressive joint degeneration and increasing valgus deformity with clinical symptoms. The range of motion was found to be reduced to E/F 0/15/90° due to contracted valgus deformity and osteophytic formations (excerpt from [19]).

j–k Stabilization of the femoral osteotomy with a LISS plate (distal femur), four locking head screws distally and three bicortical locking head screws proximally. Frontal and lateral radiographic views.

l Frontal weight-bearing view 12 weeks postoperatively. The mechanical axis runs through the center of the knee joint. The tibiofemoral angle is 2° varus, mLDFA 90° (slight overcorrection), mMPTA 88°, MJL neutral orientation, no medial joint opening. Range of motion has increased to E/F 0/0/115°.

Basically, when planning treatment for patients with pre-operative pathological alignment of the midjoint line, it must be remembered that combinations of osteotomies in the opposing direction will be required at the knee. This means that a varus deformity with medial descending midjoint line (Fig 14-6), for instance, will require a closed-wedge medial distal femoral osteotomy to normalize the distal mechanical femoral angle and the joint line. This osteotomy will, however, increase the varus deformity. An additional open-wedge medial proximal tibial osteotomy will therefore also be necessary in order to normalize the overall orientation of the leg and the alignment of the weight-bearing axis.

In cases of valgus deformity with valgus deviation of the midjoint line (MJL) (ie, the joint line is descending laterally), the authors recommend a converse procedure: lateral closed-wedge distal femoral osteotomy is combined with a medial closed-wedge proximal tibial osteotomy.

If there is a pathologically altered midjoint line of the knee with a neutral alignment of the weight-bearing axis, the combined osteotomy procedures shown in Table 14-2 can be applied.

As already mentioned, the patellofemoral alignment and the height of the patella must be given special consideration when planning double osteotomies. The femoral trochlea is displaced laterally or medially by distal femoral osteotomy [15]. On the tibial side, displacement of the tibial tuberosity depends on the osteotomy technique. In medial open-wedge osteotomy, the tuberosity shifts slightly laterally if the standard technique with proximal tuberosity osteotomy is applied (see chapter 9 "High-tibial open-wedge valgization osteotomy with plate fixator"), whereas the tuberosity shifts slightly medially if the tuberosity osteotomy cut is descending distally [15]. In closed-wedge medial tibial osteotomy with an ascending osteotomy of the tuberosity, the latter moves with the distal fragment and a lateral shift occurs. In closed-wedge medial tibial osteotomy with a distal osteotomy of the tuberosity, the latter is displaced slightly medially.

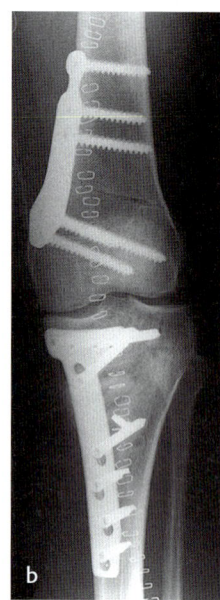 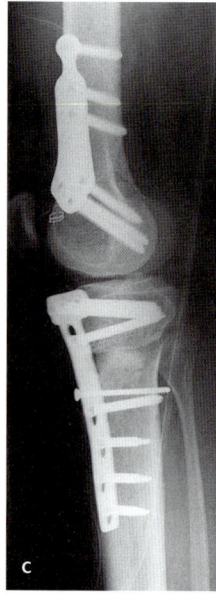

Fig 14-6a–c   24-year-old patient with a varus deformity of 10° and medial inclination of the midjoint line of 15° after failed epiphyseodesis and medial closed-wedge tibial correction osteotomy.
a   Preoperative AP x-ray.
b–c Postoperative x-rays in two planes after combined medial closed-wedge distal femoral osteotomy with medial open-wedge proximal tibial osteotomy. The joint line and the weight-bearing axis are now restored to physiological values.

Furthermore, it should be considered that an open-wedge osteotomy of the medial proximal tibia with an ascending osteotomy of the tuberosity (see chapter 9 "High-tibial open-wedge valgization osteotomy with plate fixator") is associated with a relative distalization of the tuberosity with lowering of the patella. The authors therefore prefer a distal (descending) osteotomy of the tuberosity for corrections larger than 8–10°, thus avoiding this effect [16]. If it becomes apparent during planning that the osteotomies will have an unfavorable effect on patellar height or the alignment of the patellar groove, it is recommended that a separate osteotomy of the tibial tuberosity is performed (see chapter 15 "Rotational osteotomies of the femur and the tibia", Fig 15-4e).

Today, special software programs are available for computer-assisted planning (eg, OASIS system, MediCad). With these programs it is possible to alter the desired correction parameters and to simulate different types of osteotomy on screen. The effects of altering the biomechanical parameters can be thoroughly tested prior to surgery.

5   Surgical technique

Correction osteotomies around the knee can be performed medially or laterally and in open- or closed-wedge technique, depending on the type of femoral or tibial deformity. A pendulum osteotomy is a less commonly practiced technique. A medial procedure is generally preferred at the proximal tibia where both open- and closed-wedge techniques are possible. The advantage of a medial technique over a lateral osteotomy is that a release of the proximal tibiofibular joint or a fibular osteotomy is not required, therefore, the risk of damaging the peroneal nerve is avoided.

The relative laxity of the medial collateral ligament commonly present in valgus knees has prompted the recommendation to perform additional reefing or distal transfer of the MCL attachment in closed-wedge medial HTO [21]. In the authors' experience, however, these procedures are only necessary in cases of preexisting laxity of the medial collateral ligament.

A single-shot systemic antibiotic prophylaxis is administered 30 minutes before skin incision. Arthroscopy may be performed prior to the osteotomy to confirm the indication and to address concomitant intraarticular disorders. In combined procedures any surgical repair of cartilage is completed prior to the correction osteotomy. If additional cruciate ligament replacement is planned, the osteotomies are completed first. The ligament reconstruction is performed later as a second surgery.

The patient is positioned on a radiolucent operating table. The authors utilize a radiopaque grid for intraoperative assessment of the joint line [22]. This is placed under the patient's leg and aligned on the mechanical axis (Fig 14-7). The leg is draped to the hip joint to allow for intraoperative mobility. Application of a tourniquet is possible for double osteotomy if it is placed very proximal on the thigh. Alternatively, a sterile tourniquet can be applied temporarily as required. Surgery starts with a closed-wedge procedure in order to maintain a bone wedge which can be used as an autogenous graft to fill the osteotomy gap of the subsequent open-wedge procedure. Another advantage of this sequence is that open-wedge osteotomy as a second step permits well controlled adjustment of the corrected leg axis (so-called intraoperative fine-tuning) (see chapter 9 "High-tibial open-wedge valgization osteotomy with plate fixator"). Details of the recommended osteotomy combinations are given in Table 14-2.

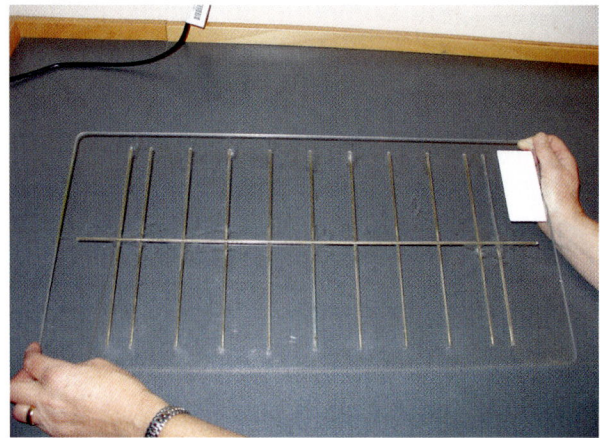

Fig 14-7   Sterile radiopaque grid placed beneath the patient's leg intraoperatively to monitor axial alignment of the leg and joint-line orientation.

Use of K-wires as described in chapter 15 "Rotational osteotomies of the femur and the tibia" simplifies intraoperative control of rotation during axial correction. A leg alignment rod is adequate for intraoperative verification of the leg alignment in the frontal plane (see chapter 9 "High-tibial open-wedge valgization osteotomy with plate fixator"), provided the operation is not performed under computer-assisted navigation. For osteosynthesis the authors use fixed-angle internal plate fixators (TomoFix). Details of the surgical technique for valgus deformity with neutral alignment of the joint line are summarized in Fig 14-5. Preoperative planning and adjustment of the joint line and mechanical axis for varus deformities are illustrated in Fig 14-4 and Fig 14-6.

Possible pitfalls and perioperative complications correspond to those of single osteotomies, whereby double osteotomies are more complex and more traumatic. For these reasons, the complication rates are higher than those for a single osteotomy.

- **Double osteotomy for varus deformity:** lateral closed-wedge femoral osteotomy combined with medial open-wedge tibial osteotomy.

  Double osteotomy for valgus deformity: medial closed-wedge femoral osteotomy combined with medial closed-wedge tibial osteotomy.

  If leg lengthening is required, this can be achieved by lateral open-wedge osteotomies of both femur and tibia taking the joint line into account. Closed-wedge osteotomy is performed first. The extracted wedge can be utilized as autogenous bone graft to fill the osteotomy gap during subsequent open-wedge osteotomy. Carefully applied adjustment of the axial correction is possible (so-called intraoperative fine-tuning) during the open-wedge procedure.

6   Postoperative management

Immediate postoperative leg positioning in 90° hip and near 90° knee flexion position is recommended as distal femur procedures tend to cause loss of range of motion in patients resting with extended leg. Mobilization on underarm crutches with partial weight bearing of 15 kg commences on postoperative day 1. Drains are removed and daily physiotherapeutic exercise to strengthen the muscles and improve mobility is allowed the first postoperative day, including coordination and gait training and manual lymph drainage. It is not generally necessary to restrict range of motion or to apply a brace. Radiological assessment in two planes is carried out on postoperative days 3–5 and after 6 weeks. The mechanical axis is documented postoperatively by weight-bearing x-ray of the leg. If clinical and radiological findings are uneventful, weight bearing can be increased from postoperative week 7. Experience has shown that patients can generally return to work after about 10–12 weeks.

7   Own first results

In the authors' own study of patients with varus and valgus deformities, planning and correction osteotomies were performed according to the method described above [2]. Six patients were treated by double osteotomies of the femur and tibia stabilized with fixed-angle systems. None of these patients presented with preoperative pathological patellar gliding pattern. Cases of varus deformity were corrected by lateral closed-wedge femoral osteotomy and medial open-wedge tibial osteotomy. Patients with valgus deformity were treated by medial closed-wedge femoral osteotomy and a medial closed-wedge tibial osteotomy. In one patient with a hypoplastic lateral femoral condyle, the authors chose to perform a lateral open-wedge femoral osteotomy combined with a medial closed-wedge tibial osteotomy in order to prevent further shortening of the extremity. Delayed bone healing was only seen in one case of lateral open-wedge femoral osteotomy. All other osteotomies healed uneventfully. Axial alignment and the pre-operatively planned correction of the joint line to ± 2° of the normal value was achieved in all patients. Short-term clinical outcomes for the presented treatment method were very good. All the patients returned to their previous activities and were capable of full employment. Despite the magnitude of the operation, the patients would undergo the same surgery again.

In another study, conducted by the senior author, eleven patients were treated with double osteotomies [15]. Preoperative patellofemoral malfunction was present in five cases (45%). Five patients with a pathological knee midjoint line in addition to varus deformity (see **Fig 14-6a**) were treated by medial closed-wedge distal femoral osteotomy and medial open-wedge high-tibial osteotomy (see **Fig 14-6b–c**). The other patients with varus deformity received a lateral closed-wedge femoral osteotomy and medial open-wedge tibial osteotomy. The cases of valgus malalignment were corrected by combined medial closed-wedge femoral osteotomy and medial closed-wedge tibial osteotomy. In one patient with a valgus deformity, the procedure involved a lateral open-wedge instead of a medial closed-wedge femoral osteotomy (see **Fig 14-5**) and, in another patient, a lateral open-wedge instead of a medial closed-wedge tibial osteotomy was performed. This was, however, an exception. In two patients, rotational correction of the femur was required in addition to the frontal plane double correction. One of these patients received a lateral open-wedge osteotomy with 10° internal rotational osteotomy of the femur combined with medial open-wedge tibial osteotomy to treat malunited femoral and tibial fractures. The other patient received a medial open-wedge femoral osteotomy with rotational correction of a malunited femoral fracture combined with medial open-wedge tibial osteotomy to correct varus malalignment. All osteotomies were stabilized with fixed-angle plate fixators.

In total, there was only one case of nonunion following a lateral open-wedge femoral osteotomy. The defect was filled with tricalcium phosphate in a secondary procedure. This patient required secondary total knee arthroplasty. In all cases, correction of the joint line to 90 ± 4° in accordance with the guidelines of the Mayo Clinic was achieved [1]. Pathological patellofemoral movement was corrected in the above-mentioned five patients. Patella baja was not observed in any patient. One patient,

however, developed lateral patellar subluxation postoperatively due to a residual valgus deformity of the femur. The residual deformity was corrected by a medial closed-wedge re-osteotomy of the femur and patellofemoral malfunction was redressed [15].

- The aim of double osteotomies of the femur and tibia around the knee for varus and valgus deformities is to restore normal anatomy or to unload an affected joint compartment and, simultaneously, to normalize knee joint angles and the orientation of the midjoint line.

  Physiological axes can be restored and a high primary stability can be achieved by thorough preoperative planning, respecting biomechanical principles, and a stable fixation with fixed-angle plate systems.

  Combined osteotomy of femur and tibia is a demanding procedure that may, however, be the only treatment option for complex deformities. The short- and mid-term outcomes following double osteotomies are very good.

8   Bibliography

[1]   **Babis GC, An KN, Chao EY, et al** (2002) Double level osteotomy of the knee: a method to retain joint-line obliquity. Clinical results. *J Bone Joint Surg Am;* 84(8):1380–1388.

[2]   **Hofmann S, Paszicneyk T, Mohajer M** (2004) *A new concept for transposition osteotomies around the knee.* Dienheim: Iatros-Verlag, 40–48.

[3]   **Arnoldi CC, Lemperg K, Linderholm H** (1975) Intraosseous hypertension and pain in the knee. *J Bone Joint Surg Br;* 57(3):360–363.

[4]   **Benjamin A** (1974) Double osteotomy of the knee. *Scand J Rheumatol;* 3(2):65.

[5]   **Schüller HM, van Dijk CN, Fidler MW** (1987) Poor results of double osteotomy for the rheumatoid knee. *Acta Orthop Scand;* 58(3):253–255.

[6]   **Pietsch M, Hofmann S** (2006) [Value of radiographic examination of the knee joint fort he orthopedic surgeon.] *Radiologe;* 46(1):55–64. German.

[7]   **Cooke TD, Pichora D, Siu D, et al** (1989) Surgical implications of varus deformity of the knee with obliquity of joint surfaces. *J Bone Joint Surg Br;* 71(4):560–565.

[8]   **Paley D, Herzenberg JE, Tetsworth K, et al** (1994) Deformity planning for frontal and sagittal plane corrective osteotomies. *Orthop Clin North Am;* 25(3):425–465.

[9]   **Müller KH, Müller-Färber J** (1985) Indications, localization and planning of posttraumatic osteotomies about the knee. *Hierholzer G, Müller KH (eds), Corrective osteotomies of the lower extremity after trauma.* Berlin Heidelberg: Springer-Verlag, 195–223.

[10]   **Cicuttini FM, Wluka AE, Stuckey SL** (2001) Tibial and femoral cartilage changes in knee osteoarthritis. *Ann Rheum Dis;* 60(10):977–980.

[11]   **Terauchi M, Shirakura K, Katayama M, et al** (2002) Varus inclination of the distal femur and high tibial osteotomy. *J Bone Joint Surg Br;* 84(2):223–226.

[12]   **Coventry MB, Ilstrup DM, Wallrichs SL** (1993) Proximal tibial osteotomy. A critical long-term study of eighty-seven cases. *J Bone Joint Surg Am;* 75(2):196–201.

[13]   **Schoettle PB, Werner cm, Romero J** (2005) Reconstruction of the medial patellofemoral ligament for painful patellar subluxation in distal torsional malalignment: a case report. *Arch Orthop Trauma Surg;* 125(9):644–648.

[14]   **Dejour H, Walch G, Nove-Josserand L, et al** (1994) Factors of patellar instability: an anatomical radiographic study. *Knee Surg Sports Traumatol Arthrosc;* 2(1):19–26.

[15]   **Wagenaar FBM, van Heerwaarden RJ** (2008) Patellar tracking in double osteotomies around the knee. (prepared for submission).

[16]   **Gaasbeek RD, Sonneveld H, van Heerwaarden RJ, et al** (2004) Distal tuberosity osteotomy in open wedge high tibial osteotomy can prevent patella infera: a new technique. *Knee;* 11(6):457–461.

[17]   **Hofmann S, van Heerwaarden RJ** (2007) General patient selection criteria and indication for double osteotomies around the knee. *Orthopädische Praxis* 43:142-146.

[18]   **Felson DT, McLaughlin S, Goggins J, et al** (2003) Bone marrow edema and its relation to progression of knee osteoarthritis. Ann Intern Med; 139(5 Pt 1):330–336.

[19]   **Van Heerwaarden RJ** (2006): Double osteotomy for valgus leg deformity due to lateral compartment osteoarthritis. In: Wagner, M., R. Frigg (eds): Internal Fixators. Thieme, Stuttgart, 611–620.

[20]   **Gaasbeek RD, Toonen HG, van Heerwaarden RJ, et al** (2005) Mechanism of bone incorporation of beta-TCP bone substitute in open wedge tibial osteotomy in patients. *Biomaterials;* 26(33):6713–6719.

[21] **Coventry MB** (1987) Proximal tibial varus osteotomy for osteoarthritis of the lateral compartment of the knee.
J Bone Joint Surg Am; 69(1):32–38.

[22] **Saleh M, Harriman P, Edwards DJ** (1991)
A radiological method for producing precise limb alignment.
J Bone Joint Surg Br; 73(3):515–516.

Authors   Ronald J van Heerwaarden, Paul Koning, Ibo B van der Haven

15   Rotational osteotomies of the femur and the tibia

1   Introduction and definition

Congenital torsion deformities of the lower extremity may be a consequence of growth disorders of the acetabulum, femur, tibia, or foot and may be the cause of substantial functional limitations and symptoms at the hip, knee, and ankle joints in adolescents and adults [1, 2]. The antetorsion of the acetabular fossa at birth remains to a large extent unchanged during growth (Fig 15-1a). Minimal changes may be seen depending on the development of the femoral head. In contrast, the femur and tibia, which are aligned in internal rotation at birth, rotate externally during childhood [3–5]. No further changes in acetabular antetorsion or femoral and tibial rotation are to be expected after the eighth year of life [3–6]. Rotational deformities of the femur may lead to pathological tibial rotation as a form of compensatory overcorrection and thus result in a rotational deformity of the lower extremity at several levels [6–8]. This must be differentiated from posttraumatic rotation deformity.

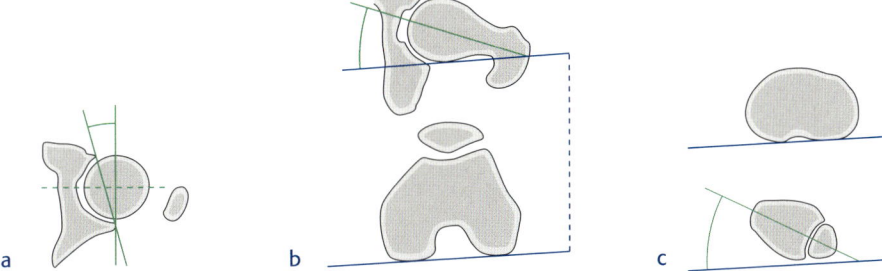

a   b   c

Fig 15-1a–c   Anteversion and torsion angles of the lower extremity measured on axial CT images.
a   Antetorsion of the acetabulum: physiological value 15–20°.
b   Femoral torsion angle. The angle between the line that runs from the center of the femoral head through the center of the femoral neck and the tangent at the posterior femoral condyles measured in the transverse plane: physiological value 15.6±6.7°.
c   Tibial torsion angle. The angle between the posterior tangent of the proximal tibial condyles and the central distal transmalleolar axis after cessation of growth: physiological value 23.5 ± 5.1°.

2   Nomenclature and standard values

The term "torsion" describes the physiological rotation of a bone segment in the longitudinal axis, eg, of long bones such as the femur and tibia. In contrast, the term "rotation" defines rotation between two bone segments and therefore describes relationships at a joint, eg, internal or external rotation of the hip joint.

The torsion angle is defined as the angle of alignment of the distal joint axis in relation to the alignment of the proximal joint in the transverse plane (internal and external rotation). Standard values and standard deviations were originally based on examination of anatomical cross sections and clinical studies [5, 9], but now more precise values have been obtained by computed tomography [4, 10–12]. Standard values differ across different ethnic groups, eg, Asians compared with West Europeans [13].

The torsion angle of the femur is the angle between the line drawn from the center of the femoral head in the transverse plane centrally through the femoral neck and the tangent at the posterior femoral condyles (see Fig 15-1b).

In relation to the distal part of the femoral shaft, the femoral neck is positioned in physiological external rotation, so-called antetorsion. The torsion angle of the femur between the distal femoral condyles and the femoral neck in adults is normally 15.6 ± 6.7° [4, 12]. The torsion angle of the tibia is the angle between the posterior tangents at the proximal tibial condyles and the central distal transmalleolar axis (see Fig 15-1c). The standard value for the tibial external torsion angle at the end of growth is 23.5 ± 5.1° [4, 12]. By definition, pathological torsion is present if the angle measured differs more than two standard deviations from the norm [8].

Congenital torsion deformities can lead to serious symptoms and cause functional limitations of all joints of the lower extremity in adolescence and adulthood. Pathological antetorsion as well as femoral retrotorsion can lead to premature coxarthrosis [9, 11]. Unphysiological femoral internal or antetorsion leads to instability of the hip joint, especially if combined with increased antetorsion of the acetabulum [14]. The joint most frequently affected is the knee since it has very little ability for rotatory compensation compared with the hip or upper ankle joint [6, 7, 9–11, 14, 15]. Torsional malalignment of the femur can result in increased patella contact pressure with secondary retropatellar cartilage damage or retropatellar joint degeneration or patellofemoral malalignment with instability of the patella, subluxation, or dislocation of the patella [2, 6, 7, 9, 16, 17]. Evidence of an increased incidence of pathological antetorsion of the femur and internal torsional malalignment of the tibia has been found in patients with tibiofemoral joint degeneration [15]. Torsion deformity of the leg affects gait pattern and heel-to-toe weight bearing and can lead to arthrotic alterations due to unphysiological load distribution at the upper ankle joint and foot [9].

- Torsion = physiological rotation of a bone segment in the longitudinal axis.
  Rotation = rotation between two bone segments, ie, joint motion.
  Torsion angle = angle of alignment of the distal joint axis of a long bone in relation to the alignment of the proximal joint in the transverse plane.
  Physiological femoral torsion angle = 15.6 ± 6.7°.
  Physiological tibial torsion angle = 23.5 ± 5.1°.
  Pathological torsion exists if the angle measured deviates more than two standard deviations from the norm.

3   Preoperative diagnostics

3.1   Clinical examination

Clinical examination must evaluate the alignment of the lower extremity in both the frontal and sagittal planes. Particular attention must be paid to the alignment of the patellae and the position of the feet. Physiologically, the feet and patellae point straight forward. A medialized patella, valgus weight-bearing axis, or internal rotation deformity of the feet may indicate increased internal torsion of the femur, so-called coxa antetorta. Similarly, a lateralized patella, varus weight-bearing axis, or external rotation deformity of the feet may indicate femoral retrotorsion or coxa retrotorta. Manifestation of a medially aligned patella combined with external rotation of the feet is defined as torsion malalignment syndrome. Its cause is pathological antetorsion of the femur that leads to secondary compensatory external torsion of the tibia [8].

The assessment protocol (rotational profile) designed by Staheli is well suited to determine the exact location and extent of a deformity [4, 5]. First, the gait pattern is analyzed and the rotational alignment of the foot is assessed. The forefoot is normally positioned in 10–35° external rotation at the moment of touchdown (Fig 15-2a). Next, the internal and external rotation capabilities at the hip are analyzed with the patient in the prone position (Fig 15-2b). According to the Neutral-0 Method, internal rotation of 45° and external rotation of 30° are possible, whereby attention must be paid to side-to-side differences. The angle between the foot axis and a straight line through the thigh is measured with the patient in the prone position, the knee in 90° flexion, and the upper ankle joint in the neutral position (norm: 10–30°) (Fig 15-2c). Here, the focus is on lower leg torsion although possible foot deformities (eg, crescent-like feet, club-foot) must be taken into account too.

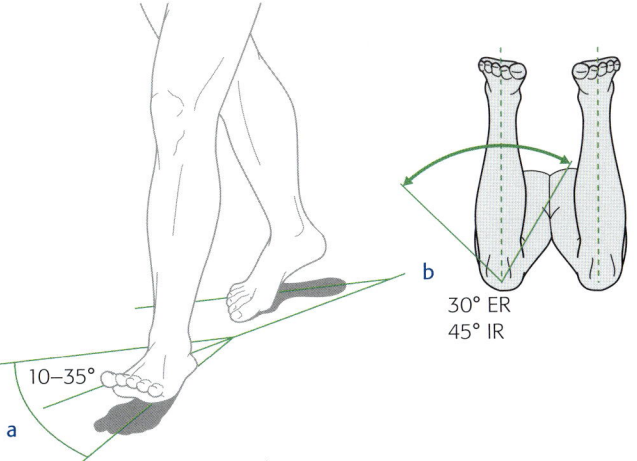

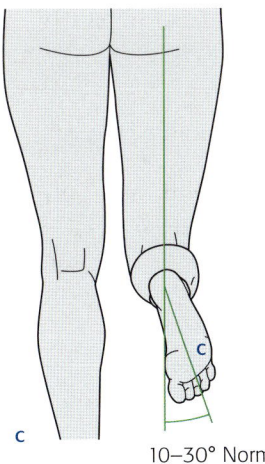

Fig 15-2a–c   Assessment protocol according to Staheli, 1985 [5].
a   Analysis of the gait pattern. At touchdown the forefoot is normally in 10–35° external rotation.
b   Analysis of external and internal rotation of the extended hip joint in prone position to assess femoral torsion. Standard value: 30° external and 45° internal rotation.
c   Measurement of the angle between a straight line through the thigh and the axis of the foot in the prone position with the knee in 90° flexion and the upper ankle joint in the neutral position to assess lower leg torsion. Standard value: 10–30°.

3.2   Diagnostic imaging

Radiological diagnostics include conventional radiographic views of the femur and tibia in both planes. If the cause of torsion deformity is probably in the region of the proximal femur or acetabulum, a pelvic overview is required in order to measure the CE angle (Wiberg angle, ie, center of the femoral head to end of acetabular roof) and the CCD angle (caput collum diaphyseal angle). Mathematical formulae can be applied to diagnose femoral and tibial torsion from conventional x-rays [7, 17]. Axial computed tomography (CT) will, however, simplify precise measurement of these angles. Imaging is performed with the patient in the supine position with the legs parallel. Scans are obtained at the level of the acetabulum with femoral head and neck, at the femoral condyles, at the tibial condyles, and at the level of the ankle joint. The method for obtaining the torsion angles is illustrated in Fig 15-1a–c. To assess patellofemoral joint alignment, the two scans showing the lowest point of the trochlea (trochlear groove, TG) and the most anterior point of the tibial tuberosity (TT) are projected onto each other (Fig 15-3). The distance between these two points is normally 10–15 mm [18], and is often pathologically enlarged or reduced in congenital torsion deformities with abnormal patellofemoral alignment as a consequence [1].

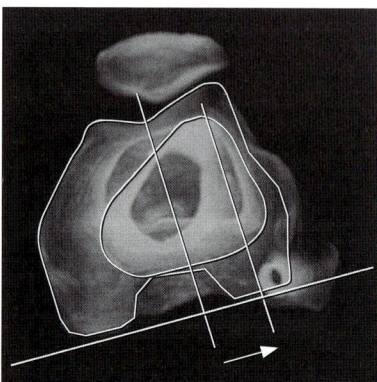

Fig 15-3   To measure the TT-TG distance, the CT scan that shows the lowest point of the trochlea (trochlear groove) and the CT scan that shows the most anterior point of the tibial tuberosity (TT) are projected onto each other. The distance between the lines (arrow) that cross the intercondylar groove and the tuberosity and run perpendicular to the tangent at the posterior condyles is the TT-TG distance. Standard value: 10–15 mm [18].

4   Patient selection

Isolated torsion deformities of the leg without clinical symptoms do not require correction. If there are clinical signs but pathological torsion is only slight (up to two standard deviations from the norm on the CT scans), conservative treatment with corrective insoles and physiotherapeutic muscle strengthening exercises (eg, isometric quadriceps exercises) is usually successful. If the measured torsion angle exceeds two standard deviations from the norm, rotational osteotomy is indicated [8] (Table 15-1). Correction should be performed at the level of the deformity since compensatory rotational osteotomy at an unaffected site will only make the deformity more complex.

	Standard value	**Indication for surgery**
Acetabular anteversion	15–20°	> 25° or < -15°
Femoral torsion angle	15.6 ± 6.7°	> 30° or < 0°
Tibial torsion angle	23 ± 5.1°	> 35° or < 10°

Table 15-1   Standard values for lower extremity torsion angles and indications for surgical treatment of torsion deformities (Caucasian population—racial differences should be taken into account).

5   General surgical technique

5.1   Osteotomy technique

The osteotomy techniques presented here aim to correct the deformity by a one-stage correction osteotomy. Multidimensional and gradual corrections with application of external fixation systems (unilateral fixator, ring fixator; [4, 17, 19]) are not the subject of this chapter. Osteotomy techniques depend on the planned fixation method. Percutaneous drill osteotomy or the use of a Gigli saw through a mini skin incision is appropriate for an intramedullary nail or external fixator [17]. Application of an intramedullary saw followed by intramedullary nail fixation can be used for osteotomy of the diaphysis of the long bones [12]. Osteotomy with the oscillating saw permits better visualization of the osteotomy plane but requires a more invasive approach and may lead to heat-induced bone necrosis.

5.2   Osteotomy level

In the treatment of congenital torsion deformities of the femur, derotation should be performed in the intertrochanteric region with an angled blade plate because of the simplicity of the approach, the excellent growth and healing potential of the metaphyseal zone, and the good fixation options. If correction in the diaphyseal or distal regions of the femur is required, osteosynthesis by intramedullary nail, angled blade plate or fixed-angle plate fixator is preferred. It is important to remember that the bone consolidation phase is longer in the diaphyseal part compared with the proximal part of the femur. Higher complication rates are reported in the literature for diaphyseal and distal femoral osteotomies [2, 20].

The proximal tibia can be osteotomized inferior or superior to the tibial tuberosity. Good bone healing can be assumed for a saw cut in the metaphyseal zone above the tuberosity, but it leaves little room for stable fixation in the proximal segment (Fig 15-4a). The disadvantage of an osteotomy below the tuberosity (Fig 15-4b) is poorer bone consolidation, but it does permit secure fixation of the proximal segment. Therefore, the authors recommend a transverse saw cut at the level of the tibial tuberosity as this will ensure good healing potential combined with stable fixation. The tuberosity can be left intact by making an anterior saw cut ascending cranially behind the tuberosity (Fig 15-4c) or a descending oblique cut (Fig 15-4d). In the latter technique a lag screw is used to prevent avulsion fracture due to the forces exerted by the patellar tendon. If a transverse osteotomy at the level of the tuberosity is combined with a separate tuberosity osteotomy (Fig 15-4e) two or three lag screws are recommended for tuberosity fixation.

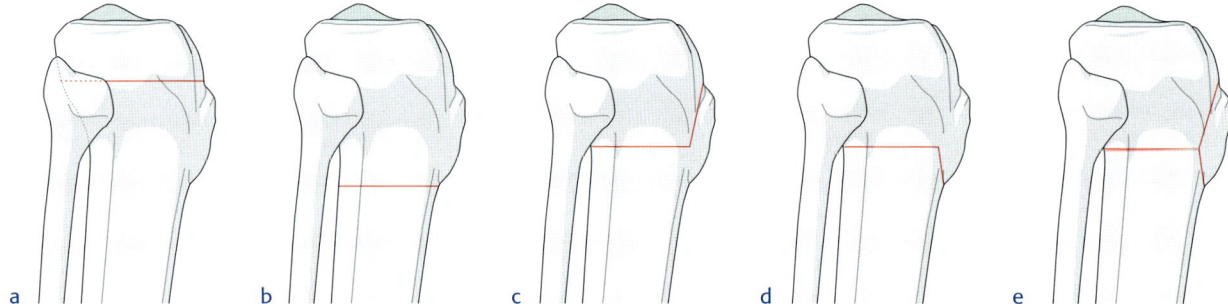

a   b   c   d   e

Fig 15-4a–e   Level of the osteotomy at the proximal tibia.
a   Transverse osteotomy proximal to the tuberosity.
b   Transverse osteotomy distal to the tuberosity.
c   Transverse osteotomy at the level of the tuberosity with anterior saw cut ascending obliquely in a cranial direction.
d   Transverse osteotomy at the level of the tuberosity with anterior saw cut descending obliquely in a caudal direction.
e   Transverse osteotomy at the level of the tuberosity with separate osteotomy of the tuberosity.

Osteotomies above the tuberosity must take into account the fact that rotation of the distal segment leads to medial or lateral translation of the tuberosity. The extent of translation can be determined by tracing it from the CT images or by mathematical calculation using the formula given in Fig 15-5. Physiological retropatellar and femoral cartilage loading and stable patellar tracking is guaranteed if the tuberosity is positioned 10–15 mm lateral to the mid-trochlea (so-called tibial tuberosity trochlea distance, TT-TG, see above) [18]. Rotational osteotomy below the tuberosity is not a problem since the tuberosity remains on the proximal segment and the distance to the femoral trochlea thus remains unchanged after rotation correction of the distal segment [2]. If it becomes apparent during preoperative planning that the rotational osteotomy will lead to a pathologically increased or decreased TT-TG distance, an alternative osteotomy level or a separate tuberosity osteotomy with appropriate lateral or medial translation of the tuberosity should be considered.

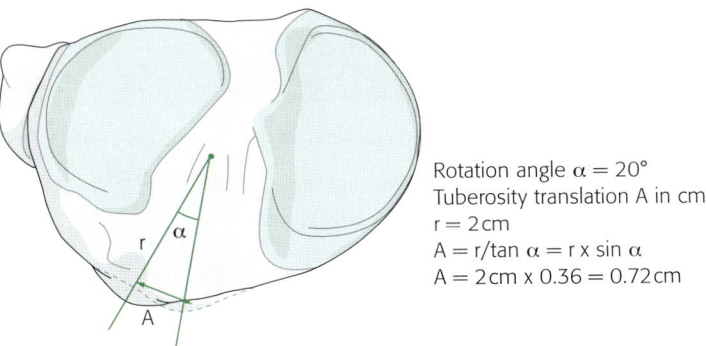

Rotation angle $\alpha = 20°$
Tuberosity translation A in cm
$r = 2\,cm$
$A = r/\tan \alpha = r \times \sin \alpha$
$A = 2\,cm \times 0.36 = 0.72\,cm$

Fig 15-5 Mathematical calculation of tuberosity translation during rotation correction. The extent of translation can be calculated preoperatively using the formula given. For an intended rotation correction of 20° and r = 2 cm (based on average normal proximal tibia diameter), the tibial tuberosity will translate 7.2 mm medially after internal rotation correction.

Due to the good bone healing potential, distal tibial rotational osteotomies should be positioned in the metaphyseal region above the tibiofibular syndesmosis. Rotation in the diaphyseal region may cause incongruence and clinical symptoms due to the triangular cross section of the tibial shaft.

- Growth and healing potential in the metaphyseal zone of the long bones is excellent, whereas the diaphyseal region has a longer bone consolidation time.

  Tibial osteotomy above the tuberosity leads to medial or lateral translation of the tuberosity after distal segment rotation.

  If a rotational osteotomy results in pathological increase or decrease of the TT-TG distance, an alternative osteotomy site or a separate osteotomy with appropriate lateral or medial tuberosity translation should be considered.

5.3   Soft-tissue problems and neurovascular structures

Depending on the level of the osteotomy, rotational osteotomy of the femur may have an important effect on the position and the direction of pull of the quadriceps femoris muscle group. By contrast, proximal tibial rotational osteotomies only have a minimal effect on the function of the lower leg muscles. Although diaphyseal and distal torsional changes of the tibia may cause twisting and elongation of the muscle compartments or a change in direction of pull of the tendons, functional limitations have not been reported as long as the correction angle is less than 45° [17].

Special attention must be paid to the neurovascular structures if more extensive torsional correction is required. Tension and compression during internal rotational osteotomy of the femur may damage the sciatic nerve. By contrast, external rotational osteotomies present no difficulties in this respect.

Since the peroneal nerve runs around the fibula, increased internal torsion of the proximal tibia during internal rotational osteotomy may result in overextension of the nerve or entrapment in the intercompartmental septum between the anterior and lateral muscle compartments. The peroneal nerve may be damaged during external rotational osteotomy due to compression within the septum or due to tension in the anterior compartmental fasciae [17]. This problem can be avoided by careful decompression of the nerve or by performing diaphyseal or distal derotation where the correction angle is greater than 20°.

Distal external rotational osteotomy of the tibia may cause overextension of the posterior tibial nerve within the posterior compartmental fasciae of the lower leg and tension in the fasciae of the abductor hallucis in the tarsal tunnel [17]. These complications can be prevented by release of both fasciae in the tarsal tunnel.

If more than a 20° rotational correction of the tibia is planned, careful decompression of the peroneal nerve is essential in proximal tibial rotational osteotomies or, alternatively, a diaphyseal or distal derotation site should be chosen. In any case, intracompartmental decompression by fasciotomy is recommended.

5.4   Fibular osteotomy

Proximal derotational osteotomy of the tibia of up to 20° does not generally require a fibular osteotomy. The proximal and distal tibiofibular joints permit compensatory rotation of the fibula. Rotation up to 16° is possible at the tibiotalar joint without incongruity at the upper ankle joint [21, 22]. If the extent of correction at the distal tibia exceeds this angle, an additional transverse osteotomy is needed in the distal fibular third. Proximal fibular osteotomy or release of the proximal tibiofibular joint will increase stability in the region of the distal

tibial osteotomy but is associated with the risk of injury to the peroneal nerve and permanent symptomatic instability of the proximal tibiofibular joint.

5.5   Instruments

Fig 15-6 shows the set of instruments needed to perform the planned rotation correction with absolute precision. The set includes threaded and unthreaded K-wires, a sterile goniometer, various triangular measuring templates, an angled tuberosity protection plate which is positioned in the cranial or caudal tuberosity cut to protect the tuberosity during the transverse tibial osteotomy, and a sterile centimeter ruler.

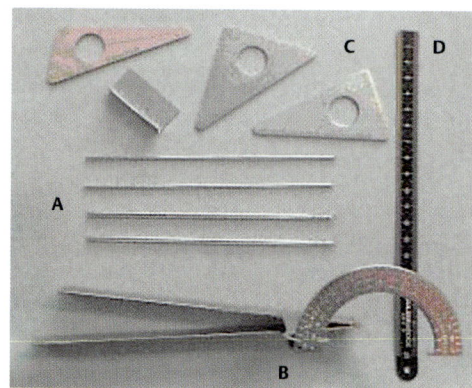

Fig 15-6   Instrument set for rotational osteotomy. Threaded and unthreaded K-wires (a), sterile goniometer (b), various triangular templates and angled tuberosity protection plate (c), sterile centimeter ruler (d).

5.6   Direction of osteotomy

When correcting purely torsional deformities of the lower extremity, it is very important that the correction is made only in the transverse plane. The transverse plane is defined as the plane perpendicular to the physiological weight-bearing axis of the leg. The fact that the anatomical and mechanical axes of the femur form a physiological angle of 7° in the frontal plane must be respected, in particular, when aligning the intertrochanteric osteotomy plane. The mechanical and anatomical axes of the tibia are almost identical. These lines run parallel, whereby the anatomical axis lies physiologically only a few millimeters medial to the mechanical axis. A long measuring rod is used to define the mechanical axes intraoperatively. This rod is positioned under image intensification over the center of the femoral head proximally and at the center of the upper ankle joint distally (see chapter 9 "High-tibial open-wedge valgization osteotomy with plate fixator", Fig 9-14). The exact angulation of the saw should also be verified under image intensification before initiating the osteotomy. A K-wire may be positioned under image intensifier view as a guide wire for exact transverse plane sawblade alignment.

Torsion deformities must be corrected in the transverse plane. When aligning the osteotomy plane at the femur it is important to remember that the anatomical and mechanical axes normally form a physiological angle of 7° in the frontal plane. The osteotomy cut is aligned transverse to the mechanical axis.

5.7   Fixation

The fixation options for rotational osteotomy include staples [6, 7, 16], external fixators [17, 19, 23], plate osteosynthesis [7], intramedullary nailing [12, 24], and internal plate fixators with fixed-angle locking head screws in accordance with the LCP and LISS principles [25]. The authors favor the use of fixed-angle internal plate fixators, since their high mechanical stability prevents secondary correction loss, periosteal vascularity is preserved, and minimally invasive insertion of screws is possible through a stab incision.

5.8   Correction loss

After correction of torsion deformity by appropriate rotation of the segments, the cortices are frequently seen to be incongruent at the level of the osteotomy, which hinders application of a rigid plate. Advancing the plate towards the shaft can then lead to correction loss, especially if bicortical screws are inserted. This can be prevented by careful smoothing of the cortex of the distal segment. It has also proven worthwhile to smooth out any incongruity distal to the saw cut. This can be achieved, for example, by wedging short K-wires or short saw blades between plate and cortex like a palisade that prevents correction loss when the plate is moved toward the bone. Instead of reduction forceps, the osteotomy can temporarily be stabilized with K-wires prior to insertion of the plate. Incongruity is not a problem if osteosynthesis involves application of staples, intramedullary nails or external fixators.

5.9   Multilevel osteotomies and multiplanar rotational osteotomies

Patients with so-called torsion malalignment syndrome not only have pathological femoral internal torsion, but also compensatory pathological external torsion of the tibia [6, 7, 8] (see subchapter 3.1 "Clinical examination") (Fig 15-7a–c). External rotational osteotomy of the femur alone would aggravate tibial pathology. Therefore, a combined procedure with additional internal rotational osteotomy of the tibia is required in these cases (Fig 15-7d–e). Growth disorders and posttraumatic malalignment, in particular, often cause deformities in the frontal plane (varus/valgus) and in the sagittal plane (procurvatum/recurvatum) in addition to the torsion deformity. Surgical treatment of such complex deformities of the weight-bearing axis requires thorough deformity analysis and planning. Oblique osteotomies are highly effective in the correction of multiplanar deformities [4, 17, 19]. Nevertheless, it should be remembered that rotation of the two oblique surfaces may cause or worsen deformity in the frontal and sagittal planes.

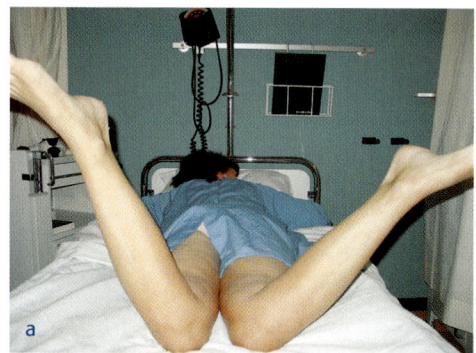
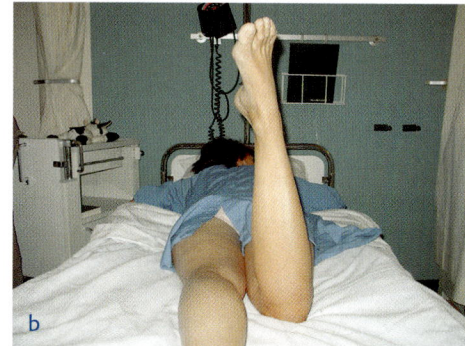
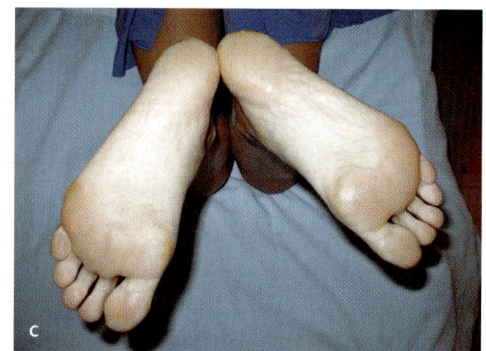

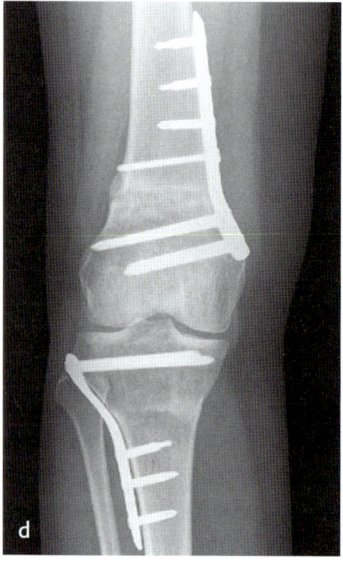
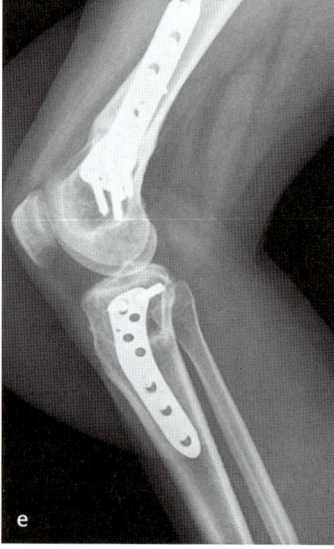

Fig 15-7a–e   Patient with torsion malalignment syndrome.
a   Excessive internal rotation of the right hip in side-to-side comparison.
b   External rotation of the right hip is clearly limited.
c   Compensatory external torsion deformity of the right tibia.
d–e Postoperative x-rays in both planes after bone consolidation of a combined external rotational osteotomy of the distal femur and internal rotational osteotomy of the tibia stabilized with fixed-angle plate fixators.

6   Rotational osteotomy of the femur

A 90° angled blade plate with U-profile is utilized to stabilize a transverse, intertrochanteric osteotomy of the femur [25]. Blade length is determined with reference to the AP x-ray, whereby an offset of 10 mm is sufficient since neither lateralization nor medialization of the femoral diaphysis is intended.

Position

The operation is performed with the patient in the supine position, whereby the buttock of the affected side is positioned on a foam wedge. Sterile draping goes as far as the iliac crest to allow free intraoperative mobility of the leg and facilitate evaluation of the clinical outcome after correction. Fig 15–8a shows the position of the leg. The leg is held with the hip in internal rotation and the knee flexed. The surgeon is seated.

Surgical technique

Skin incision begins at the greater trochanter and runs 10–15 cm in a distal direction. After longitudinal incision of fascia lata, an L-shaped detachment of vastus lateralis from the innominate tubercle is performed. The femur and the intertrochanteric region are exposed by insertion of two Hohmann elevators (Fig 15-8b). The location for the transverse osteotomy is marked directly cranial to the lesser trochanter using the electrocautery or a chisel. The planned position of the angled-blade plate on the femur is determined under image intensification, whereby the lower bend in the plate should lie at the level of the planned osteotomy. The plate blade is thus situated in the femoral neck. The blade insertion site at the greater trochanter is likewise marked using the electrocautery or a chisel. A threaded K-wire is inserted bicortically cranial to the osteotomy mark. Similarly, a bicortical threaded wire is placed caudal to the osteotomy mark and is aligned so that it forms the preoperatively calculated correction angle with the first wire (Fig 15-8c). Both wires must lie perpendicular to the mechanical axis of the

femur. In terms of the anatomical axis an angle of 7° downwards must be observed to align the osteotomy transverse to the mechanical axis (see above). Another wire is inserted and advanced into the femoral neck in direct contact with the bone and under image intensification. This marks the position and antetorsion of the femoral neck. A seating chisel with U-profile is carefully hammered in parallel to this wire to prepare the insertion site and blade bed (Fig 15-8d). Rotation of the chisel can be controlled by advancing it into the bone with a slotted hammer. Correct orientation of the chisel blade in the frontal plane and sagittal plane is achieved by aligning the tongue of the guiding angle parallel to the femoral shaft in both planes. After reaching the desired blade depth, the chisel is left in position to act as a guide and the leg is positioned in full extension on the operating table. It is recommended that the blade now be hammered back out by 1–2 cm to facilitate extraction of the seating chisel after the osteotomy. Under the protection of two Hohmann retractors, the osteotomy is now done with the oscillating saw under constant cooling (Fig 15-8e–f). As described in section 12.5.6, the osteotomy is at 90° to the mechanical axis. Consequently, the saw blade must lie in the same plane as wires 1 and 2. Afterwards, the chisel is withdrawn and the blade plate is carefully hammered into the prepared implant bed (Fig 15-8g). The distal segment is rotated until the second K-wire lies exactly parallel to the first K-wire so that the planned correction angle is achieved (Fig 15-8h–i). The angled blade plate should be stabilized temporarily with Verbruggen clamps. Compression can be applied to the osteotomy gap either by application of the plate compression device or by eccentric screw placement in the plate holes distal to the osteotomy. After insertion of the bicortical screws, radiological documentation of the surgical outcome (Fig 15-8l) and insertion of Redon drains followed by wound closure in layers is performed.

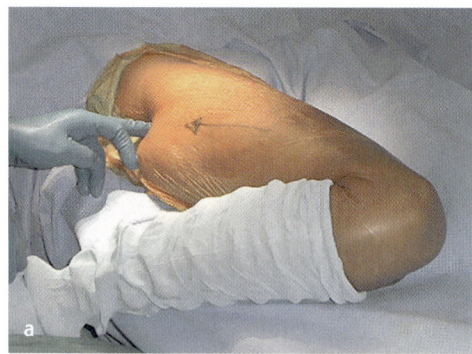
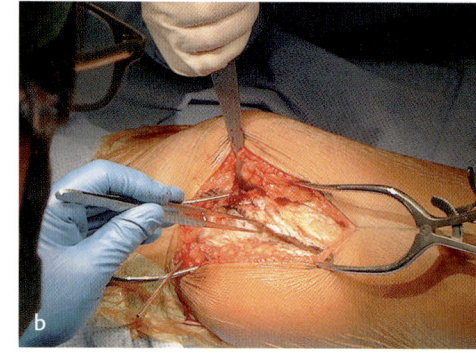
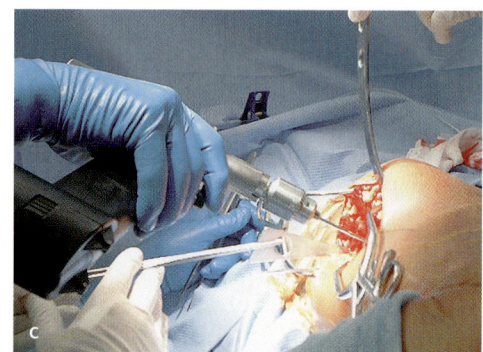
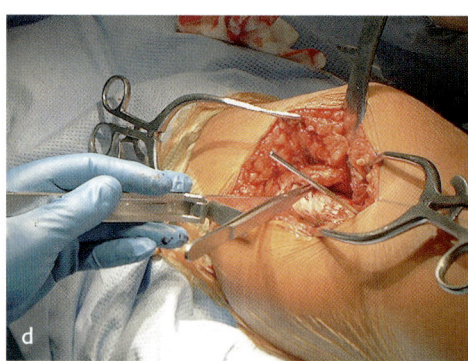
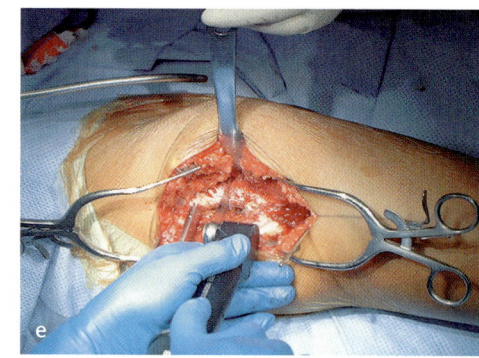
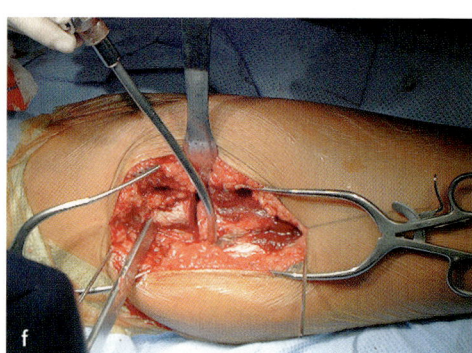
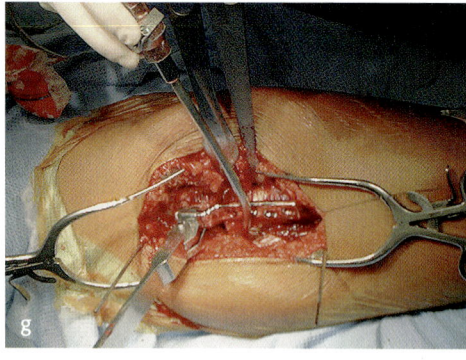

Fig 15-8a–l Intertrochanteric rotational osteotomy of the femur.
a   Positioning the leg.
b   Longitudinal incision of fascia lata and L-shaped release of vastus lateralis from the innominate tubercle.
c   Bicortical insertion of threaded K-wires inferior and superior to the marked osteotomy site. The angle between the two wires corresponds to the correction angle calculated preoperatively. Both wires must lie perpendicular to the mechanical femoral axis.
d   Preparation of the bed for the blade plate by insertion of a seating chisel.
e–f Intertrochanteric osteotomy with the oscillating saw.
g   Careful advancement of the blade plate.

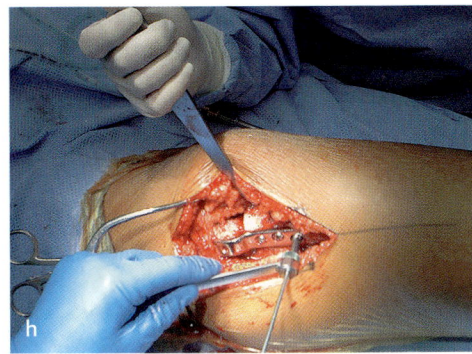

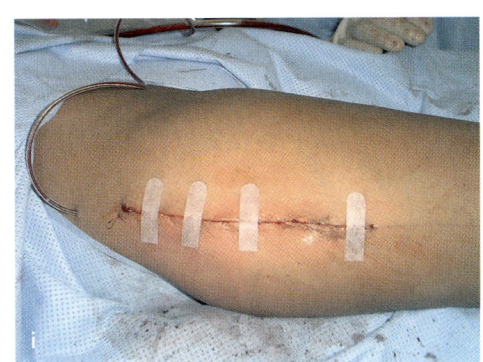

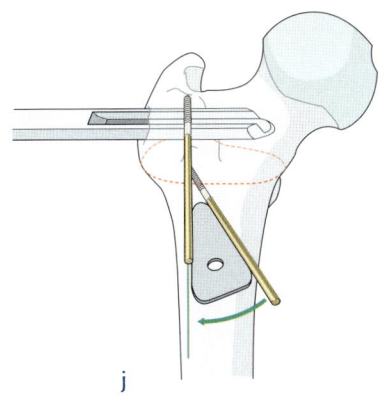

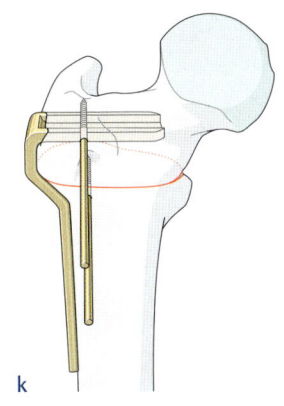

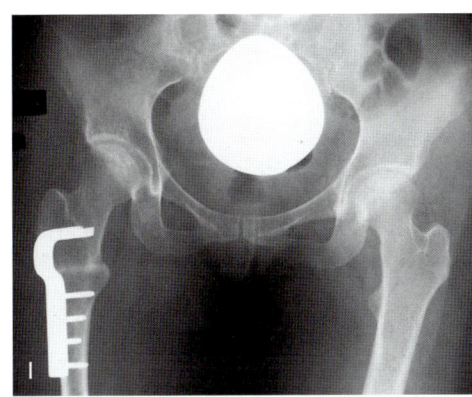

Fig 15-8a–l (cont)   Intertrochanteric rotational osteotomy of the femur.

h   Plate fixation by eccentric bicortical insertion of screws to compress the osteotomy.

i   Status after wound closure.

j–k Schematic representation showing rotation of the distal segment. The angle between the two K-wires corresponds to the planned correction angle. The distal segment is rotated until the second wire is exactly parallel to the first K-wire at which point the planned correction has been achieved.

l   Postoperative pelvic overview after intertrochanteric rotational osteotomy stabilized with an angled blade plate.

Postoperative management

Dressings are changed and the Redon drains removed on the first postoperative day. Mobilization commences at 10–15 kg partial loading on underarm crutches. Passive motion of the hip is not restricted, however, active motion against resistance should be avoided. Radiological follow-up on postoperative day 3 and after postoperative week 6. Depending on clinical and radiological findings, weight bearing can be increased from postoperative week 7.

7 Rotational osteotomy of the tibia

7.1 Proximal rotational osteotomy of the tibia

Proximal tibial osteotomy (with or without osteotomy of the tibial tuberosity) is stabilized with an internal fixed-angle plate fixator.

The degree of corrective rotation required and the extent of medialization or lateralization of the tibial tuberosity, if relevant, is determined preoperatively from the CT images. The level of the tibial osteotomy and any relevant translation of the tuberosity are defined with reference to the physiological TT-TG distance (see subchapter 5.2 "Osteotomy level" and subchapter 5.3 "Soft-tissue problems and neurovascular structures").

Positioning

Surgery is performed with the patient in the supine position. As for the femoral rotational osteotomy, sterile draping should go as far as the iliac crest to ensure free intraoperative mobility of the leg for clinical evaluation of the mechanical axis. A sterile tourniquet can be applied to the thigh but is not generally necessary in our experience.

Surgical technique

The knee is placed in extension but slightly flexed on a towel roll. An anterolateral curved approach (Fig 15-9a) or a 5–7 cm longitudinal skin incision anterior to the tuberosity are standard procedure. The fascia of the tibialis anterior is dissected longitudinally from about 1 cm lateral to the tibial attachment, whereby the fascia will be reattached later to the residual medial part. About 5 cm of the tibial anterior muscle is detached to expose the proximal lateral tibia. After longitudinal incision of the periosteum medial to the tuberosity, a bone rasp is passed beneath it and it is detached from the tibia until a Hohmann retractor can be placed behind the posteromedial edge of the tibia. After this the medial collateral ligament and the tendons of the pes anserinus are protected (Fig 15-9b). It is helpful to mark the joint line by percutaneous insertion of two small cannulae beneath the medial and lateral menisci. The tibial axis is identified under image intensification using a measuring rod. The image intensifier is also utilized to mark the direction of the saw cut with a K-wire. The mark for the level of the osteotomy is made perpendicular to the mechanical tibial axis about 1 cm distal to the cranial margin of the tuberosity with the electrocautery. The internal plate fixator is positioned under image intensification on the lateral tibia and the two proximal screw holes are predrilled (Fig 15-9c). The plate is withdrawn and the mark is made for the cranially ascending or inferior oblique descending osteotomy. If there is no need to rotate the tuberosity, the saw cut runs distally. If the tuberosity needs to be rotated with the distal segment, the anterior osteotomy must be cranial so that the tuberosity remains part of the distal segment. As for valgus open-wedge tibial correction osteotomy, the angle between the transverse osteotomy and the oblique osteotomy should be about 100° and the tuberosity segment should be about 10–15 mm in width (see chapter 9 "High-tibial open-wedge valgization osteotomy with plate fixator").

First, the anterior oblique osteotomy is made with a thin saw blade (Fig 15-9d). It is important to ensure that the saw cut is strictly in the frontal plane and that the patellar tendon is protected by a retractor. Threaded K-wires are inserted bicortically parallel to each other, one proximal and one distal to the planned osteotomy and both perpendicular to the tibial axis in order to monitor the extent of derotation. Next, the transverse tibial osteotomy is performed under image intensification, likewise from lateral to medial and perpendicular to the mechanical tibial axis (Fig 15-9e). To protect the tibial tuberosity, a saw blade or an angled protection plate should be left in the osteotomy cut while the transverse tibial saw cut is made. After removing the protective saw blade from the tuberosity osteotomy cut, a small amount of bone is removed from the tibia behind the tuberosity so that rotation is possible (Fig 15-9f). This is followed by immediate verification of whether the segment can be rotated easily without resistance since it may be necessary to cut carefully through any residual bone bridges with a chisel. Next, the distal segment is rotated in relation to the proximal segment until the planned correction is achieved which can be verified the sterile goniometer (Fig 15-9g–h). It is essential to ensure correct alignment of the foot in relation to the patella and the tibial tuberosity. The correction may be stabilized temporarily with two K-wires without impeding application of the fixed-angle plate fixator. The plate is now positioned so that the two proximal plate holes are aligned with the two predrilled holes in the proximal tibial segment (Fig 15-9i). Two locking head screws of appropriate length as measured are inserted bicortically. Stable fixation requires insertion of three monocortical locking screws into the plate holes distal to the osteotomy (Fig 15-9j).

If the derotational osteotomy creates a pathological distance between the tibial tuberosity and the trochlea (TT-TG > 15 mm or < 10 mm), a separate osteotomy of the tuberosity must be planned to achieve corrective medialization or lateralization to within normal limits. In these cases, the complete tuberosity osteotomy is performed first from a lateral approach perpendicular to the sagittal plane over a length of 6 cm with a thin saw blade, and then the transverse tibial osteotomy follows (see Fig 15-4e). If the entire tuberosity needs to be detached and translated, it should be stabilized by bicortical insertion of two or three small fragment screws.

The authors' experience has shown that a derotation of up to 20° does not require decompression of the peroneal nerve or osteotomy of the fibula or release of the proximal tibiofibular joint (see subchapter 5.3 "Soft-tissue problems and neurovascular structures" and subchapter 5.4 "Fibular osteotomy"). It is however recommended that the fasciae of the anterior compartment be split to prevent pressure increase as a result of postoperative hematoma formation (Fig 15-9k). Finally, refixation of the muscle, insertion of Redon drains and wound closure in layers.

Postoperative management

The dressing is changed and Redon drains removed on postoperative day 1. Mobilization is allowed on underarm crutches with partial weight bearing to half bodyweight for 6 weeks postoperatively. Passive and active motion at the knee is unrestricted, active motion against resistance should however be avoided. Radiological follow-up is performed on postoperative day 3 and after postoperative week 6. Depending on the clinical and radiological findings, full weight bearing can commence from postoperative week 7. If separate medial or lateral repositioning of the tibial tuberosity was performed, a removable splint is prescribed for 6 weeks after surgery to reduce quadriceps pull on the tuberosity during walking.

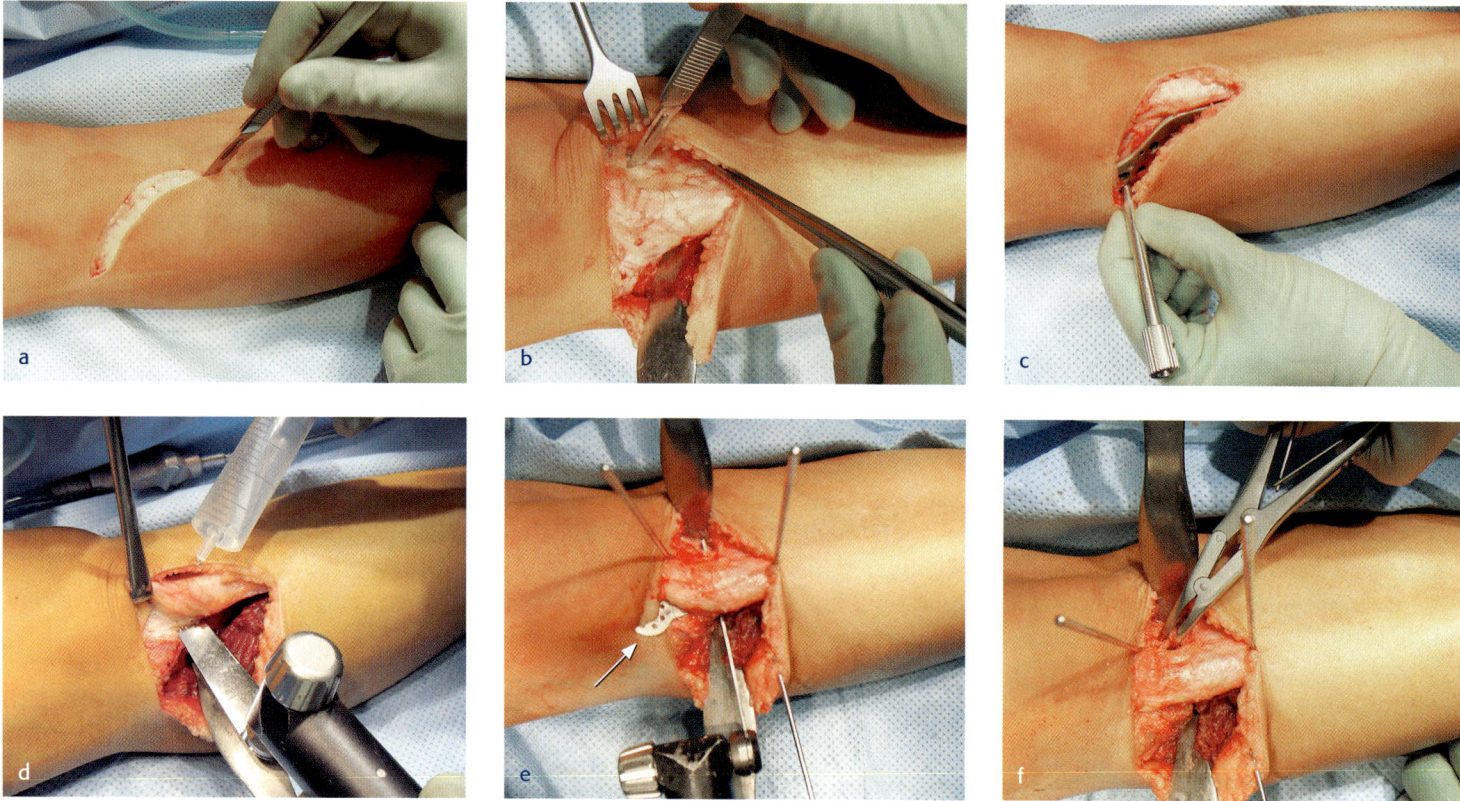

Fig 15-9a–k   Proximal rotational osteotomy of the tibia with cranial tuberosity osteotomy.

a   Anterolateral curved approach to the proximal tibia.

b   Longitudinal incision of the periosteum medial to the tuberosity, undertunneling of the periosteum, insertion of a Hohmann retractor behind the posteromedial margin of the tibia to protect the medial ligament and the tendons of pes anserinus.

c   After positioning the internal plate fixator on the proximal lateral tibia.

d   Cranial tuberosity osteotomy.

e   Transverse osteotomy perpendicular to the tibial axis. A narrow saw blade is left in the tuberosity osteotomy cut (see arrow) to protect the tuberosity. Two threaded K-wires are inserted, one proximal and one distal to the osteotomy.

f   A small amount of bone is removed behind the tuberosity so that rotation is possible.

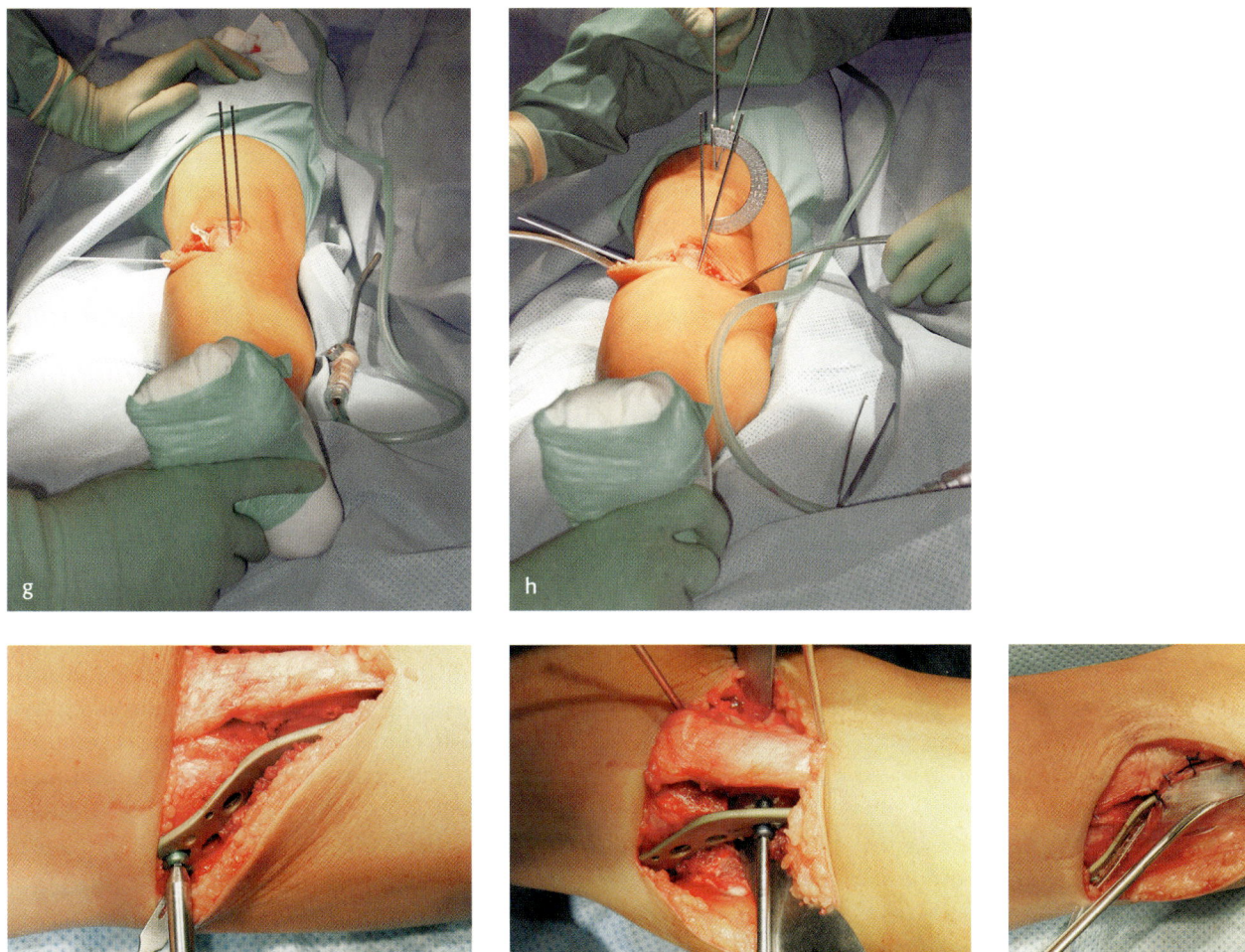

Fig 15-9a–k (cont)   Proximal rotational osteotomy of the tibia with cranial tuberosity osteotomy.

g–h The planned correction is achieved by rotation of the distal segment in relation to the
proximal segment, and can be verified with the sterile goniometer.

i   The plate fixator is inserted after the two proximal plate holes are aligned with the two
predrilled holes in the proximal tibial segment.

j   Monocortical locking head screws are inserted into the screw holes distal to the osteotomy.

k   Incision of the fascia of the anterior compartment.

7.2 Distal rotational osteotomy of the tibia with fibular osteotomy

An LCP T-plate is utilized to stabilize the distal rotational osteotomy of the tibia. The size of the plate, plate and screw position, and the level of the fibular osteotomy are planned on the basis of the AP and lateral x-rays of the tibia. In very slim patients, or if the soft-tissue situation is precarious, the less bulky small fragment T-plate is recommended instead of the LCP. The tibial osteotomy is located in the metaphyseal region cranial to the tibiofibular syndesmosis.

Positioning

With the patient in the supine position, a thigh tourniquet is applied followed by sterile draping of the leg proximal of the knee so that the mechanical axis of the lower leg can be evaluated intraoperatively.

Surgical technique

First, a transverse osteotomy of the fibula is performed through a small longitudinal incision in the mid to lower third of the fibular diaphysis with an oscillating saw (Fig 15-10a–b). The peroneal muscles and nerve are protected during this procedure by two small Hohmann retractors that are inserted around the fibula in direct contact with the bone at the level of the osteotomy. The approach to the distal tibia is through an approximately 4 cm long, slightly oblique skin incision medial to the tibialis anterior tendon. The line of the incision depends on the planned direction of rotation. If external rotation correction is required, the incision should be made slightly on the posteromedial side. If the correction involves internal rotation, the incision lies slightly laterally. After derotation the oblique incision will become longitudinal. The great saphenous vein is carefully dissected and mobilized so that it will not be damaged during the osteotomy. Now the T-plate can be inserted. It is advisable to slide the plate shaft cranially along the bone first (Fig 15-10c) and then to position the T-part above the malleolus under image intensification so that the distal locking screws lie just above the tibial joint line. When the implant is in the correct position it is properly fixed by the assistant and the drill sleeve for the two distal plate holes are mounted. In addition to bicortical predrilling of the two distal screw holes with the help of the drill sleeves, the first screw hole proximal of the T-arm is predrilled in one cortex only (Fig 15-10d). The level of the osteotomy on the distal tibia is marked with the electrocautery between the first and second plate holes on the plate shaft. The next step is to withdraw the LCP T-plate and to insert threaded K-wires perpendicular to the tibial axis proximal and distal to the planned transverse osteotomy. The K-wires are placed in an offset corresponding to the angle of correction as measured with the goniometer, ie, the angle between the two wires represents the degree of correction as planned preoperatively (Fig 15-10e). At the mark for the tibial osteotomy, the periosteum is incised and a threaded K-wire is inserted under fluoroscopic view in the exact transverse direction relative to the tibial mechanical axis. After subperiosteal insertion of the two Hohmann retractors, the transverse saw cut is made with the oscillating saw below the K-wire that acts as a guide (Fig 15-10f). After complete osteotomy, the foot can be rotated until the two K-wires are parallel to each other and the correction is complete (Fig 15-10g–h). Prior to clinical and radiological verification of the axes, the segments may temporarily be stabilized with two K-wires. Attention must be paid to correct alignment of the foot in relation to the patella and tibial tuberosity. In addition, radiological assessment with a measuring rod must show physiological alignment of the mechanical axis. The T-plate is again positioned on the distal tibia and is stabilized by application of one monocortical and two bicortical locking head screws inserted into the corresponding predrilled holes. Now, a temporary lag screw is placed in the first plate hole proximal to the osteotomy. This allows the LCP T-plate to be pulled nearer to the bone surface of the distal tibia. The osteotomy can also be compressed by application of the dynamic compression principle. Monocortical locking bolts are inserted into the other holes in the plate shaft through stab incisions (Fig 15-10i). The

K-wires can now be withdrawn. The final step of the operation is to replace the lag screw by a bicortical locking head screw. As in the proximal technique, intracompartmental decompression by incision of the fascia is also important in the distal tibial osteotomy. To conclude, the surgical outcome is documented radiologically (Fig 15-10j–k). Redon drains are inserted and the wound is closed in layers.

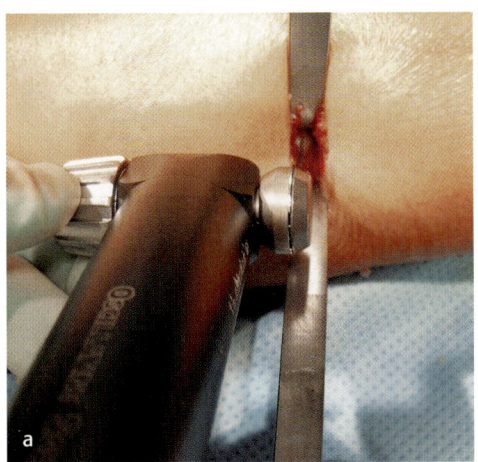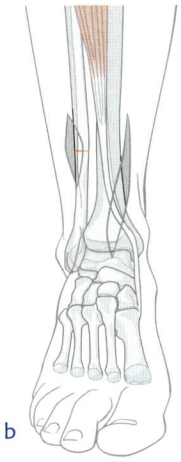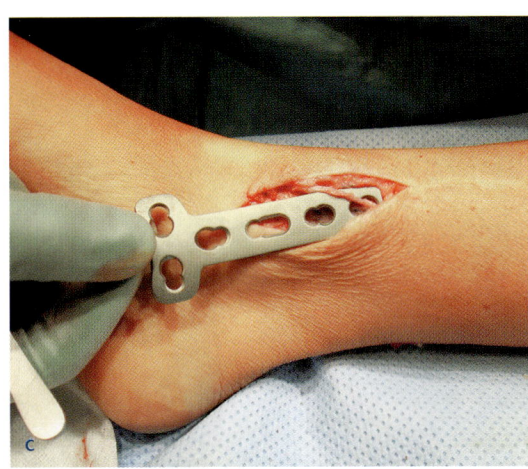

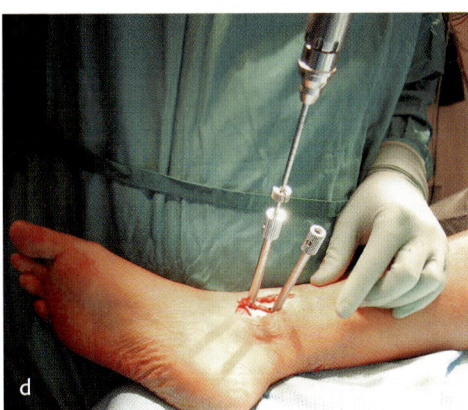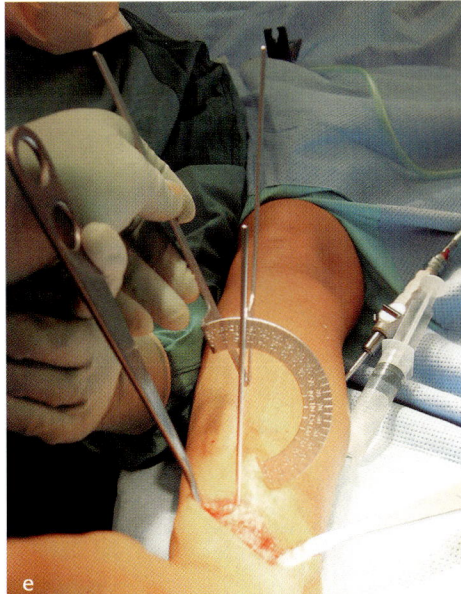

Fig 15-10a–k Distal rotational osteotomy of the tibia.

a–b Transverse osteotomy of the fibula in the mid to lower diaphyseal third protected by two Hohmann retractors.

c   Slide insertion of the plate fixator.

d   After positioning the implant, bicortical predrilling of the two distal screw holes through the drill sleeve.

e   Marking the correction angle with two threaded wires inserted proximal and distal to the osteotomy with the help of the sterile goniometer.

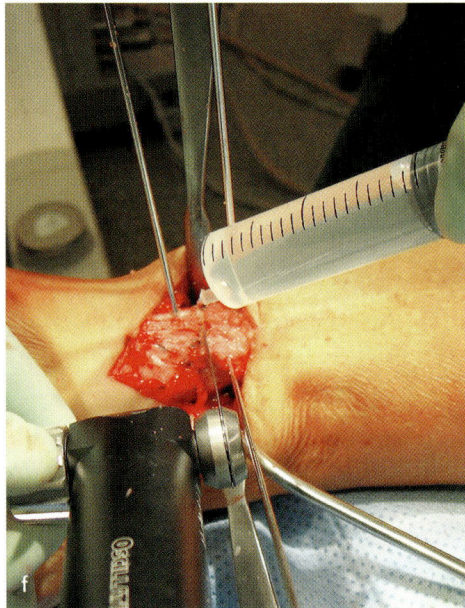

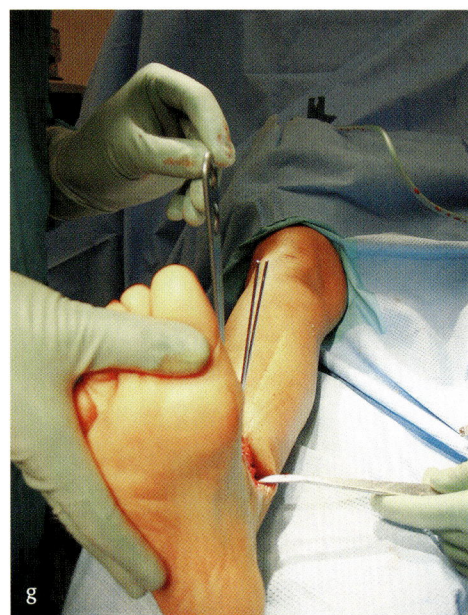

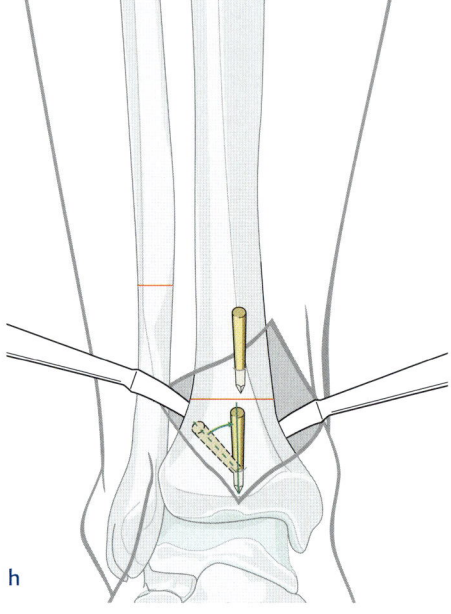

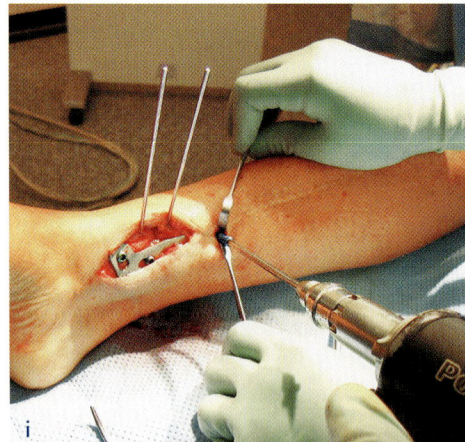

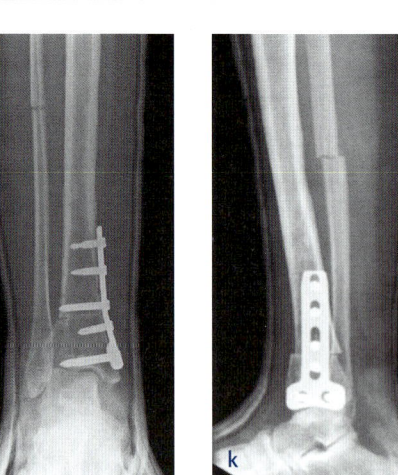

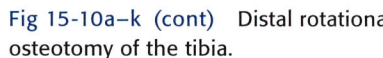

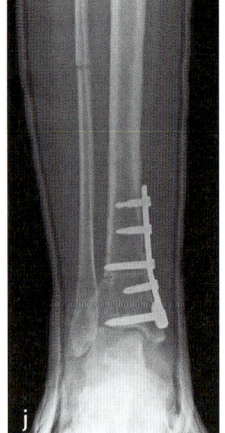

Fig 15-10a–k (cont)   Distal rotational osteotomy of the tibia.

f   Transverse osteotomy of the distal tibia with the oscillating saw under continuous irrigation.

g–h Rotation of the distal segment until the two K-wires are parallel and the correction angle is achieved (clinical image and schematic representation).

i   The T-plate is stabilized distally with two bicortical and one monocortical locking head screw. Monocortical locking bolts stabilize the plate shaft and may be inserted through small stab incisions.

j–k Postoperative x-rays in two planes after distal rotational osteotomy of the tibia and application of a plate fixator showing correct alignment with the talus centered in the ankle mortise.

Postoperative management

The postoperative regime for change of dressing and postoperative radiological follow-up is the same as for proximal tibial rotational osteotomy. Partial loading on underarm crutches at 10 kg bodyweight should be adhered to until the end of the sixth week after surgery. Range of motion at the upper ankle joint must not be restricted.

8   Results

The results achieved after derotational osteotomy as a treatment for torsion deformities of the lower extremities are encouraging. In 1999 Tönnis and Heinecke [14] reported a significant improvement in function after acetabular osteotomy for pathological anteversion of the acetabulum. Good outcomes were also achieved after pelvic osteotomy in twelve patients with isolated retroversion of the acetabulum greater than 15° [10]. Other studies also showed that intertrochanteric femoral rotational osteotomy for pathological ante- or retroversion of the femur brought pain relief and improved mobility of the hip [11, 20].

In their investigation in 1996, Server et al [16] recorded 88.5% good to excellent outcomes in a sample of 35 patients who required rotation correction to treat chronic patellofemoral subluxation as a consequence of pathological external torsion of the tibia. There was residual instability of the patella in only 5% of the cases. Cook et al [6] reported similarly good results for proximal tibial rotational osteotomy with additional tuberosity translation and lateral retinaculum release in 1990.

The authors have conducted a follow-up study to evaluate the outcomes of 23 limbs of 18 patients treated with a proximal tibial derotational osteotomy for isolated external tibial torsion [26]. Preoperatively, external tibial torsion averaged 50° (range 42–68°). All limbs were corrected about 15–20° of internal rotation. 14 proximally ascending biplanar osteotomies, six distally descending biplanar osteotomies and three complete transverse tuberosity osteotomies were performed (see Fig 15-4). Perioperative complications were reported in only one patient, in whom malunion resulted in an abnormal slope that required revision surgery. Fixation stability was excellent; there was no loss of correction in the other patients. Bone healing time was normal in all patients but one; delayed bone healing was seen in only one case, which consolidated uneventfully within five months postoperatively. No neurovascular (peroneal nerve) complications were observed.

Preoperatively, most common complaints were knee pain (19 knees) and patellar subluxations (13 knees). Average duration of complaints was 14 years (range 6–22 years). Seven patients had previous surgeries (eg, arthroscopies, extensor apparatus realignment) which did not relieve the complaints.

Average follow-up was 50 months (range 20–92 months). On follow-up examination, a little less than half of the patients still had some mild degree of discomfort of the knee not interfering with activities of daily life. However, in all but one patient the pain was significantly less than preoperatively. Persistent but less frequent patellar subluxations were reported by three patients (4 knees). 14 out of 18 patients said that they would have the surgery performed again.

In young patients with torsion malalignment syndrome, femoral distal external rotational osteotomy combined with internal rotational osteotomy to correct the proximal or distal

tibia led to a significant reduction in knee symptoms and to a pedographically assessed improved gait pattern [7]. Distal rotational osteotomy of the tibia with and without fibular osteotomy has proven to be a safe and effective method of treating pathological torsion of the tibia [22, 27].

9   Possible complications

Complications that may occur in association with femoral and tibial rotation surgeries include over- and undercorrection as a consequence of poor preoperative planning, malalignment in the frontal or sagittal planes, secondary loss of correction and implant fatigue failures, fractures, and postoperative infections [6, 16, 20, 22, 28–30]. Ischemic femoral head necrosis after intertrochanteric femoral osteotomy has been reported [28, 29].

Reports of complications after rotational osteotomy of the lower extremity refer mainly to pediatric surgery. For information on possible neurovascular complications see subchapter 5.3 "Soft-tissue problems and neurovascular structures" and the relevant literature [1].

■ Symptomatic torsion deformities of the lower extremity require careful clinical examination and precise evaluation of the radiological findings. Rotational osteotomy is only indicated after exact localization and definition of the deformity. Osteotomy should be performed at the level of the pathology taking the neurovascular structures, the tibial tuberosity trochlea distance (TT-TG), and the healing potential of the bone into account. Application of internal plate fixators to stabilize the correction guarantees high primary mechanical stability, permits functional postoperative rehabilitation, and reduces the risk of secondary correction loss.

10   Bibliography

[1] **van Heerwaarden RJ, van der Haven I, Kooijman M, et al** (2003) Derotation osteotomy for correction of congenital rotational lower limb deformities in adolescents and adults. *Surg Tech Orthop Traumatol;* 55-575-A-10: 10.

[2] **Teitge R A** (1994) Treatment of complications of patellofemoral joint surgery. *Op Techn Sports Med;* 2:317–334.

[3] **Crane L** (1959) Femoral torsion and its relation to toeing-in and toeing-out. *J Bone Joint Surg Am;* 41(3):421–428.

[4] **Shtarker H, Volpin G, Stolero J, et al** (2002) Correction of combined angular and rotational deformities by the Ilizarov method. *Clin Orthop Relat Res;* 402:184–195.

[5] **Staheli LT, Corbett M, Wyss C, et al** (1985) Lower-extremity rotational problems in children. Normal values to guide management. *J Bone Joint Surg Am;* 67(1):39–47.

[6] **Cook TD, Price N, Fischer B, et al** (1990) The inwardly pointing knee. An unrecognized problem of external rotational malalignment. *Clin Orthop Relat Res;* 260:56–60.

[7] **Delgado ED, Schoenecker PL, Richmm, et al** (1996) Treatment of severe torsional malalignment syndrome. *J Pediatr Orthop;* 16(4):484–488.

[8] **Staheli LT** (1989) Torsion--treatment indications. *Clin Orthop Relat Res;* 247:61–66.

[9] **Eckhoff DG** (1994) Effect of limb malrotation on malalignment and osteoarthritis. *Orthop Clin North Am;* 25(3):405–414.

[10] **Reynolds D, Lucas J, Klaue K** (1999) Retroversion of the acetabulum. A cause of hip pain. *J Bone Joint Surg Br;* 81(2):281–288.

[11] **Tönnis D, Heinecke A** (1991) Diminished femoral antetorsion syndrome: a cause of pain and osteoarthritis. *J Pediatr Orthop;* 11(4):419–431.

[12] **Winquist R A** (1986) Closed intramedullary osteotomies of the femur. *Clin Orthop Relat Res;* 212:155–164.

[13] **Cheng JC, Chan PS, Chiang SC et al** (1991): Angular and rotational profile of the lower limb in 2630 Chinese children. *J Pediatr Orthop* 11:154–161.

[14] **Tönnis D, Heinecke A** (1999) [Decreased acetabular anteversion and femur neck antetorsion cause pain and arthrosis. Part 1: Statistics and clinical sequelae and part 2: Etiology, diagnosis and therapy. *Z Orthop Ihre Grenzgeb;* 137(2):153–167. German.

[15] **Yagi T, Sasaki T** (1986) Tibial torsion in patients with medial-type osteoarthritic knees. Clin Orthop Relat Res; 213:177–182.

[16] **Server F, Miralles RC, Garcia E, et al** (1996) Medial rotational tibial osteotomy for patellar instability secondary to lateral tibial torsion. *Int Orthop;* 20(3):153–158.

[17] **Paley, D** (2002) Rotation and Angulation -Rotation Deformities. Length Considerations. Hardware and Osteotomy Considerations. *Paley D (ed) Principles of deformity correction.* Berlin Heidelberg, Springer-Verlag, 235–410.

[18] **Dejour H, Walch G, Nove-Josserand L, et al** (1994) Factors of patellar instability: an anatomic radiographic study. *Knee Surg Sports Traumatol Arthrosc;* 2(1):19–26.

[19] **Herzenberg JE, Smith JD, Paley D** (1994) Correcting torsional deformities with Ilizarov's apparatus. *Clin Orthop Relat Res;* 302:36–41.

[20] **Payne LZ, DeLuca PA** (1994) Intertrochanteric versus supracondylar osteotomy for severe femoral anteversion. *J Pediatr Orthop;* 14(1):39–44.

[21] **Lundberg A, Svensson OK, Bylund C, et al** (1989) Kinematics of the ankle/foot complex--Part 3: Iinfluence of leg rotation. *Foot Ankle;* 9(6):304–309.

[22] **Manouel M, Johnson LO** (1994) The role of fibular osteotomy in rotational osteotomy of the distal tibia. *J Pediatr Orthop;* 14(5):611–614.

[23] **Schrock RD Jr** (1969) Peroneal nerve palsy following derotation osteotomies for tibial torsion. *Clin Orthop Relat Res;* 62:172–177.

[24] **Kempf I, Grosse A, Abalo C** (1986) Locked intramedullary nailing. Its application to femoral and tibial axial, rotational, lengthening and shortening osteotomies. *Clin Orthop Relat Res;* 212:165–173.

[25] **Rüedi TP, Murphy WM** (2000) AO Principles of Fracture Management. New York, Stuttgart: Thieme Verlag.

[26] **Koning P, Hoefnagels E, van Heerwaarden RJ** (2008) Proximal tibia derotation osteotomies for patellofemoral pain and instability. In preparation.

[27] **Dodgin DA, De Swart RJ, Stefko RM, et al** (1998) Distal tibial/fibular derotation osteotomy for correction of tibial torsion: review of technique and results in 63 cases. *J Pediatr Orthop;* 18(1):95–101.

[28] **Staheli LT, Clawson DK, Hubbard DD** (1980) Medial femoral torsion: experience with operative treatment. *Clin Orthop Relat Res;* 146:222–225.

[29] **Svenningsen S, Apalset K, Terjesen T, et al** (1989) Osteotomy for femoral anteversion. Complications in 95 children. *Acta Orthop Scand;* 60(4):401–405.

[30] **Staheli LT** (1987) Rotational problems of the lower extremities. *Orthop Clin North Am;* 18(4):503–512.

Authors   Koen C Defoort, Gijs G van Hellemondt, Ronald J van Heerwaarden, Alex E Staubli

16   Total knee arthroplasty after osteotomy around the knee

1   Introduction

High-tibial osteotomy (HTO) and distal femur osteotomy (DFO) are widely applied and accepted methods for treating unicompartimental osteoarthrosis, especially in the relatively young and active patient. When the deformity is mainly situated in the proximal tibia, HTO is an excellent technique with good pain relief and improvement in function. Even though an initial success rate of 80–90% has been reported, results are known to deteriorate with time to 45–65% at 7–10 years [1–4]. Insall reported that, because of progression of the osteoarthritis, 23% of HTO patients will be converted to a total knee arthroplasty (TKA) [5]. The average time to conversion to TKA is approximately 6 years. Therefore, an HTO should be seen as a means to gain time before the need for a TKA arises. For DFO the probability of survival at 10 years was reported 64% as determined with use of the Kaplan-Meier method [6].

Progression of the osteoarthritic process is the most common cause for failure of an osteotomy around the knee. Apart from this progression, there are other causes of failure, eg, severe over- or undercorrection, nonunion at the osteotomy site, and infection. There are several mechanisms to enhance the accuracy of the osteotomy procedure—and prevent over- or undercorrection—like intraoperative control mechanisms, computer-assisted surgery, and angular stable fixation devices.

This chapter will provide a practical guide for the management of a patient with persisting or recurring pain after an osteotomy around the knee, requiring secondary total knee arthroplasty (TKA). It is fundamental for a successful outcome to understand the indications and contraindications of such a procedure. TKA after osteotomy confronts the surgeons with a set of technical peculiarities, which will be discussed.

2   Preoperative work-up

In the management of a patient with persistent or recurring pain after an osteotomy around the knee, a good history and clinical examination is of paramount importance.

2.1   History

A complete history should include a characterization of the pain. Were the patient's symptoms completely resolved after the correction? How long was the pain-free interval? Where is the localization of the pain? The pain history should also exclude other sources of pain, like referred pain from a hip or spinal disease. Bursitis or tendinitis are other sources of

extraarticular knee pain. An intraarticular injection with a local anesthetic might help to differentiate knee pain from other sources of pain. The most important questions are summarized in Table 16-1.

Also of great importance is the patient's social history. Are there issues of litigation or worker's compensation? Mont et al have already described factors such as worker's compensation, reflex sympathetic dystrophy, pain relief of less than 1 year, multiple surgical procedures, and employment as a laborer to be associated with poor outcome [7].

History of patient with failed osteotomy around the knee

Are there previous knee surgeries other than HTO/DFO

Is there a history of previous knee joint infection?

Was there a previous knee injury?

What is the character of the pain?

Is the pain localized in the knee or are there other sources of pain?

Table 16-1   Important questions in the history of a patient with failed knee osteotomy.

Clinical examination

Gait pattern: antalgic—varus/valgus thrust—Trendelenburg ?

Alignment: varus/valgus—flexion/recurvatum—rotational deformity?

Soft tissues: scars—previous infection—reflex sympathetic dystrophy?

Knee effusion?

Ligament laxity?

Examine hip and spine.

Table 16-2   Clinical examination of a patient with failed knee osteotomy.

2.2   Clinical examination

The patient's gait pattern, eg, antalgic gait or a varus thrust during stance, must be observed (Fig 16-1). A Trendelenburg gait points to hip pathology.

The alignment of the lower limb in stance and the soft-tissue condition including previous scars must be examined. Knee effusion suggests intraarticular pathology. The ligamentous laxity of the knee must be evaluated. In knees with a gross malalignment or gross laxity a more constrained type of knee prosthesis might be indicated. Also, one should check for signs of reflex sympathetic dystrophy, like skin temperature changes and skin hypersensitivity (Table 16-2).

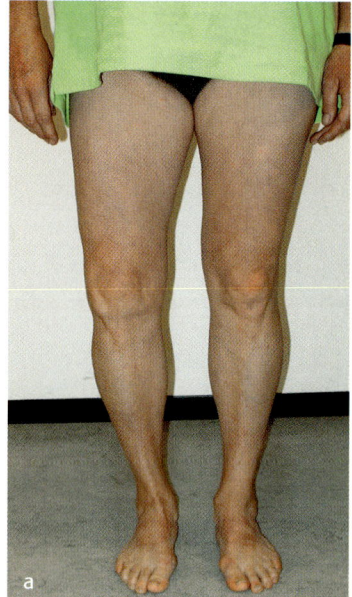
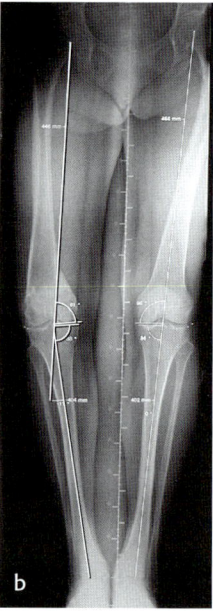

Fig 16-1a–b   Patient with failed overcorrected DFO. Due to the 11° varus leg alignment a varus thrust is found during stance and gait.

2.3   Radiographical work-up

Radiographic examination includes standard standing AP and lateral x-rays, and also a patellar view (Fig 16-2a–c, 16-3a–b). The alignment of the leg is evaluated on a weight-bearing AP view of the whole leg (Fig 16-2d, 16-3c). In case of suspected ligamentous laxity, stress x-rays can be of use.

On the AP x-ray the progression of the osteoarthritic process can be assessed. At the site of the osteotomy the presence of a nonunion must be excluded. One should look for the presence of (stress) fractures. The tibiofemoral alignment should be assessed regarding over- or undercorrection. Also the presence of hardware should be noted.

Other radiographic peculiarities will be discussed in the surgical technique section.

It is important to determine whether the radiographic findings can explain the patient's complaints.

2.4   Further preoperative diagnostics

Occasionally, other investigations can be of use. A scintigraphy may be useful in the diagnosis of infection or neoplasm. Magnetic resonance imaging (MRI) can be employed if an intraarticular pathology is suspected, eg, loose bodies or a meniscal tear. In case of a suspected nonunion, a computed tomography (CT) scan is mandatory.

In case of a suspected infection, a blood analysis with ESR, CRP, and white cell count can be useful. A culture sample should also be obtained either through tissue biopsy or knee punction aspirate. Infection scan (eg, IgG, labelled white blood cells) is indicated in these cases.

Diagnostic arthroscopy can be useful to determine the progression of the osteoarthritis or to treat meniscal tears or loose bodies.

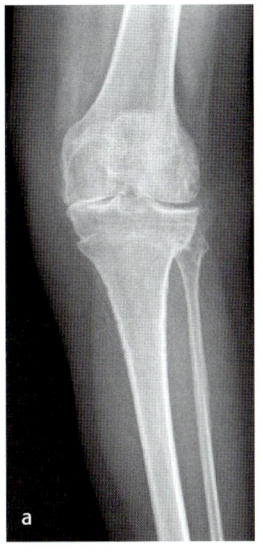
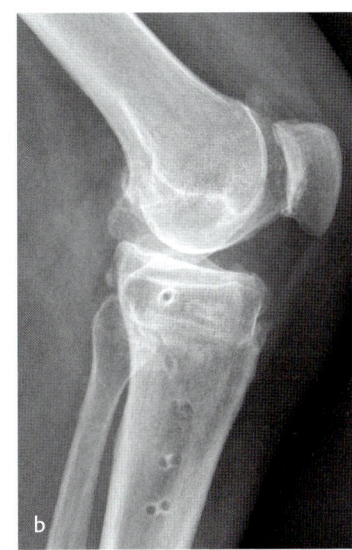
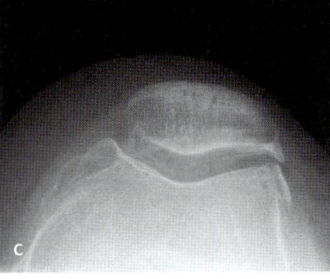
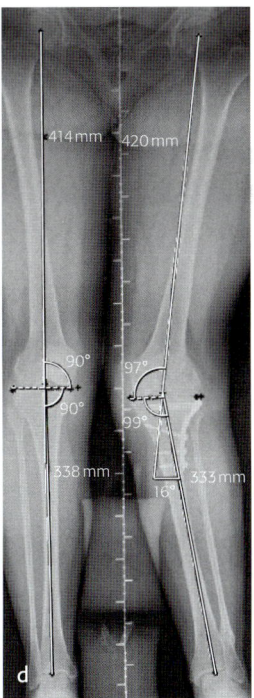

Fig 16-2a–d Standard radiographic work-up in a patient with valgus overcorrection after HTO.
a   AP view.
b   Lateral view.
c   Patella view.
d   Weight-bearing view of both legs.

If patient history, physical examination, and radiographic views do not explain the patient's symptoms, a conservative management is preferable. Only when conservative treatment is insufficient and the patient's complaints are caused by progressive degenerative changes, TKA is indicated.

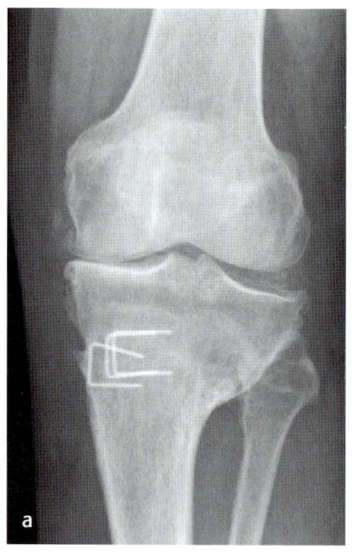

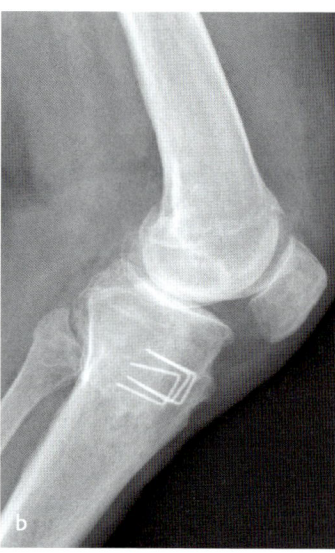

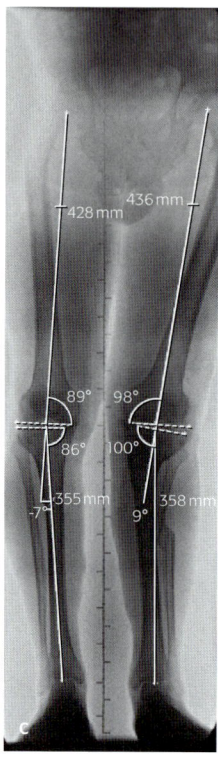

Fig 16-3a–c   Severe valgus overcorrection after HTO due to malunion. Note the oblique joint line and the reduced tibial slope.
a–b AP and lateral view.
c   Weight-bearing view of both legs.

3   Surgical considerations

The aims of a TKA after failed osteotomy around the knee are to obtain pain-relief and to restore the neutral alignment of the lower limb. Restoration of a neutral alignment means creating a tibiofemoral mechanical axis of 180° with a horizontal joint line that is perpendicular to the femoral and tibial mechanical axis. Achieving these neutral axes and angles poses the main problem after osteotomy around the knee.

In case of severe valgus or varus alignment, one can expect problems in properly balancing the knee prosthesis. It might be necessary to use more constrained implants with (offset) stems or to retension the ligaments in these cases. In case of extreme extraarticular deformities, revision osteotomy to correct the extraarticular deformity can be performed prior to the TKA procedure. For planning of the surgical strategy a flowchart might be helpful. In Table 16-3 a flowchart on decision making for TKA after HTO is shown.

Decision making

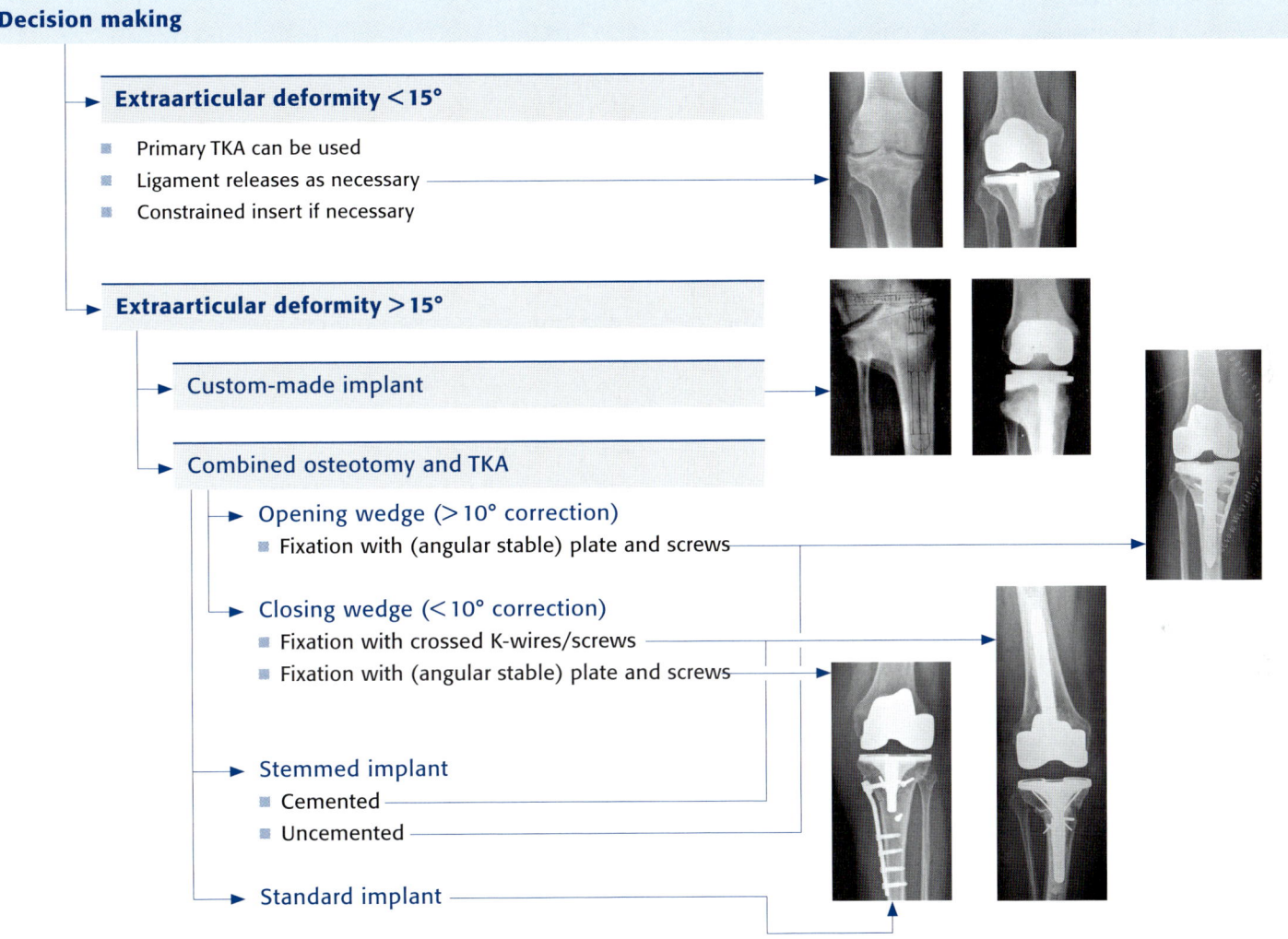

► **Extraarticular deformity < 15°**

- ▪ Primary TKA can be used
- ▪ Ligament releases as necessary
- ▪ Constrained insert if necessary

► **Extraarticular deformity > 15°**

► Custom-made implant

► Combined osteotomy and TKA

  ► Opening wedge (> 10° correction)
    ▪ Fixation with (angular stable) plate and screws

  ► Closing wedge (< 10° correction)
    ▪ Fixation with crossed K-wires/screws
    ▪ Fixation with (angular stable) plate and screws

  ► Stemmed implant
    ▪ Cemented
    ▪ Uncemented

  ► Standard implant

Table 16-3 Flowchart of decision making for TKA with or without osteotomy based on deformity after failed HTO and choice of implant.

3.1   Preoperative planning

On examining the knee x-rays after HTO, three major changes in anatomy can be observed. In the AP plane there is an increased valgus angulation of the proximal tibia, resulting in a higher medial plateau and a relative "depression" of the lateral plateau (Fig 16-4). Due to this anatomy the lateral plateau cannot be used as a reference for the position of the joint line. Especially after a lateral closed-wedge HTO, the tibial shaft is displaced medially relative to the tibial plateau. This step-off can cause problems in fitting the tibial component since the tibial stem might interfere with the lateral cortex. In cases of severe depression of the lateral tibial plateau, tibial augments are needed.

On the lateral x-ray, a decrease of the tibial slope or even a negative slope after HTO is sometimes observed (Fig 16-5). This influences balancing of the TKA, as the tibial slope needs to be corrected to obtain equal flexion and extension gaps.

The third anatomical change is the presence of a patella infera in up to 80% of patients after HTO (Fig 16-6) [8–10]. This causes problems with exposure and impingement of the patella against the prosthesis.

In the authors' experience these anatomical changes are not present or are less severe after a medial open-wedge HTO than after lateral closed-wedge techniques. Patella infera is less frequent when combining a medial open-wedge HTO with a distal tuberosity osteotomy [11].

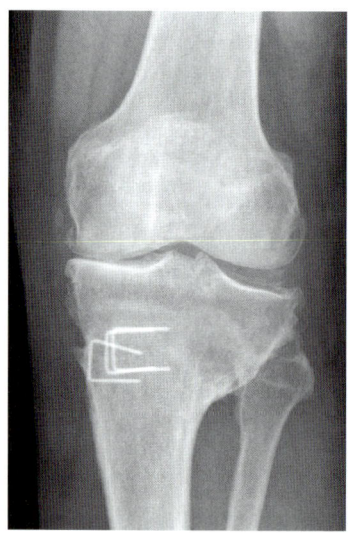

Fig 16-4   Severely overcorrected proximal tibia after HTO requiring large medial resection and minimal lateral resection of the tibial plateau for the TKA.

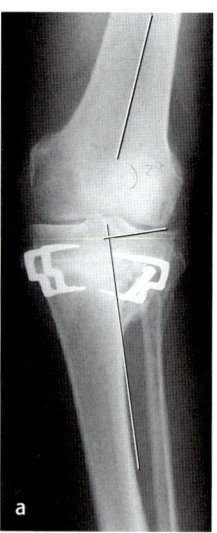

Fig 16-5a–b   Negative tibial slope in the sagittal plane after HTO which requires a high amount of resection in the posterior aspect of the tibial plateau.

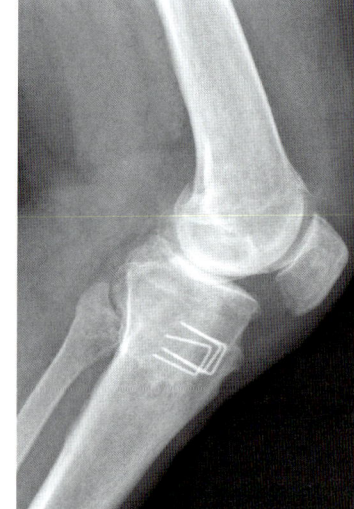

Fig 16-6   Patella infera after lateral closed-wedge HTO.

On AP x-rays the tibial resection needs to be planned to restore the anatomical tibial angle. Note that in most cases there is a very small amount of bone to be resected on the lateral side (see Fig 16-4, Fig 16-7). In case of a severe lateral depression, augments should be used rather than lowering the level of resection and consecutively the joint line. Also consider the medial displacement of the tibial shaft. One might need to place the component slightly more medial to prevent impingement of the tibial stem on the lateral cortex. In order to prevent overhang on the medial side sometimes a smaller tibial metal back must be implanted. In cases of severe medial displacement

one might use offset stems or even a custom-made prosthesis. On the lateral x-ray the tibial slope and patellar height must be evaluated to be aware of overresection of the posterior tibia and difficulties of exposure.

The presence of gross ligament laxity might need for more constrained implants or ligament retensioning procedures. Open- wedge procedures can be used to tighten the ligaments at the medial or lateral side of the knee, obviating the need for a constrained implant (Fig 16-8).

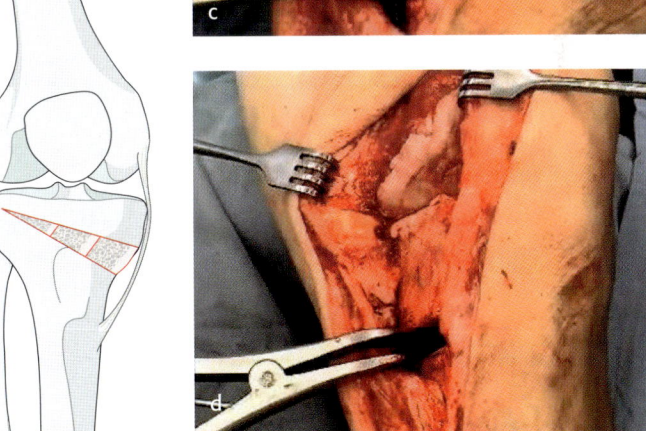

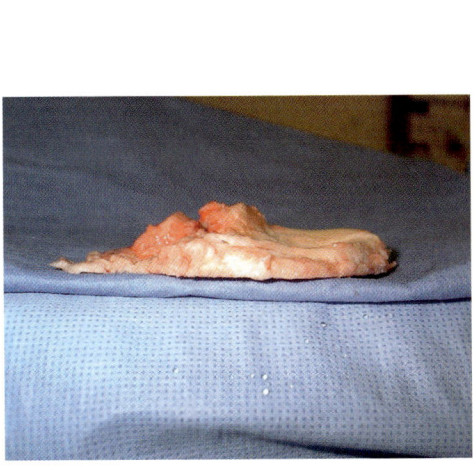

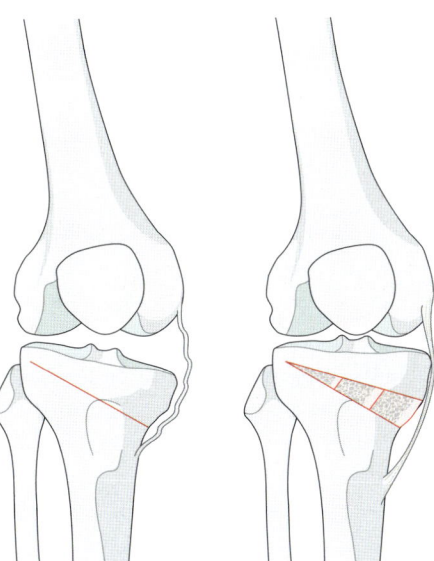

Fig 16-7   Asymmetrical tibial resection for TKA after HTO. Minimal resection of the lateral plateau (left), high amount of resection at the medial aspect (right).

Fig 16-8a–d   Open-wedge HTO used to retension a slack medial collateral ligament (MCL). Schematic presentation (a–b) and clinical pictures (c–d) before and after tensioning of the MCL.

3.2   Surgical approach

The condition of the soft tissues and previous incisions must be examined carefully. Higher complication rates in TKA after HTO due to soft-tissue problems have been described [12]. Previous transverse incisions at the proximal tibia can be ignored, and a standard midline incision can be used. If there still is hardware in place laterally, a full-thickness flap should be created to reach this hardware and remove it. If a previous lateral longitudinal incision is present, a more medial incision should be used for the TKA. A medial approach has been described by Krackow for these cases [13]. However, it is recommended to leave a skin bridge of 7cm between both incisions, in order to preserve the blood supply of the soft tissues. Alternatively, the surgeon can use the previous lateral incision and perform a lateral approach employing a tibial tubercle osteotomy.

It is advisable to remove any hardware that was used to stabilize the osteotomy first and to implant the prosthesis as a secondary procedure. In the authors' experience this results in less hematoma and fewer postoperative wound complications.

Because of soft-tissue scarring, the subperiostal exposure of the tibia might be more difficult and the dissection might be more demanding than in a primary procedure.

As there is a high incidence of patella infera after HTO, patellar eversion might be difficult during TKA surgery. In order to facilitate exposure and to avoid avulsion of the patellar ligament a release of the lateral retinaculum should be performed prior to the eversion maneuver. If this is not sufficient, a quadriceps snip technique or a quadriceps V-Y plasty should be considered. The authors prefer performing the tibial tubercle osteotomy with a step-cut to obtain adequate exposure [14].

3.3   Tibial resection

Especially after lateral closed-wedge HTO, the reduction of bone stock in the proximal tibia is significant. Therefore, special care should be taken when performing the tibial resection. The least possible amount of bone should be resected to obtain an adequate surface for fixation of the tibial component.

As already stated, the goal is to achieve a component that is placed perpendicular to the mechanical axis of the tibia. As the anatomy of the proximal tibia is altered after HTO, the tibial cut should be performed using an extramedullary reference system. It is not uncommon to have a minimal tibial resection on the lateral side, opposite to the normal situation in a varus knee (see Fig 16-7). In case of a severe lateral depression, the defect can either be bone-grafted or augmented with a unilateral tibial wedge.

Attention must be paid to the rotational alignment of the tibial component. In a primary TKA procedure the rotational alignment can be referred to the tibial tubercle. In some HTO patients the tibial tuberosity has been displaced and therefore is a less reliable landmark for rotational alignment. In these cases it is more accurate to refer to the anterior tibialis tendon or the second ray of the foot for correct rotational alignment of the tibial component.

If the tibial slope is altered and especially when a negative slope has been induced by the HTO, the tibial resection is impeded. A minimal resection anteriorly might result in a large resection posteriorly as one tries to overcorrect a negative slope. This results in a relatively oversized flexion gap, causing flexion instability of the prosthesis (Fig 16-9). In these cases the flexion-extension gap mismatch must be corrected by either increasing the distal femoral resection and using a thicker insert or by upsizing the femoral component and inserting posterior femoral augments. The first technique results in a raise of the joint line, which might lead to patella impingement, especially in the presence of patella infera.

In case of a medial displacement of the tibial shaft, the stem of the tibial component might impinge on the lateral cortex counteracting proper positioning of the implant. This can be avoided by positioning the component slightly more medial and by using a smaller component. In total knee systems providing an anatomical metal back (ie, left and right version), a right component can be implanted in a left knee and vice versa (Fig 16-10). Offset stems present an alternative method. In case of a severe shift of the shaft, the use of a custom-made implant might be indicated. In these cases especially, preoperative templating of the tibial component is of utmost importance.

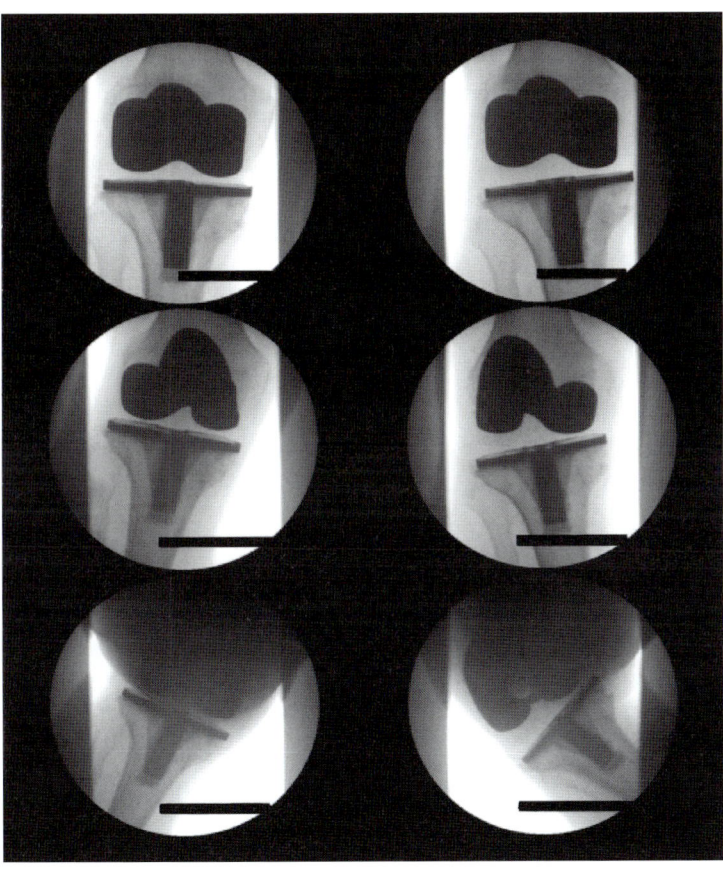

Fig 16-9   Fluoroscopic imaging of a flexion instability after TKA.

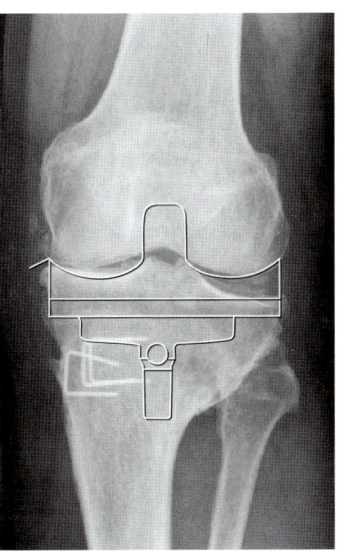

Fig 16-10   Planning insertion of a right-sided tibia component in a left knee after HTO using a total knee system with an anatomical metal back.

3.4 Ligament balancing

The distal femoral cut should be performed after the tibial cut has been made according to the above mentioned recommendations. After the distal femoral cut has been accomplished, it is possible to assess ligament balance in extension using either spacer blocks or a ligament tensioner. As the knee is balanced in extension, the obtained extension gap can be referred to the flexed position using spacer blocks or a ligament tensioner. This spacer block or tensioner can be used to guide the rotation of the femoral component, thus creating a balanced flexion gap.

In case of severe imbalance, ie, medial ligament laxity, it is recommended to apply a more constrained prosthesis or combine the TKA procedure with an additional osteotomy, especially if severe overcorrection to a valgus angle of more than 15° is present (see Fig 16-8, Table 16-3). With a normal medial ligament complex and a tight lateral complex common ligament balancing ("pie-crusting" of the posterolateral capsule and/or iliotibial tract) can be performed.

Due to postoperative scarring and possible alteration of the joint-line height and tibial slope, the posterior cruciate ligament function is less predictable after HTO. Therefore, it is recommended to use a posterior stabilized implant to provide anterior-posterior stability. When a cruciate-retaining implant is chosen, one should carefully asses the posterior cruciate ligament (PCL) function.

3.5 Patella function

As already mentioned, patella infera might be present after HTO depending on the osteotomy technique. This can be due to the fact that the tibial tubercle has been distalized in relation to the tibiofemoral joint line. Also, the patellar ligament can become scarred and contracted after the osteotomy procedure resulting in a patella infera. When performing a TKA after HTO, the patella function must be carefully evaluated during the procedure in order to recognize patellofemoral problems.

Apart from difficulties in exposure and the risk of avulsion of the patellar ligament, a patella infera can have a negative effect on the postoperative function of the knee prosthesis. A low patella might contact the tibial insert before it engages the femoral groove, resulting in a limited flexion and pain.

When considering patella resurfacing, it is advisable to choose a small patella implant and to place it as proximal in the retropatellar surface as possible. The distal patella can be thinned to create sufficient space for the anterior rim of the tibial insert. Care should be taken not to damage the patellar tendon. Another technique is to prepare the anterior edge of the tibial insert, as is already done in some total knee systems. In severe cases, the tibial tubercle should be proximalized or the patella tendon should be lengthened. However, these procedures are often disappointing since they do not restore the patella height completely. It is not advisable to distalize the femoral component using augments as this creates an unphysiological joint-line height and abnormal knee kinematics.

3.6 TKA combined with osteotomy

Osteotomies can be used as a separate procedure prior to TKA (Fig 16-11). The advantages of a two-stage approach are that the osteotomy and the TKA as single surgeries are standard procedures, and as less exposure is needed, the risk of infection is smaller. After realignment of the leg, however, the osteoarthritic symptoms may significantly decrease and postpone a TKA for a long time. The disadvantages of a two-stage procedure are the necessity of two anesthesiologic procedures, two rehabilitation periods, and two times the risks of infection, thrombosis etc. Performing the osteotomy as the second part of the two-stage procedure is only necessary if surgery attempted to correct a deformity by TKA failed to correct leg alignment sufficiently.

Combining osteotomy and TKA in a single surgery is a demanding procedure that potentially prevents the disadvantages of the two-stage procedure. Furthermore, it is easier to preserve the joint level, the PCL and the patellar height. In open-wedge osteotomies the gap can be filled with resected bone of the bone cuts for the TKA.

As already mentioned above, in cases with severe varus or valgus overcorrection after HTO it is often difficult to achieve a proper ligament balance. In case of an extraarticular deformity of 15° or more, the authors recommend a combination procedure of TKA surgery with corrective osteotomy. The different options are presented in Table 16-3. Stability of the osteotomy can be obtained by using crossed K-wires or screws and by bypassing the osteotomy with the tibial stem of the prosthesis. However, the authors prefer to use a plate or plate fixator and to implant a standard tibial component (Fig 16-12).

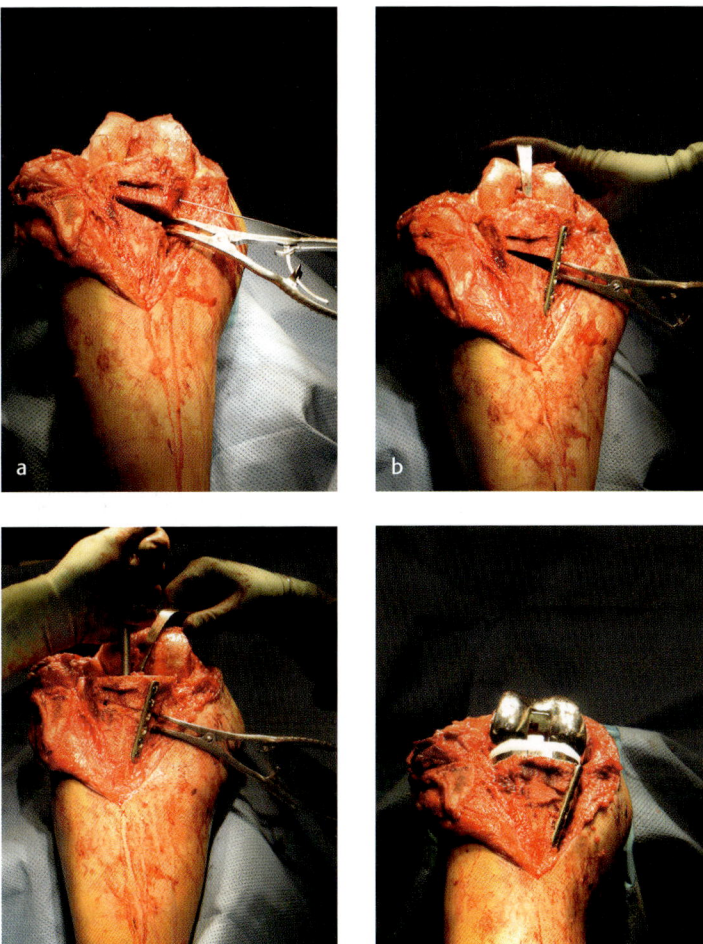

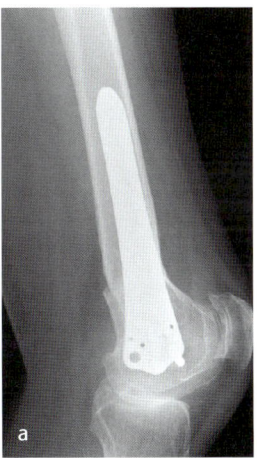 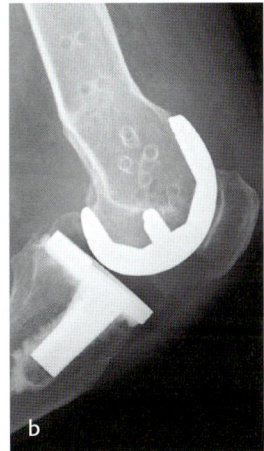

Fig 16-11a–b   Two-stage procedure in a patient with knee osteoarthritis and extension deficit.
a   First an extending DFO was performed.
b   After consolidation and plate removal a TKA was implanted.

Fig 16-12a–d   Combined corrective osteotomy and TKA.
a   Medial open-wedge osteotomy of the proximal tibia to restore physiological alignment.
b   Fixation of the osteotomy with an angular stable plate.
c   Preparation of the tibial plateau for the prosthesis. Note the bone graft in the osteotomy gap.
d   Result after osteotomy and TKA.

For femoral deformities, the same recommendations (see Table 16-3) apply as mentioned before. It should be noted that after osteotomy fixation intramedullary guiding of the sawguides is often prohibited (Fig 16-13). Extramedullary guiding using fluoroscopy and leg alignment rods, specific extramedullary guiding devices or computer navigation will help the surgeon to implant the TKA.

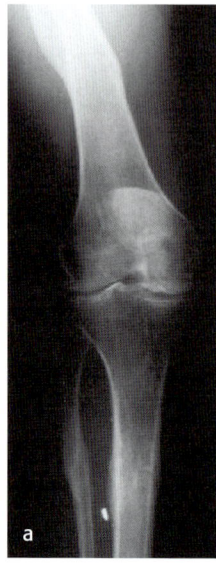 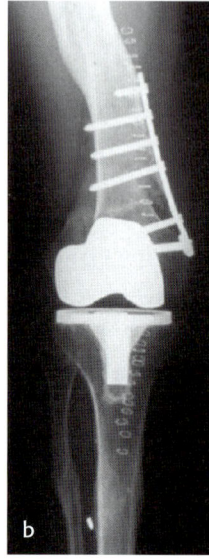 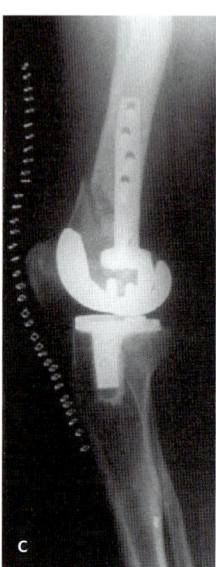

Fig 16-13a–c   Combined biplane DFO and TKA in a patient with a malunited femur fracture requiring translation and varization of the distal femur.
a   Preoperative AP view.
b   Postoperative AP view.
c   Postoperative lateral view.

4   Results of TKA after osteotomies around the knee

There is still controversy in the literature regarding to the outcome of TKA after HTO. Several reports state that the results of postosteotomy TKA are comparable to the results after primary TKA [15–17]. Other studies indicate poorer results for TKA after HTO and show results comparable to revision TKA [7, 10, 18]. A recent long-term study by Haslam et al has shown slightly poorer results of TKA after HTO with more patients with poor results and also less knee flexion compared to a matched control group [19]. An interesting conclusion in this study is that patients who do poorly after HTO might also do less well after TKA.

The problem in comparing these studies is the fact that the patient group that underwent a proximal tibial osteotomy is a very heterogeneous group. Patients that require a TKA after HTO range from cases with minimal malalignment with mild progression of the osteoarthritis to cases with severely over- or undercorrected limbs with multiple scars and soft-tissue problems. It is obvious that a patient with TKA will show better outcome than a patient with severe varus or valgus malalignment and ligament instability.

For TKA after DFO the reports also differ from a technically more difficult procedure [20, 21] as no technical difficulties encountered [6, 22]. The use of an extramedullary guide to check alignment was recommended.

For combined osteotomies and TKA very little can be found in the literature. Open-wedge HTO performed simultaneously with TKA for varus osteoarthritis had a good result in four patients with osteoarthritis and severe congenital knee varum deformity of more than 15° [23]. As correction of the extraarticular deformity was obtained by the osteotomy, in none of the cases was it necessary to perform extensive soft-tissue release or advancement to restore alignment. It was concluded that TKA associated with high-tibial valgization osteotomy seems to be a technically satisfying alternative in patients with osteoarthritis and severe congenital varus deformity of the tibia. At mean follow up of 46 months simultaneous femoral osteotomy and TKA for severe extraarticular femoral deformity resulted in a series of eleven patients in a mean function score of 81 and mean knee score of 87, respectively, according to the "Knee society score" [24]. It was concluded that this combined procedure is technically difficult but effective and it was recommended that the femoral osteotomy site be secured with a plate or a locked intramedullary nail, depending on the location of the deformity.

5   Bibliography

[1]   **Coventry MB** (1985) Upper tibial osteotomy for osteoarthritis. *J Bone Joint Surg Am;* 67(7):1136–1140.

[2]   **Coventry MB, Ilstrup DM, Wallrichs SL** (1993) Proximal tibial osteotomy. A critical long-term study of eighty-seven cases. *J Bone Joint Surg Am;* 75(2):196–201.

[3]   **Healy WL, Riley LH Jr** (1986) High tibial valgus osteotomy. A clinical review. *Clin Orthop Relat Res;* 209:227–233.

[4]   **Ritter MA, Fechtman RA** (1988) Proximal tibial osteotomy. A survivorship analysis. *J Arthroplasty;* 3(4):309–311.

[5]   **Insall JN, Joseph DM, Msika C** (1984) High tibial osteotomy for varus gonartrosis. A long-term follow-up study. *J Bone Joint Surg Am;* 66(7):1040–1048.

[6]   **Finkelstein JA, Gross AE, Davis A** (1996) Varus osteotomy of the distal part of the femur. A survivorship analysis. *J Bone Joint Surg Am;* 78(9):1348–1352.

[7]   **Mont MA, Antonaides S, Krackow KA, et al** (1994) Total knee arthroplasty after failed high tibial osteotomy. A comparison with a matched group. *Clin Orthop Relat Res;* 299:125–130.

[8]   **Amendola A, Rorabeck CH, Bourne RB, et al** (1989) Total knee arthroplasty following high tibial osteotomy for osteoarthritis. J Arthroplasty; 4 Suppl:S11–S17.

[9]   **Scuderi GR, Windsor RE, Insall JN** (1989) Observations on patellar height after proximal tibial osteotomy. *J Bone Joint Surg Am;* 71(2):245–248.

[10]   **Windsor RE, Insall JN, Vince KG** (1988) Technical considerations of total knee arthroplasty after proximal tibial osteotomy. *J Bone Joint Surg Am;* 70(4):547–555.

[11]   **Gaasbeek RD, Sonneveld H, van Heerwaarden RJ, et al** (2004) Distal tuberosity osteotomy in open wedge high tibial osteotomy can prevent patella infera: a new technique. *Knee;* 11(6):457–461.

[12]   **Jackson M, Sarangi PP, Newman JH** (1994) Revision total knee arthroplasty. Comparison of outcome following primary proximal tibial osteotomy or unicompartmental arthroplasty. *J Arthroplasty;* 9(5):539–542.

[13] **Krackow KA, Holtgrewe JL** (1990) Experience with a new technique for managing severely overcorrected valgus high tibial osteotomy at total knee arthroplasty. *Clin Orthop Relat Res;* 258:213–224.

[14] **van den Broek CM, van Hellemondt GG, Jacobs WC, et al** (2006) Step-cut tibial tubercle osteotomy for access in revision total knee replacement. *Knee;* 13(6):430–434.

[15] **Staeheli JW, Cass JR, Morrey BF** (1987) Condylar total knee arthroplasty after failed proximal tibial osteotomy. *J Bone Joint Surg Am;* 69(1):28–31.

[16] **Haddad FS, Bentley G** (2000) Total knee arthroplasty after high tibial osteotomy: a medium-term review. *J Arthroplasty;* 15(5):597–603.

[17] **Bergenudd H, Sahlström A, Sanzén L** (1997) Total knee arthroplasty after failed proximal tibial valgus osteotomy. *J Arthroplasty;*12(6):635–638.

[18] **Katz MM, Hungerford DS, Krackow KA, et al** (1987) Results of total knee arthroplasty after failed proximal tibial osteotomy for osteoarthritis. *J Bone Joint Surg Am;* 69(2):225–233.

[19] **Haslam P, Armstrong M, Geutjens G, et al** (2007) Total knee arthroplasty after failed high tibial osteotomy: long-term follow-up of matched groups. *J Arthroplasty;* 22(2):245–250.

[20] **Beyer CA, Lewallen, DG, Hanssen AD** (1994) Total knee arthroplasty following prior osteotomy of the distal femur. *Am J Knee Surg;* 7:25–30.

[21] **Nelson CL, Saleh KJ, Kassim RA, et al** (2003) Total knee arthroplasty after varus osteotomy of the distal part of the femur. *J Bone Joint Surg Am;* 85-A(6):1062–1065.

[22] **Cameron HU, Park YS** (1997) Total knee replacement after supracondylar femoral osteotomy. *Am J Knee Surg;* 10(2):70–71.

[23] **Zanone X, Ait Si Selmi T, Neyret P** (1999) [Total knee prosthesis and simultaneous corrective tibial osteotomy, for osteoarthritis and severe congenital tibia varum deformity.] *Rev Chir Orthop Réparatrice Appar Mot;* 85(7):749–756. French.

[24] **Lonner JH, Siliski JM, Lotke PA** (2000) Simultaneous femoral osteotomy and total knee arthroplasty for treatment of osteoarthritis associated with severe extra-articular deformity. *J Bone Joint Surg Am;* 82(3):342–348.

Authors   Mellany Galla, Philipp Lobenhoffer

17   Management of complications after high-tibial open-wedge osteotomy

1   Introduction

Performing open-wedge osteotomies around the knee the surgeon must be aware of complications that might occur and must be able to manage these.

2   Overcorrection

Overcorrection in medial open-wedge osteotomy of the proximal tibia leads to a severe valgus deformity of the leg. Besides being cosmetically unacceptable, this overcorrection results in overload of the lateral joint compartment.

2.1   Treatment

If overcorrection is noticed intraoperatively, the osteotomy gap can be corrected by adjusting the arthrodesis spreader before inserting the angular locking head screws ("fine tuning" see chapter 9 "High-tibial open-wedge valgization osteotomy with plate fixator", subchapter 5 "Surgical technique", and Fig 9-12).

If the overcorrected axis is observed during the early postoperative phase (week 1–12), it is sufficient to remove the distal locking bolts and to readjust the osteotomy opening. In some cases it might be necessary to remove the granulation tissue in the osteotomy gap (see chapter 12 "Radiological examination of bone healing after open-wedge tibial osteotomy", subchapter 2 "Evaluation of magnetic resonance imaging") and to weaken the lateral hinge with a 2.0 mm drill to close the osteotomy. After achieving the correct alignment the distal fixation of the TomoFix implant should be performed with bicortical locking head screws. The authors would like to stress that in primary high-tibial open-wedge osteotomy (HTO) procedures monocortical locking head screws should be used in holes 2–4 of the plate fixator. If a revision is necessary, the opposite cortex is intact and secure fixation can be achieved using bicortical locking head screws (Fig 17-1).

During the late postoperative phase (after 3 months) bone healing of the osteotomy has advanced. In order to achieve correction the implant must be removed completely and a medial closed-wedge osteotomy of the proximal tibia is necessary. The result is stabilized by reapplying the TomoFix fixator with bicortical locking head screws (Fig 17-2).

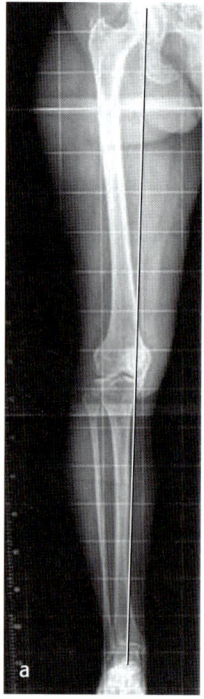
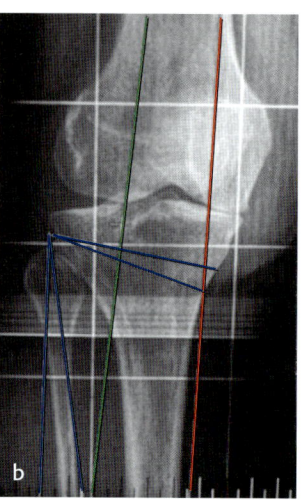
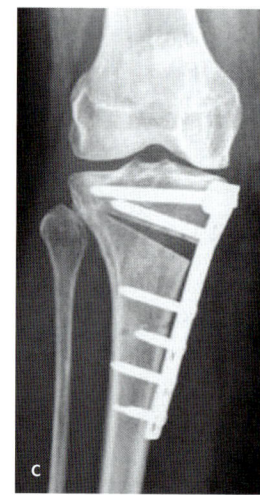
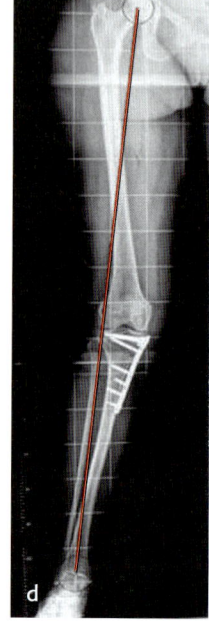
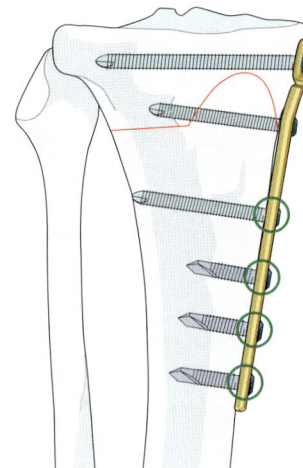
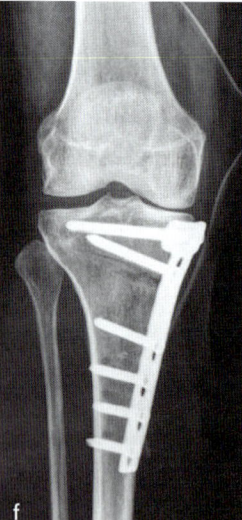

Fig 17-1a–f   Patient with early recognized valgus overcorrection after high-tibial open-wedge osteotomy (HTO).

a   Preoperative long-leg weight-bearing x-ray showing the varus deformity of the leg (red line = mechanical weight-bearing line).

b   Preoperative planning (red line = preoperative mechanical axis, green line = corrected axis, blue lines = corrective osteotomy).

c   Postoperative AP x-ray after HTO.

d   Postoperative long-leg weight-bearing x-ray showing the severe overcorrection to a valgus deformity (red line = mechanical weight-bearing line).

e   The four distal locking head screws are removed in order to achieve the recorrection.

f   Postoperative x-ray after recorrection osteotomy. The plate is fixed with four distal bicortical locking head screws.

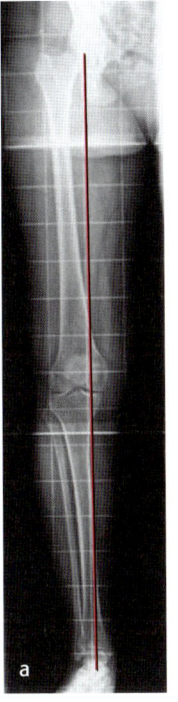
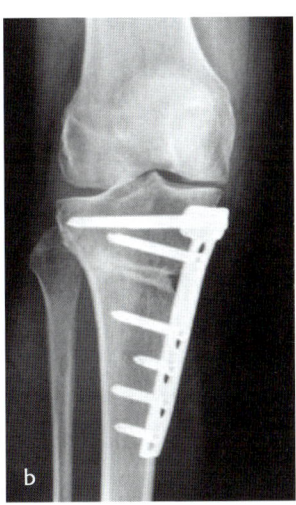
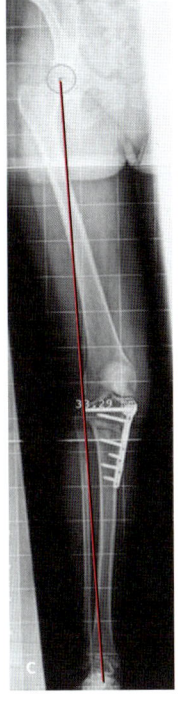
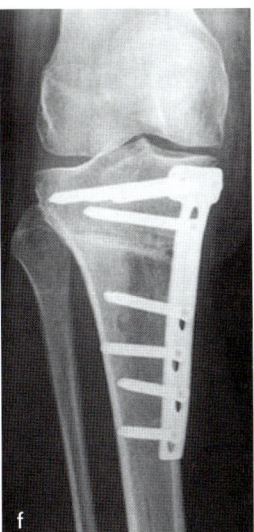
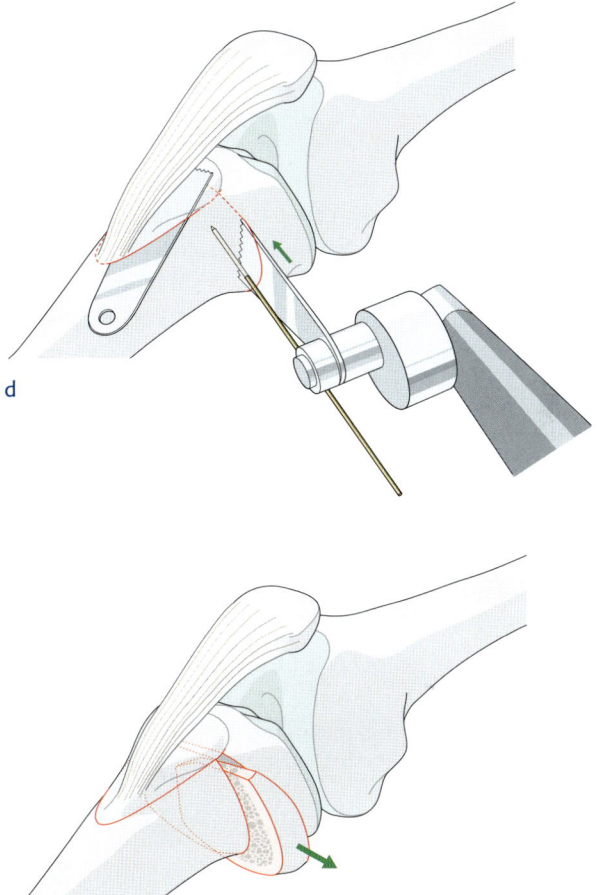

Fig 17-2a–f   Patient with valgus overcorrection several months after HTO.

a   Preoperative long-leg weight-bearing x-ray showing the varus deformity of the leg (red line = mechanical weight-bearing line).

b   Postoperative AP x-ray after HTO.

c   Postoperative long-leg weight-bearing x-ray showing the severe overcorrection to a valgus deformity. The mechanical axis (red line) runs through the lateral compartment.

d–e Due to advanced bone healing a medial closed-wedge osteotomy needs to be performed. A bone wedge is removed and the osteotomy is closed.

f   Postoperative x-ray after recorrection osteotomy. The plate is fixed with four distal bicortical locking head screws.

2.2 Prevention

Valgus overcorrection can be prevented by correct preoperative planning. Projection errors on the long-leg weight-bearing x-ray must be detected, eg, the patella must be located exactly anteriorly on the AP view, the knee must be completely extended and both legs should be loaded symmetrically. Before planning the osteotomy on the radiographic workstation, a calibration must be performed. The problem of asymmetric joint line opening must be addressed either by graphic or mathematical correction (see chapter 5 "Detailed planning algorithm for high-tibial osteotomy"). To assess the mechanical axis during surgery, the entire leg should be draped including the iliac crest. Before stabilizing the osteotomy the corrected axis must be checked using a metal rod (see chapter 9 "High-tibial open-wedge valgization osteotomy with plate fixator", **Fig 9-14**) which is more reliable than an electrocautery cable. Correct positioning in full extension of the knee joint and exact rotation is mandatory in this step. Weight bearing should be simulated to balance asymmetric joint opening by applying dosed axial pressure to the foot sole.

- Drape entire leg and iliac crest.
  Be aware of projection errors.
  Correct asymmetric joint opening during preoperative radiographic planning.
  Check corrected mechanical axis intraoperatively.
  Simulate weight bearing and balance asymmetric joint opening.

3 Joint-line obliquity

When correcting the leg axis of the lower limb, the osteotomy must be performed at the site of the deformity. Frontal plane correction can result in a pathological alteration of the joint line if the correction is not performed at the site of the bone deformity (**Fig 17-3**), therefore leading to subsequent loading on an incorrectly aligned plane (see chapter 14 "Double osteotomies of the femur and the tibia", **Fig 14-2a–c**). Studies have proven that only 31% of patients with varus degeneration of the knee have osseous deformity at the tibia, whereas in 59% the varus deformity is located at the femur and in 10% both femur and tibia are affected [1]. This means that in 69% of patients with varus deformity a valgization osteotomy at the tibia will result in an unphysiological joint line. Joint-line divergence more than 8° from normal will definitively lead to significant pain under loading [2, 3] and must be avoided under all circumstances.

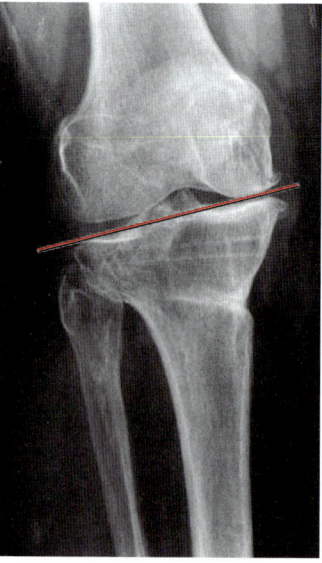

Fig 17-3 Unphysiological oblique joint line (red line) due to incorrect preoperative planning.

3.1   Prevention

All axes and angles must be analyzed preoperatively (see chapter 1 "Physiological axes of the lower limb", Fig 1-1a–b) and the level of the deformity must be identified (see chapter 1 "Physiological axes of the lower limb", Fig 1-5a–b). In case of a pathological mechanical lateral distal femoral angle (mLDFA >87 ± 3°) and a normal mechanical medial proximal tibial angle (mMPTA = 87 ± 3°) the correction must be performed at the femoral side as a lateral closed-wedge osteotomy.

■ Analyze all axes and angles preoperatively. Identify level of deformity.

4   Pseudarthrosis

Pain under loading at the lateral proximal tibia more than 8 weeks after a medial high-tibia open-wedge osteotomy indicates delayed bone healing respectively pseudarthrosis. During the early postoperative phase a callus at the lateral hinge in the AP x-ray points to instability due to delayed healing (Fig 17-4) and the CT scan shows a fracture of the lateral hinge.

During the later postoperative phase, pseudarthrosis becomes evident when the osteotomy gap remains radiolucent, and the CT scan will show a failure of bone regeneration in the gap (Fig 17-5). If the osteotomy has been performed with the correct technique and the TomoFix plate has been applied correctly the implant will not fail. However, the pain will persist over several months.

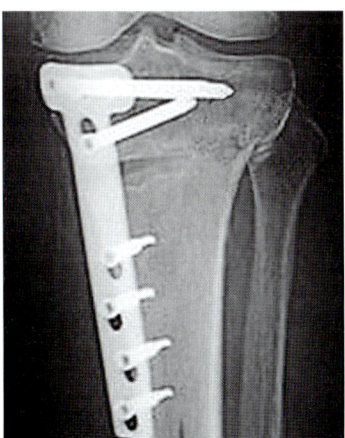

Fig 17-4   Fracture and callus formation of the lateral hinge 6 weeks after HTO.

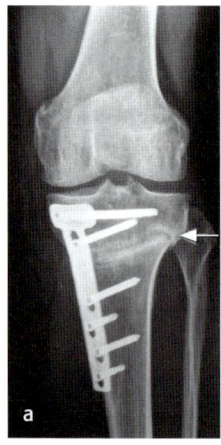

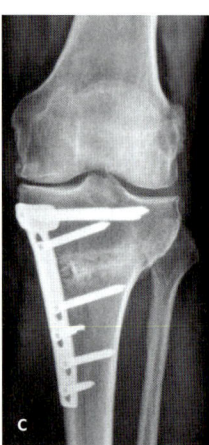

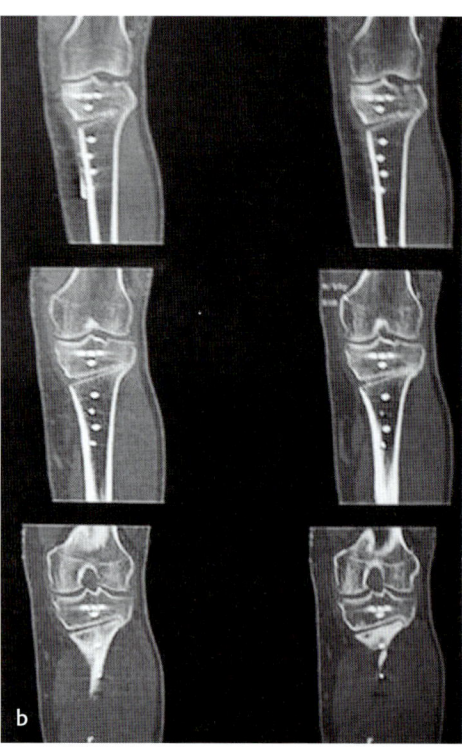

Fig 17-5a–c Patient with persisting pain at the lateral proximal tibia 6 months after HTO due to pseudarthrosis.
a   AP x-ray. Note the fracture of the lateral hinge and the bone resorption (arrow).
b   CT scan showing failure of bone healing in the osteotomy gap.
c   AP x-ray after revision surgery with curettage of the osteotomy gap and insertion of cancellous bone graft harvested from the iliac crest.

4.1   Treatment

If delayed bone healing or pseudarthrosis is suspected, autogenous bone grafting from the iliac crest is indicated. Cancellous bone is harvested from the iliac crest via a cortical window. It is not necessary to use bone wedges and to remove any cortical bone. A limited exposure of the osteotomy is made and the osteotomy gap is curetted. The cancellous bone graft is inserted especially in the posterior aspect of the osteotomy. In the authors' experience the osteotomy will then heal uneventfully in 4–6 weeks. Weight bearing is allowed postoperatively.

4.2   Prevention

Bone healing is impaired by heat during sawing. Therefore it is advisable to rinse the saw blade continuously during the bone cut, eg, with a 24G cannula attached to an arthroscopy pump. It is important to apply the plate fixator correctly: the distance holders must be inserted and temporary lag screw should be used to compress the lateral hinge by pulling the distal osteotomy segment towards the plate fixator. Potential fissures within the lateral bone bridge are brought under elastic preload and any distraction on the lateral side is eliminated (see chapter 9 "High-tibial open-wedge valgization osteotomy with plate fixator", Fig 9-17). In the sagittal plane the surfaces of the ascending osteotomy of the tibial tuberosity must have close contact. This is usually achieved by extension of the leg during the fixation of the implant. This maneuver induces compression on the ascending osteotomy plane. In rare cases the authors use a reduction clamp to adapt these bone planes temporarily. If the anterior biplanar cut is performed distally, it is mandatory to compress the two planes by one or two small-fragment lag screws (Fig 17-6). In this situation the extensor apparatus will distract the osteotomy planes postoperatively when the patient regains his quadriceps function, and there is a risk of pseudarthrosis caused by the motion between the two segments.

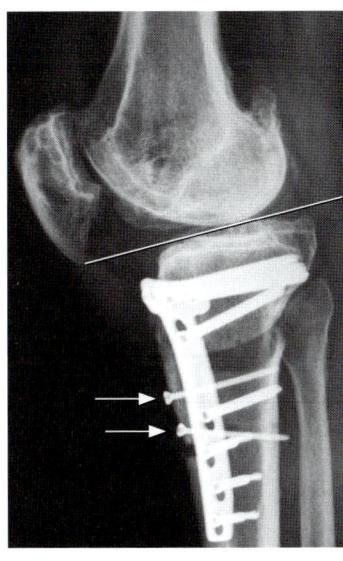

Fig 17-6   Descending osteotomy of the tibial tuberosity fixed with two small-fragment lag screws (arrows).

Care must be taken in patients with nicotine abuse (see chapter 9 "High-tibial open-wedge valgization osteotomy with plate fixator", subchapter 11 "Nicotine abuse"). Open-wedge osteotomies should not be performed in smokers. If the surgeon wishes to apply open-wedge osteotomy despite nicotine abuses, we recommend insertion of an autogenous bone graft even in small osteotomy gaps.

- Rinse saw blade.
  Use distance holders and temporary lag screw.
  Watch ascending part of the osteotomy.
  Care in patients with nicotine abuse.

5   Infection and hematoma

As in all surgical procedures, early and late infections might occur postoperatively after high-tibial osteotomy.

5.1   Treatment

Early infections (postoperative week 1–3) are usually correlated with hematoma and can be treated by evacuation of the hematoma, debridement, jet lavage, and eventually antiseptic lavage. It is important to clean the space under the plate fixator since the implant does not press on bone and there is dead space beneath. A local antibiotic carrier may be applied. The implant is left in situ. Repetitive lavage procedures may be necessary. In the authors' experience most cases will heal uneventfully with this regime and implant removal will not be necessary except in selected cases.

A late postoperative infection (after 3 months) is more difficult to treat. First of all, the bone healing of the osteotomy needs to be assessed either on plain x-rays or CT scans. If the osteotomy is consolidated, the implant is removed and the revision procedure described above for the early infections is performed. In case the osteotomy has not healed yet, the implant should be left in situ during revision as described above. If the infection cannot be cured, the implant must be removed during a second revision and a medial external fixator must be applied to stabilize the osteotomy until sufficient bone healing is achieved (Fig 17-7).

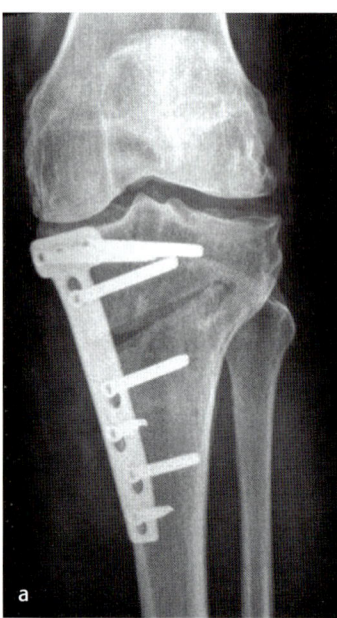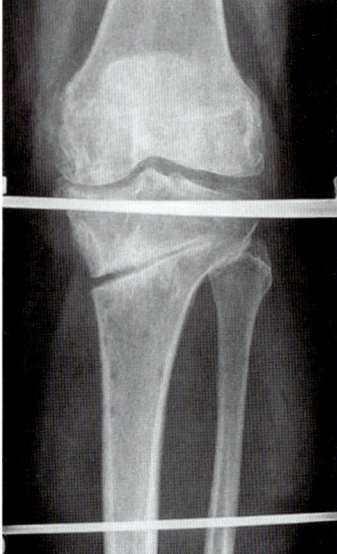

Fig 17-7a–b   Patient with infection 8 weeks after HTO.
a   AP x-ray 8 weeks after HTO procedure. The osteotomy has not
     healed yet.
b   During revision surgery including debridement, jet lavage, and
     antiseptic lavage a medial external fixator was applied and the plate
     was removed.

5.2   Prevention

Hematoma can be prevented by accurate hemostasis. The osteotomy gap should be covered with a collagen fleece (see chapter 9 "High-tibial open-wedge valgization osteotomy with plate fixator", subchapter 5 "Surgical technique"). An overflow drain that exits proximally should be inserted. The skin must be closed meticulously to ensure sufficient coverage of the implant. The authors advise against the use of skin staples because of the thin soft tissues in this area. Any wound that shows secretion after the third postoperative day should be surgically revised.

- Accurate hemostasis and skin closure.
  Do not use skin staples.
  Insert collagen fleece to cover osteotomy gap.
  Use an overflow drain.
  Revise secretion from wounds early.

Implant failure occurs very seldomly with the angular stable TomoFix plate when the correct technique has been followed. In the authors' experience with over 15,000 medial open-wedge osteotomies less than five fixator failures were seen. When failure occurs with other implants, the plate should be removed, the osteotomy should be reperformed and an angular stable plate fixator should be applied including autogenous bone grafting (**Fig 17-8**).

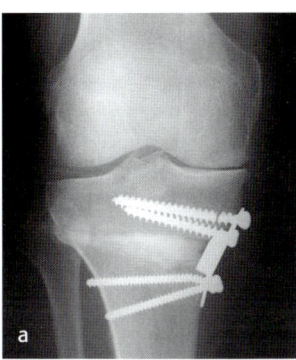

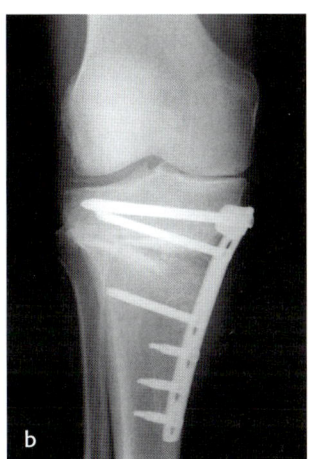

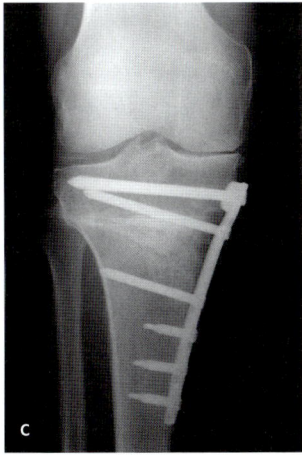

Fig 17-8a–c   Patient with implant failure after HTO with a spacer plate.
a   AP x-ray. Two screws of the spacer plate are broken.
b   Radiographic result 6 weeks after revision surgery with removal of the spacer plate, refixation with an angular locked plate fixator (TomoFix) and cancellous bone grafting.
c   AP view after 12 weeks. Bone healing has progressed rapidly.

6.1   Prevention

Implant failure using the TomoFix plate can be avoided by inserting a locking bolt into hole D (**Fig 17-9**) in all cases since this increases the torsional and bending stiffness of the plate significantly (see chapter 7 "Principles of angular stable fixators", subchapter 3 "Application of angular stable plate fixators in open-wedge tibial osteotomy"). We would like to stress that due to the unidirectional locking principle of the TomoFix implants, the predrilling must be performed with the drill sleeve mounted exactly in the threads of the plate hole, and the locked head screws must be inserted in the correct direction to ensure optimum holding strength. The limited torque screwdriver should be used in any case to lock the screws in the plate, or implant removal will become extremely difficult.

- Insert locking head screw into hole D in all cases.
  Use drill sleeve for pre-drilling and mount drill sleeve and screws with great accuracy in the threads of the plate hole.
  Use limited torque screwdriver to lock the screws.

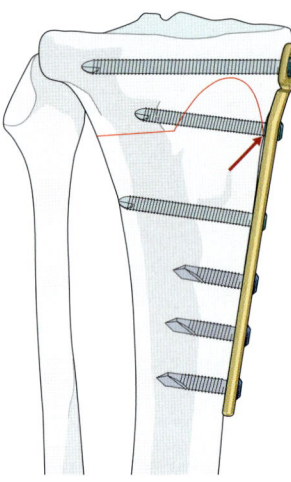

Fig 17-9   A locking head screw must be inserted in plate hole D (red arrow) in all cases to increase stiffness of the implant and to prevent implant breakage.

7   Bibliography

[1]   **Strecker W, Keppler P** (2002) [Analysis and correction of leg deformities. 1: Analysis.] *Unfallchirurg;* 105(9):811–829. German.

[2]   **Strecker W, Keppler P** (2002) [Analysis and correction of leg deformities. 2: Correction.] *Unfallchirurg;* 105(10):901–917. German.

[3]   **Keppler P, Suger G, Kinzl L, et al** (2002) [Osteotomies in malalignment of the lower extremities.] *Chirurg;* 73(10):982–989. German.

Authors   Robert A Teitge, Ronald J van Heerwaarden

18   Osteotomies for failed osteotomies around the knee

1   Introduction

A failed osteotomy can be defined as an osteotomy of which the goal aimed at preoperative planning of correction was not reached as a result of intraoperative or postoperative complications. Although osteotomies around the knee are the most frequently performed osteotomies in the limbs, only few references can be found in the literature regarding failed osteotomies treated with recorrective osteotomies [1–3]. The complications that may lead to a failed high-tibial osteotomy (HTO) have been described [4–8]. In a previous publication the complications in a large series of high-tibial osteotomies were presented [4]. These complications include the following:

(1)   Undercorrection
(2)   Overcorrection
(3)   Fracture of the medial cortex with opening medially in closed-wedge HTO
(4)   Nonunion or delayed union
(5)   Loss of fixation
(6)   Peroneal palsy
(7)   Instability
(8)   Shortening
(9)   Recurvatum
(10) Flexion contracture
(11) Late plateau fracture
(12) Rotational deformity
(13) Fibular nonunion
(14) Patellar problems
(15) Infection
(16) Deep venous thrombosis

Almost all of these complications also apply to the distal femur osteotomies (DFO).

Malunited osteotomies may have been caused by many [1–5, 7–12] of the above mentioned complications. Depending on the time of presentation of a patient with a malunited osteotomy around the knee, there still may be the possibility of performing a recorrective osteotomy. However, in some patients joint-preserving surgery is not possible and the deformity can only be corrected during total knee replacement. The treatment of total knee replacement after osteotomies is discussed in chapter 16 "Total knee arthroplasty after osteotomy around the knee". In this chapter the bone corrections of failed osteotomies around the knee by recorrective osteotomies is described.

2   Causes of failure

Malunited osteotomies can result from inaccurate preoperative planning, intraoperative technical errors, and failure of fixation of the osteotomy [5]. In addition, mistakes can be made in postoperative rehabilitation jeopardizing the stability after the correction and the bone healing (eg, functional aftertreatment and early full weight bearing after osteotomies fixed with less stable implants).

Preoperative planning of osteotomies is mandatory and has been discussed in chapter 4 "Basic principles of osteotomies around the knee" and chapter 5 "Detailed planning algorithm for high-tibial osteotomy". Failed osteotomies due to inadequate planning may be caused by planning of correction in the wrong bone, ie, a HTO is performed to correct varus in a leg where (part of) the deformity is localized in the femur. Deformity

Clinical applications

analysis included as part of the preoperative planning will help to find whether the correction should be performed in the femur or the tibia or in both (Fig 18-1) [9, 10].

Another cause of failure that can be attributed to preoperative planning is the increased joint-line obliquity (see also chapter 14 "Double osteotomies of the femur and the tibia").

Intraoperative technical errors include imprecise intraoperative measurements, improper use of instrumentation, and errors in performing bone cuts [5]. In addition, specific pitfalls of the osteotomy technique chosen may increase the risk of failure. Imprecise intraoperative measurements can be reduced by using fluoroscopy, rigid alignment bars, fluoroscopy grids, rulers and goniometers, or use of computer navigation during surgery. Improper use of instrumentation and errors in performing bone cuts must be attributed to the skills of the surgeon. Saw guides that allow for guiding of the saw blade have been suggested as very helpful in improving the accuracy of bone cuts. Instead of K-wires used as guides for bone cuts it is advisable to use drill bits as these maintain a straight line through the bone as opposed to K-wires.

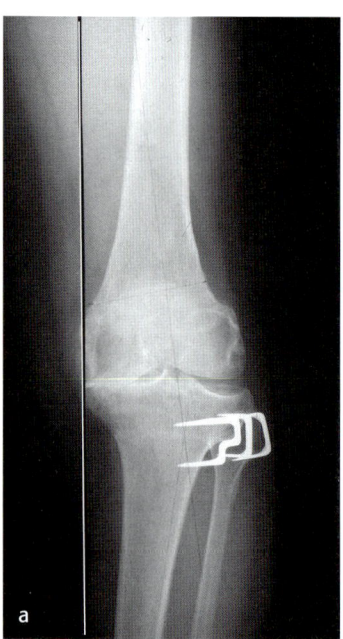
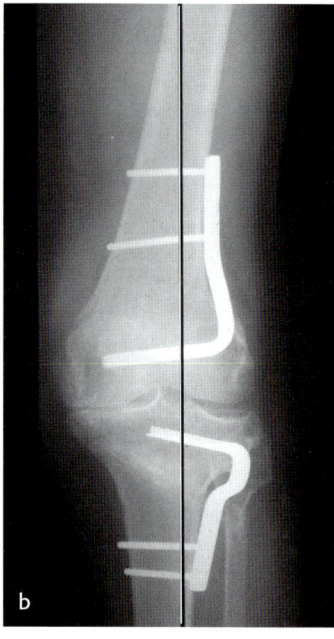
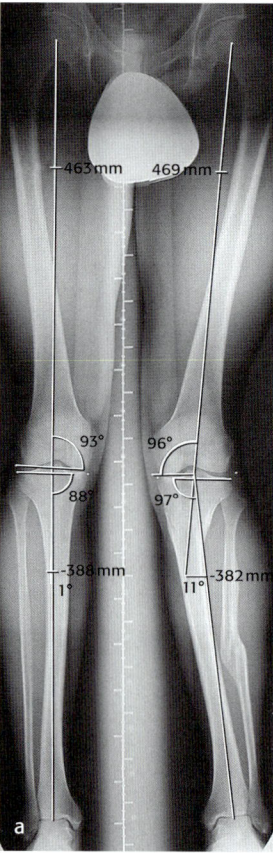
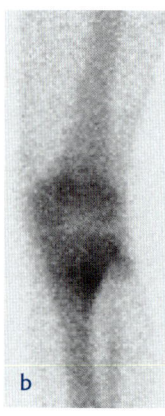

Fig 18-2a–b Weight-bearing full-leg view (a) and scintigram (b) of a patient complaining of lateral tibial head bone pain after overcorrected HTO. The hotspot in the lateral tibial head identifies overloading of subchondral and metaphysial bone.

Fig 18-1a–b
a   Failed lateral closed-wedge HTO due to wrongful preoperative planning not identifying distal femur varus deformity and insufficient staple fixation.
b   A double osteotomy combining lateral closed-wedge DFO and lateral closed-wedge HTO fixed with blade plates aimed for recorrecting the leg alignment.

Specific pitfalls of the closed-wedge as well as open-wedge osteotomy techniques are frequently found as causes of failure. In closed-wedge osteotomies the position of the hinge point near the contralateral cortex is critical. If the hinge point is not chosen close enough to the cortex the remaining bridge of bone will be broken rather than bent, thus creating an unstable fracture [4]. If the opposing cortex breaks, not only is stability lost but it may spring open after wedge closing, thus increasing the correction greatly over what was planned. This is an important cause of overcorrection in closed-wedge osteotomies. Loss of cortical contact may be a cause of undercorrection as well as overcorrection. If there is loss of cortical contact on the opposite side, the distal cortex may drop inside the proximal cortex when it settles into the cancellous bone, thus losing correction. However, if the distal cortex falls inside of the proximal cortex on the other side an increase in correction is caused after closing and compression of the osteotomy. Inadequate medial

buttress of the fixation material inserted may lead to collapse of the opposite cortex after weight bearing is started and result in undercorrection (Fig 18-3).

In open-wedge osteotomies integrity of the opposite cortex is equally important. If the opposite cortex cracks during opening of the wedge, there is no bone stability because there is only point contact [11]. As the wedge is opened the osteotomy may become unstable in rotation as Hohmann retractors inserted to facilitate exposure cause rotation forces in the distal femur as well as the proximal tibia. A specific problem may be encountered regarding plate positioning. When the plate is positioned too anterior or too posterior, flexion respectively extension may be introduced in the osteotomy (Fig 18-4). In addition, a specific problem may be encountered when blade plates are used during wedge opening in osteoporotic bone: during distraction the plate instead of pushing open the osteotomy may sink into

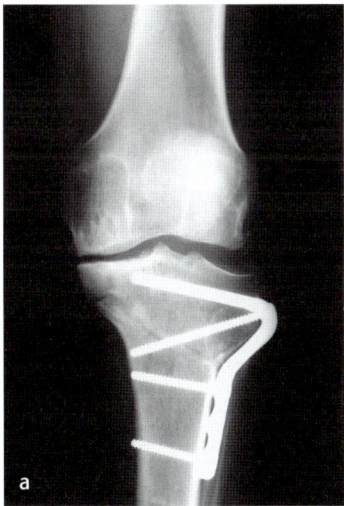
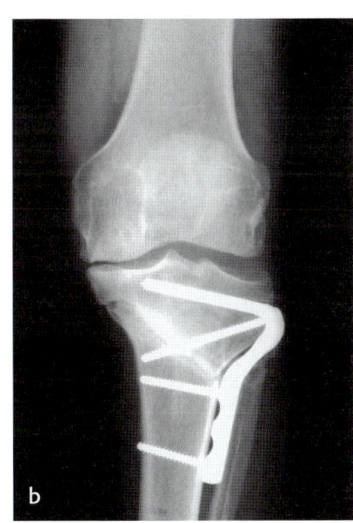

Fig 18-3a–b Undercorrection after lateral closed-wedge HTO due to inadequate medial buttress resulting into varus collapse.

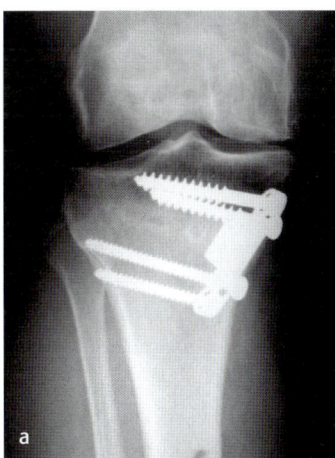
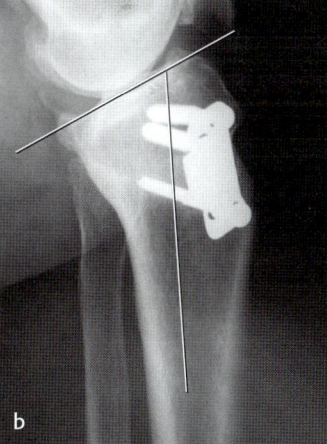

Fig 18-4a–b Anterior positioning of the wedge plate in an open-wedge HTO resulted in an inadvertent change in tibial slope and knee extension loss.

the osteoporotic fragment preventing further opening of the wedge. After fracture of the opposite cortex, stability can be regained by bone grafting and compression of the grafted osteotomy. However, if the bone graft is compressed back beyond the planned correction, the wedge must be reopened and more graft inserted and recompressed until enough graft is added under compression to give stability at the desired position.

Failure of fixation as a cause of a failed osteotomy may be due either to insufficiency of the fixation material or weakness of the bone, or a combination of both. During closed-wedge osteotomies, a secondary breakage of the opposite cortex can occur when the distal cortical screws in tibial osteotomies or the proximal femoral screws are tightened. The cause could be a shift of the distal part of the tibia respectively the proximal part of the femur towards the plate if the blade were not advanced far enough into the metaphyseal fragment. Furthermore, the

surgeon should be well aware of the fixation strength of the fixation material chosen to stabilize the osteotomy after correction. Less stable fixation constructs necessitate application of additional stability through casting or bracing and adjustments in postoperative rehabilitation regarding functional aftertreatment and start of full weight bearing. Osteoporotic bone may cause fixation material to sink in after which correction is lost. Important advantages of plate fixators are not only the superior mechanical strength but also the specific fixation stability even when applied in osteoporotic bone.

The gathering of documentation, preoperative x-rays (if available) planning drawings, surgical reports, fluoroscopy pictures and x-rays taken immediately postoperatively, documentation on postoperative rehabilitation, and x-rays taken at postoperative follow-ups will allow the reconstructive surgeon to gain insight in the causes of failure.

3   Symptoms, clinical findings, and planning for recorrection

Depending on the cause of failure, the patient with a malunited osteotomy presents with a wide array of complaints. It should be remembered that complaints may only develop after compensation mechanisms fail. The importance of a mobile subtalar joint to compensate for overcorrected or under-corrected frontal plane osteotomies is well known [9, 12] Generally, valgus deformity is more acceptable than varus deformity because inversion in the subtalar joint is greater than eversion [12]. In Fig 18-5 the compensatory motions in the subtalar joint are displayed.

Malunions in the sagittal plane may be compensated for by stretching or contracture of soft tissues around the knee joint. Transverse plane malunions are not well tolerated by the knee

joint as essentially the knee joint acts as a hinge and has very limited compensatory mechanisms for malrotations. Pain after a malunited osteotomy may have several causes: stretching of capsule and ligaments, overload of cartilage, subchondral and metaphyseal bone (see Fig 18-2), or referred pain in the knee caused by abnormal loading of a hip joint, leg-length difference, low back pain, etc.

In patients who complain about persistent pain localized at the osteotomy side, the surgeon should always rule out the existence of a nonunion as this calls for a different preoperative work up and operative treatment. In undercorrected failed osteotomies a patient presents with persistent joint pain not or only slightly improved by the osteotomy that has been performed. Persistent stretching of ligaments or created overtension of ligaments, eg, because of lack of release during open-wedge osteotomies may also cause pain. Failure of fixation material and protrusion of screws or plates is not an infrequent cause of pain. Soft-tissue scarring may be another cause of pain in the osteotomy area.

The cosmetic aspect of a failed osteotomy may pose a serious problem for the patient and should not be overlooked (Fig 18-6). Generally, patients are unhappy with the cosmetic appearance of correction of more than 3–4° varus or valgus beyond neutral. Although as a general rule osteotomies should not be performed only for the purpose of cosmesis, an indication may be present for a recorrection in a patient presenting with a multiply malunited osteotomy.

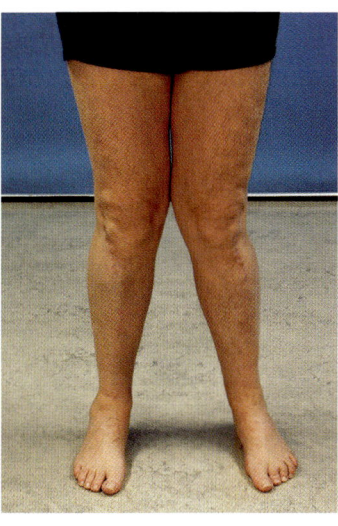

Fig 18-6   Cosmetic appearance of overcorrected left leg after valgization HTO in both legs.

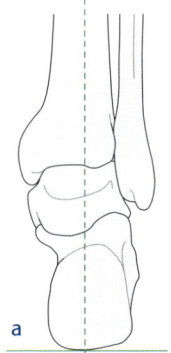 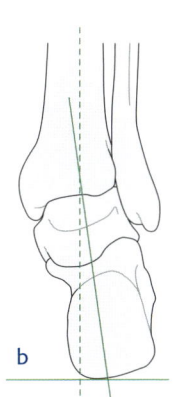 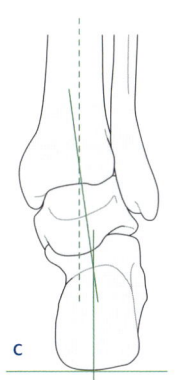 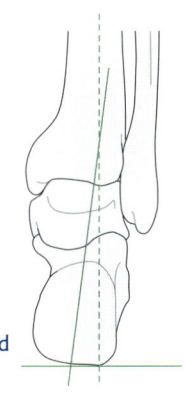 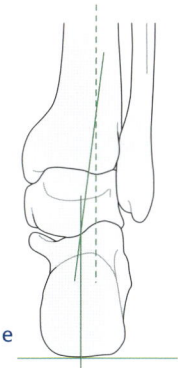

a   b   c   d   e

Fig 18-5a–e   Effects of limb malalignment on subtalar joint position (taken from [9]).
a   Physiological alignment.
b   Valgus malalignment.
c   Subtalar compensation for valgus malalignment.
d   Varus malalignment.
e   Subtalar compensation for varus malalignment.

On clinical examination specific findings can be noted in patients with malunited osteotomies. Gait and stance abnormalities can be inspected. A varus thrust gait (Fig 18-7), antalgic limping, limping due to leg-length difference, or instability may all be found. Leg-length difference should be measured in stance and documented. Shortening always exists when bone is removed, yet with a valgization osteotomy this almost never poses a problem. Shortening is often seen when the osteotomy has sheared and when the apex of the wedge for correction has been medial to the medial cortex. Shortening is a greater clinical problem when a varization osteotomy is performed.

The position of scars around the knee should be documented as well as areas of sensory loss related to the location of the osteotomy. Calluses on the feet point at abnormal loading. Muscle atrophy may be caused by disuse or neurological deficit related to complications of the osteotomy. The range of motion of the knee joint and in most cases also of the hip joint and upper and lower ankle joints should be documented. This information will, for example, help the surgeon to find out whether a hyperextension of the knee can only be attributed only to a malunited osteotomy resulting in a negative tibial slope or is also partly caused by a stretched posterior capsule of the knee.

The rotation profile should be assessed as described in chapter 15 "Rotational osteotomies of the femur and the tibia" to document or rule out transverse plane deformities.

The laxity of the knee ligaments should be carefully examined and documented as new ligamentous laxities may be caused by the osteotomy performed or the malunited position of the bones. A special mention should be made of the laxities that can be caused by severely depressed knee compartments after closed-wedge osteotomies around the knee. Stress x-rays will help to diagnose these laxities (see Fig 18-8) Instability causes a major problem in these patients. Any surgical procedure that compromises the lateral ligament will compromise the result. The lateral ligaments are not easily tensioned and the proximal fibula must not be compromised. Resection of the fibular head and reattachment of the ligaments or disarticulation of the proximal tibiofibular joint allowing the tibia to slide proximally, and is a source of catastrophic failure. For salvage in these cases, the fibula may be shortened and the fibular head pulled distally to regain tension (see Fig 18-8).

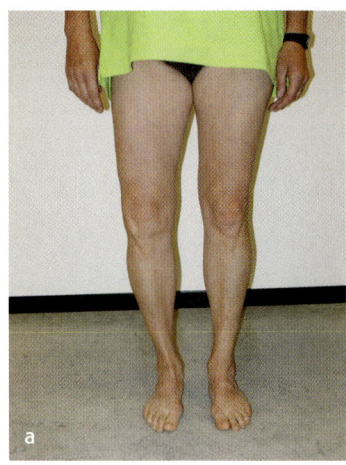
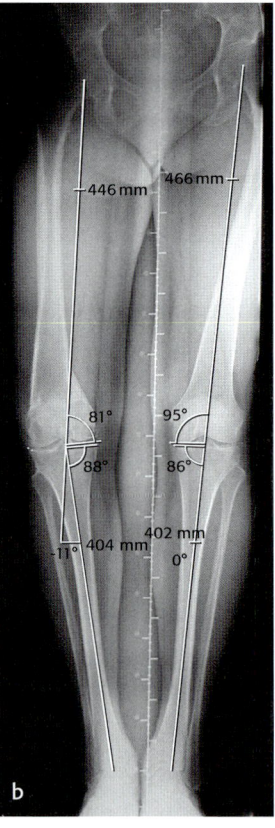

Fig 18-7a–b   Patient with failed overcorrected DFO. Due to the 11° varus leg alignment a varus thrust is found during stance and gait.

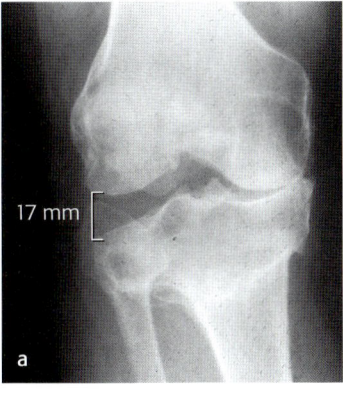

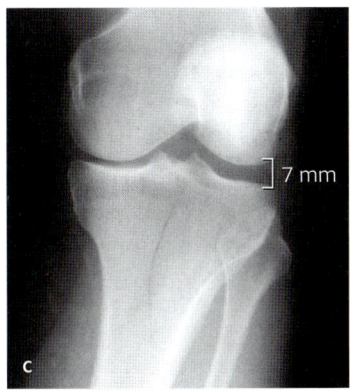

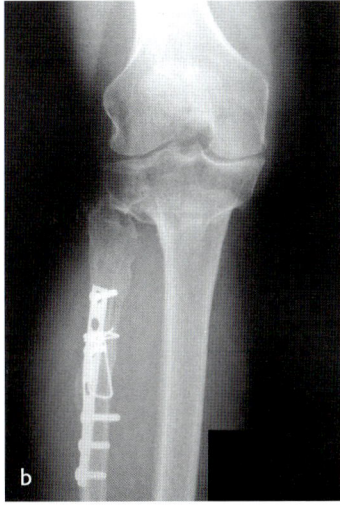

Fig 18-8a–c   Instability and recurrent varus due to lateral collateral ligament laxity after lateral closed-wedge HTO.

a   Stress x-rays show a 17 mm lateral opening with proximal position of the fibular head in the operated knee.

b   Lateral opening of the contralateral normal knee is 7 mm with normal fibular head position.

c   Correction by shortening the fibula to retension the lateral collateral ligament.

4   Radiological work-up

The radiological work-up for malunited osteotomies does not essentially differ from a radiologic analysis used for primary osteotomies (see chapter 4 "Basic principles of osteotomies around the knee", chapter 5 "Detailed planning algorithm for high-tibial osteotomy", chapter 9 "High-tibial open-wedge valgization osteotomy with plate fixator", and chapter 13 "Supracondylar varization osteotomy of the femur with plate fixation"). Stress x-rays are added if increased laxity is found to confirm diagnosis and quantify laxity relative to the contralateral knee (see Fig 18-8) In addition, a scintigram may be added to rule out nonunion, persistent bone infection or diagnose bone overload and stress reactions (see Fig 18-3). CT scans may be used to analyze bone healing, bone consistency, and bone deformity including rotational leg alignment. It should be anticipated that a great number of deformities after failed osteotomies are multiplane deformities necessitating whole-bone x-rays for deformity analysis. The measurements that can be made on these x-rays are equally important to find out how much of the deformity found during clinical examination can be attributed to the bone deformity [9].

5 Preoperative planning

Preoperative planning for correction of malunited osteotomies should follow the guidelines described in the formation of a surgical plan (see chapter 4 "Basic principles of osteotomies around the knee"). As recorrective procedures often need to be performed in the area of the primary correction, similarities to osteotomies for posttraumatic deformities can be found [13]. The preoperative planning for posttraumatic deformities has been described including anticipation on soft-tissue damage and scarring in the area approached [9]. As described above, deformity analysis is of major importance to identify where the deformity or deformities to be corrected are located. For single-plane reconstructions the planning methods described in chapter 5 "Detailed planning algorithm for high-tibial osteotomy" are used after definition of the aim of correction. In case of multiplane deformities mathematical formulas or graphical methods may help to calculate the angles and direction for single cut corrections. Alternatively, external fixators can be used for multiplane corrections as will be described at the end of this chapter.

6 Surgical techniques

For the correction of failed osteotomies, surgical techniques similar to primary osteotomy techniques may be used. However, often the cause of failure leading to the malunion may pose specific new problems (eg, bone defects and bone loss, broken screws, soft-tissue scarring) limiting the possibilities for reconstruction. Creative thinking and inclusion of all osteotomy and fixation options will help the surgeon to find the best option for a specific deformity correction.

Depending on the time of presentation, bone healing may not be complete and therefore a recorrection may be possible by manipulating the healing bone without performing an osteotomy. Retensioning of inserted plates and application of extra screws reinforce the initial fixation construct and enable realignment providing that grip of the fixation material in the bone is secure (Fig 18-9).

In cases of overcorrection caused by breakage of the opposite cortex in closed-wedge osteotomies the other cortex is no longer under tension. When the bone is still malleable a tension band wiring can be performed to reinforce and compress the opposite cortex (Fig 18-10). Alternatively, a lag screw or staples can be used to compress the opposite cortex. In general no repositioning of the initial fixation is necessary.

Most patients with failed osteotomies present or are referred after full bone healing. Some patients only present years after the failed osteotomy with new complaints related to the malaligned limb. It is important to define the aim of recorrection together with the patient as the patient may have lost confidence in osteotomies as a treatment and the goal of the patient may differ from the plan of the surgeon (Fig 18-11).

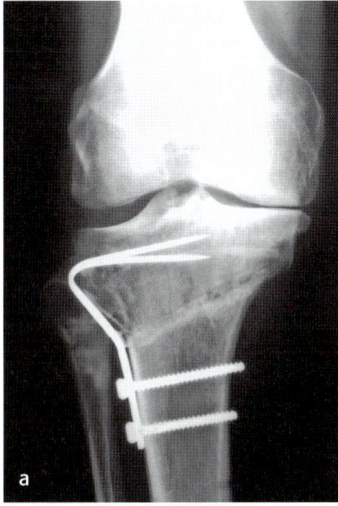
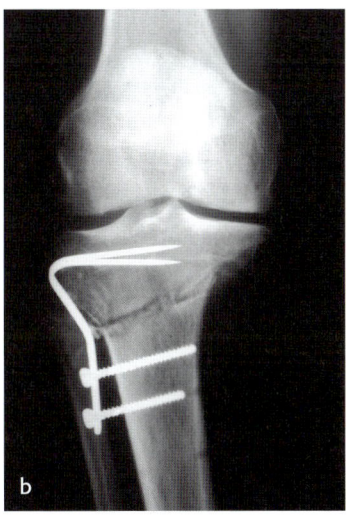
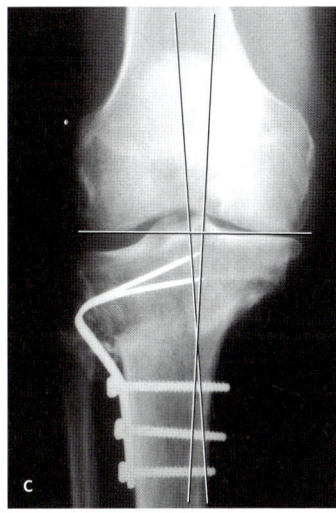

Fig 18-9a–c
a–b Varus collapse 3 months after lateral closed-wedge HTO.
c   Recorrection by retensioning of the plate resulting in full consolidation in planned corrected alignment.

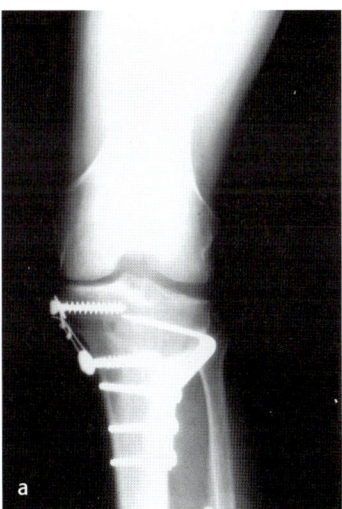
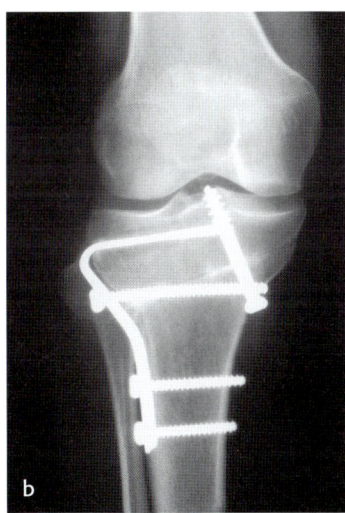

Fig 18-10a–b   Medial tension band wiring (a) and medial lag screw (b) to reduce medial opening and overcorrection after lateral closed-wedge HTO.

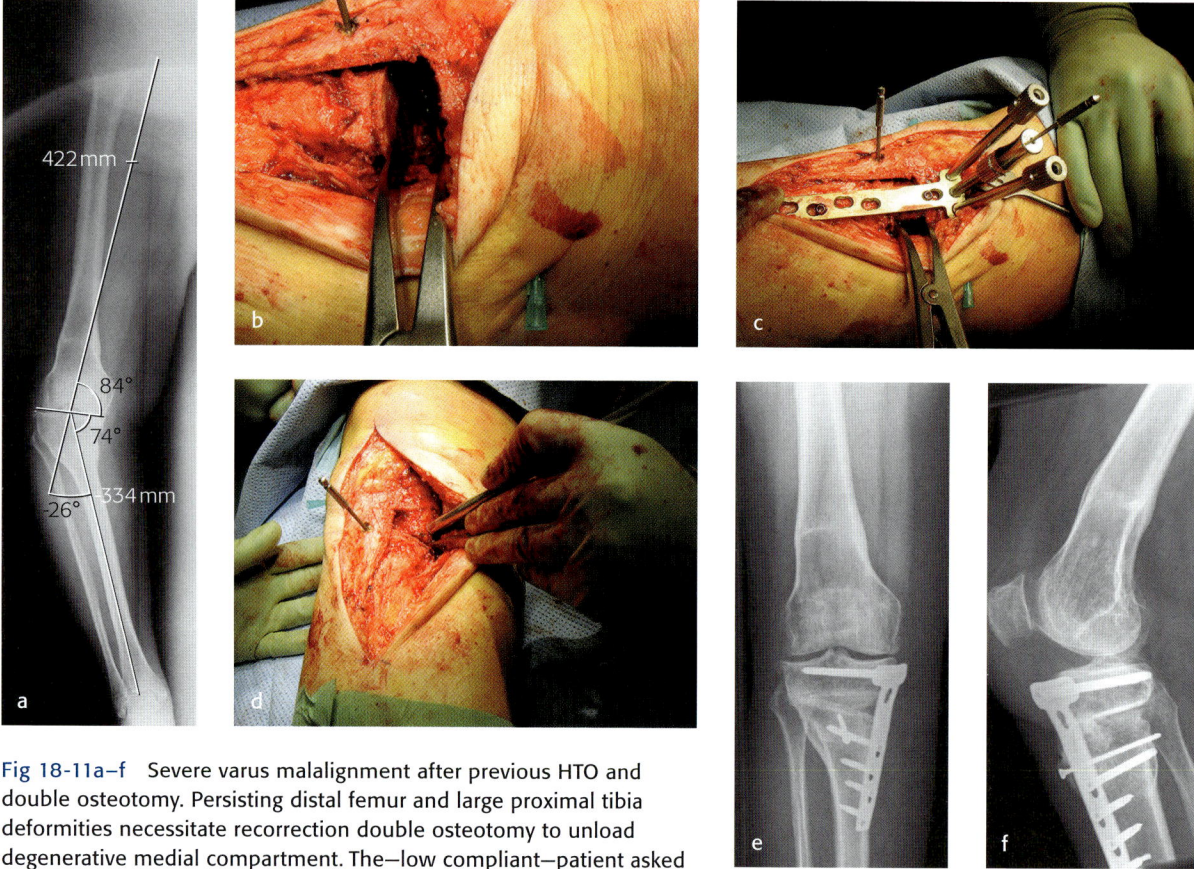

Fig 18-11a–f   Severe varus malalignment after previous HTO and double osteotomy. Persisting distal femur and large proximal tibia deformities necessitate recorrection double osteotomy to unload degenerative medial compartment. The—low compliant—patient asked for a simple correction to decrease leg malalignment. A large medial open-wedge HTO with distal tuberosity osteotomy and bone grafting was performed.

An important factor in the choice of recorrective technique is the amount of bone left in the distal femur or proximal tibia after the initial correction. After a failed closed-wedge osteotomy a large amount of bone may be lost and addition of bone by open-wedge techniques and bone grafting is preferred over closed-wedge techniques that further decrease the bone stock (Fig 18-12). In this respect a future total joint replacement and the problems with extensive bone loss should be kept in mind. The decision whether or not to remove remnants of broken screws may also be viewed in relation to joint replacement.

In failed open-wedge corrections and in patients with sufficient remaining bone stock after planning the recorrection, a closed-wedge technique may be chosen. Often the wedge can best be removed at the site where new bone was formed during bone healing of the open-wedge correction as this is the location of maximum deformity (CORA) (Fig 18-13).

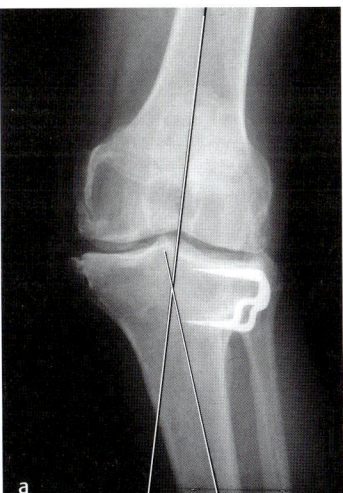
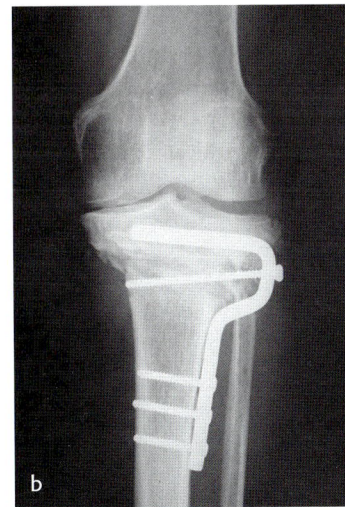

Fig 18-12a–b   Overcorrection of lateral closed-wedge HTO (a) treated by lateral open-wedge HTO bone grafting and blade plate fixation (b).

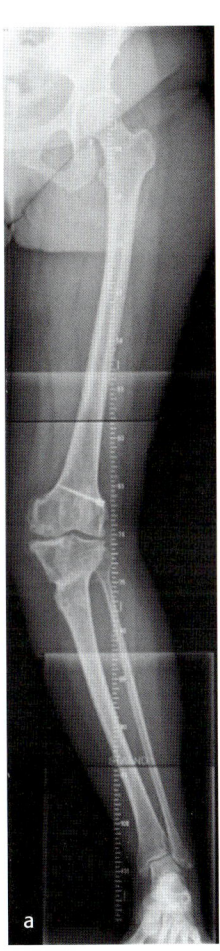
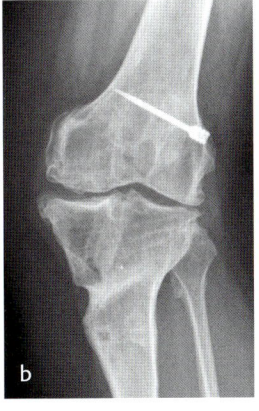
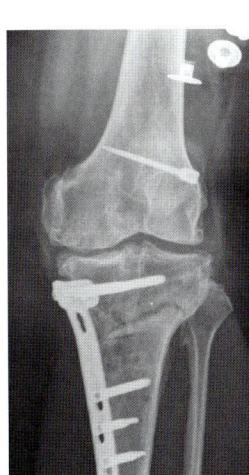
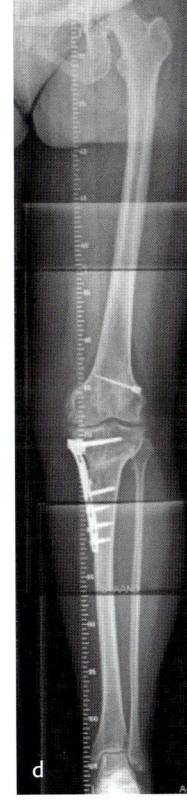

Fig 18-13a–d   Varus overcorrection of 20° after combined open-wedge HTO and anterior cruciate ligament reconstruction (a–b), treated by medial closed-wedge HTO fixed with plate fixator (c–d).

Even more important in the distal femur than the proximal tibia is the accuracy of correction. This is due to the longer distance to the foot causing small deviations of the planned correction which can result in recurrence of malalignment after correction. The longer lever arm including the knee joint also asks for a stronger fixation and specific rehabilitation. As bone healing is also slower in the distal femur compared to the proximal tibia, it is strongly advised to use bone grafts in open-wedge techniques. Often closed-wedge techniques are preferred for recorrections in the distal femur to prevent osteotomy related causes of failure as described above (Fig 18-14).

In patients with multiplane deformities after failed osteotomy a strategy that enables full correction of all planes during one surgical procedure is preferred. In general, acute corrections are much more appreciated by the patient than gradual corrections for which an external fixator must be applied. Depending on the combination of deformities in the different planes and bones a multiplane deformity may be corrected by a single level osteotomy (Fig 18-15) or a double osteotomy.

In multiplane deformity correction external fixators may be a useful tool. After measurement of the deformities in all planes an external fixator frame can be build that integrates all deformities, and which can be mounted on the deformed bone before the osteotomy is performed. Depending on the location of the CORA, hinges should be positioned that enable correction in all planes. During surgery the frame is mounted on the bone with pins that on one side are positioned at angles that combine all deformities and on the other side pins are fixed in a normal part of the bone. After the osteotomy the external fixator is straightened to normal bone alignment after which all planes are corrected and the pins proximal and distal of the osteotomy become parallel. After that, a temporary fixation (eg, with crossed K-wires) can stabilize the realigned bone before plate fixation (Fig 18-16). This corrective method with temporary external fixation can also be used in combination with intramedullary nail fixation [14]. Alternatively, the external fixator can be left in place after the correction if the patient has no objections to walking with an external fixator until full bone healing.

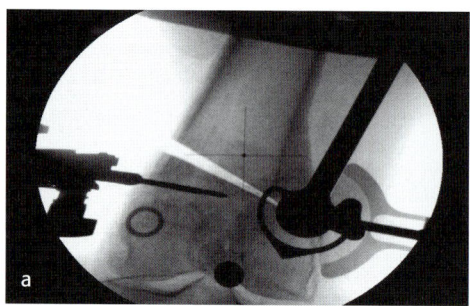
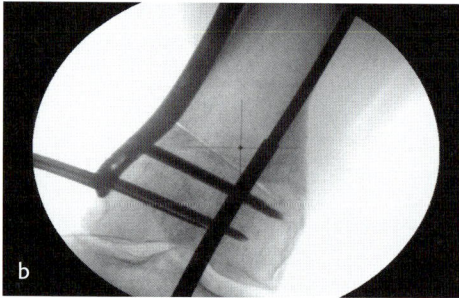
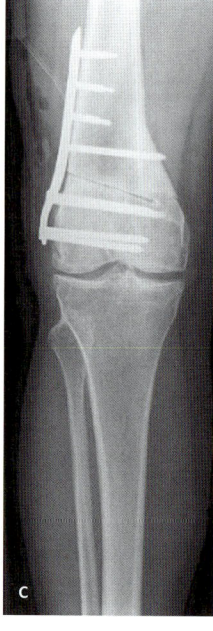

Fig 18-14a–c   Closed-wedge lateral DFO for recorrection of varus overcorrected DFO in the patient presented in Fig 18-4. Intraoperative pictures after wedge resection using a calibrated saw guide (a), and after wedge closing, distal plate fixation, and leg-alignment check (b). Postoperative x-ray with lateral distal femur plate fixator (c).

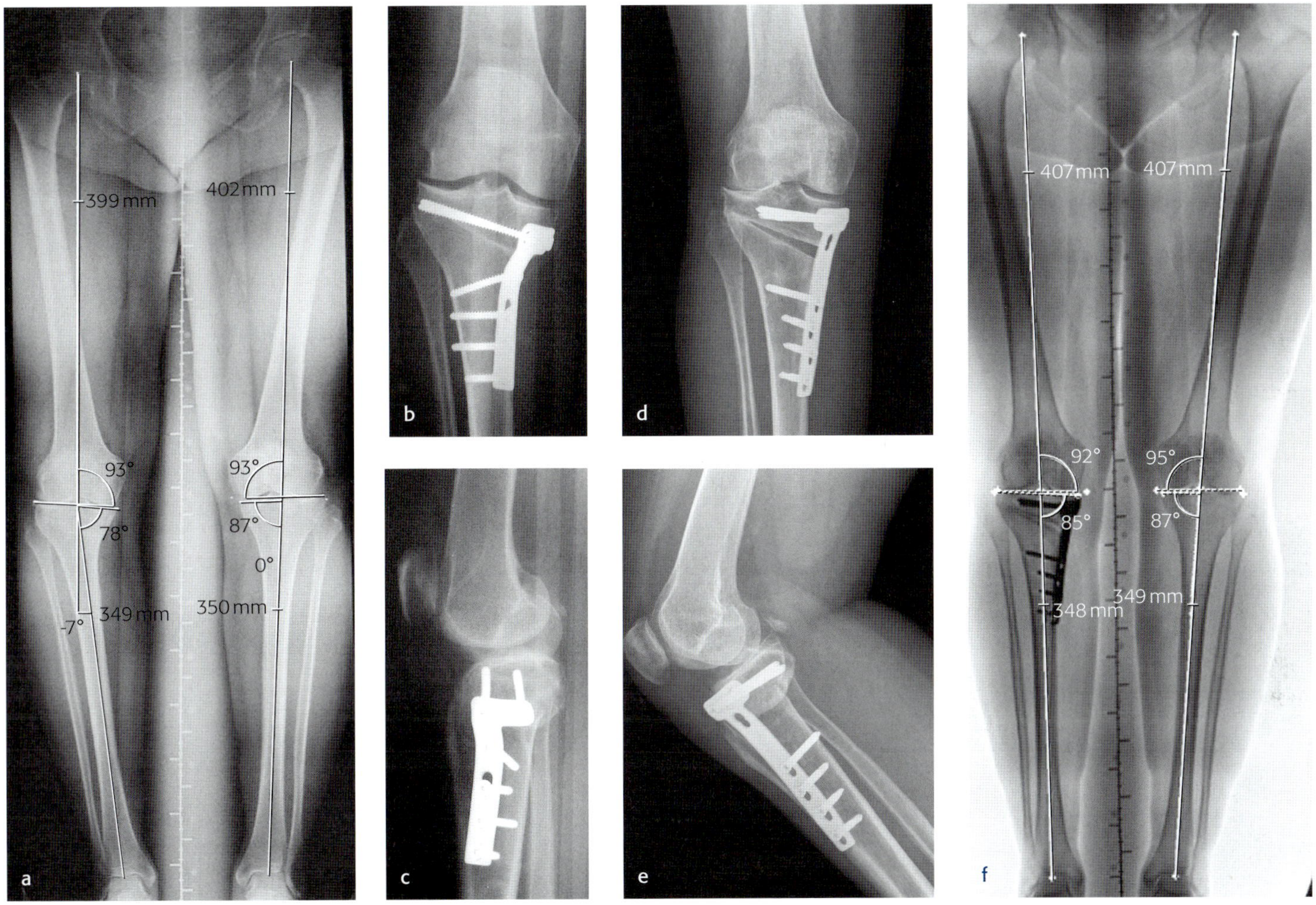

Fig 18-15a–f   Overcorrection in varus and recurvatum after medial closed-wedge HTO resulting in varus joint-line obliquity and negative tibial slope (a–c). A medial open-wedge flexion HTO was performed to recreate normal knee joint line orientation and neutral alignment in frontal and sagittal plane (d–f).

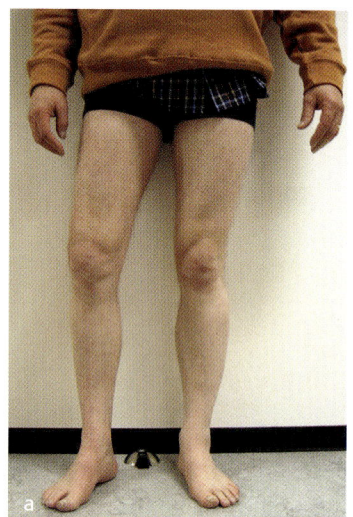

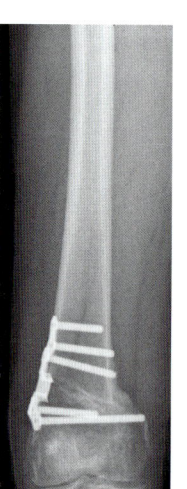

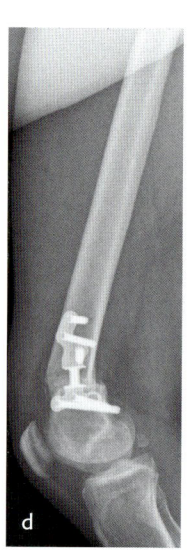

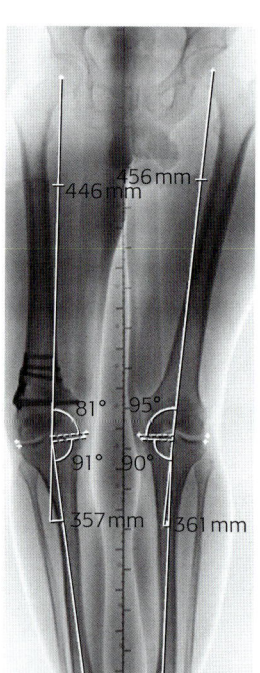

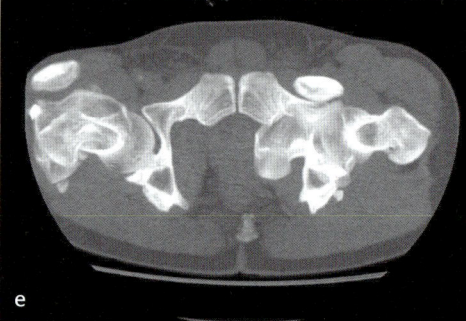

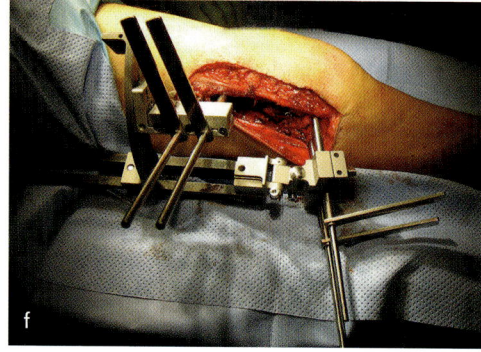

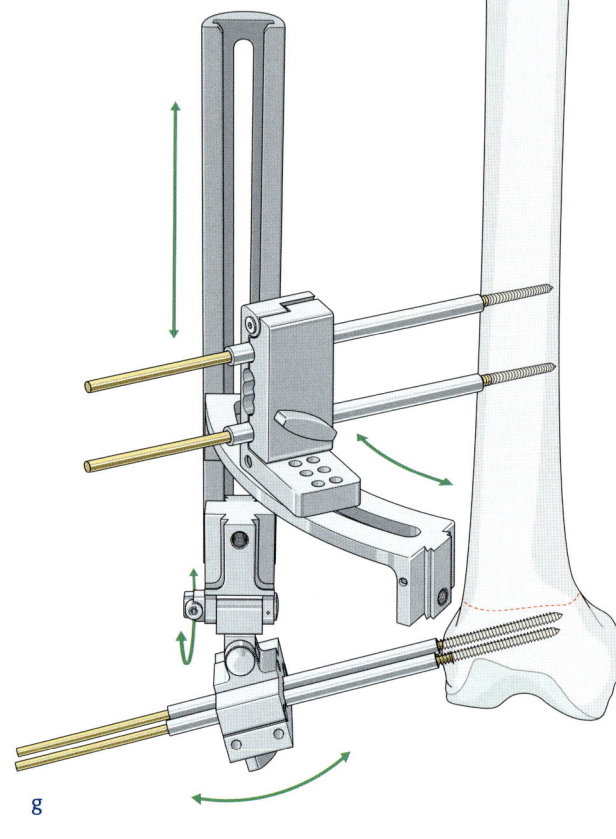

Fig 18-16a–o   Correction of a multiplane distal femur deformity after failed lateral open-wedge DFO. Preoperative analysis, recorrective osteotomy with use of temporary external fixation, and postoperative result.

a   Varus, external rotation position of the right leg with 15° knee extension loss.

b   9° varus leg alignment in weight-bearing full-leg view.

c–d   AP and lateral view of the knee show a distal femur varus and flexion deformity.

e   Transverse CT scan shows a 30° external rotation malalignment.

f–g   Intraoperative view of external fixator mounted on the distal femur before correction and schematic presentation illustrating hinge points for 3-D corrections.

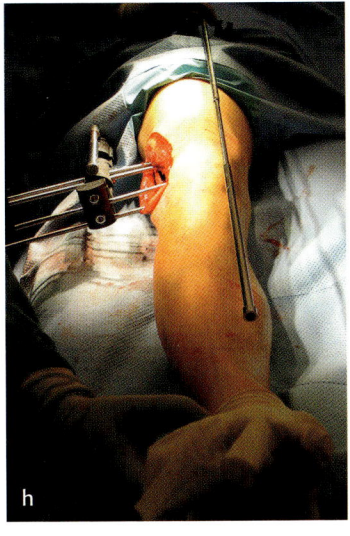

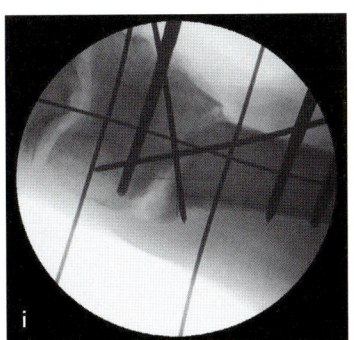

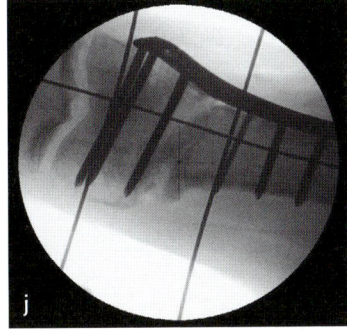

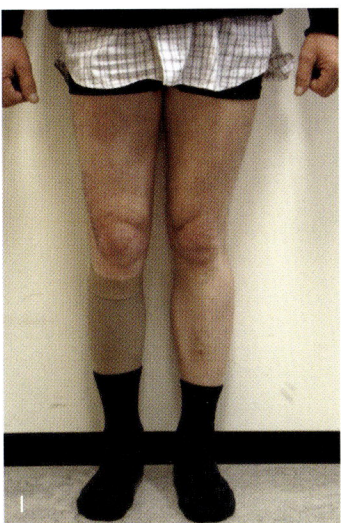

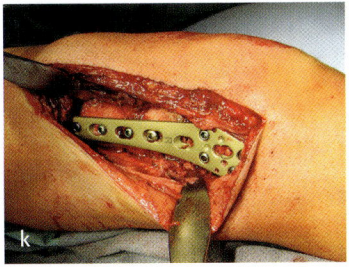

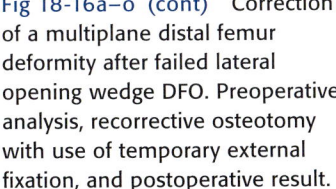

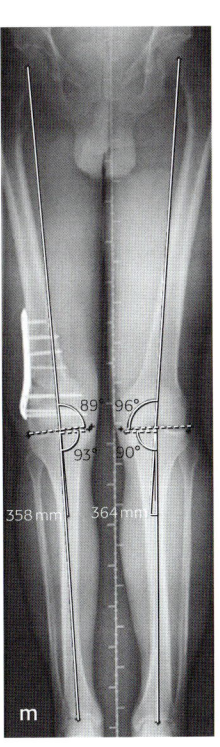

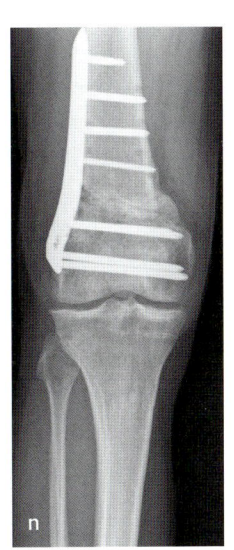

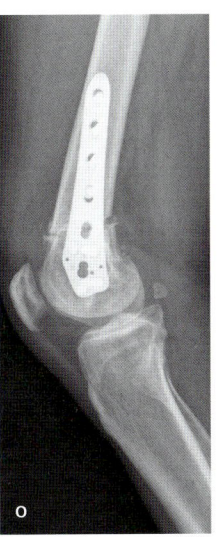

Fig 18-16a–o (cont)   Correction of a multiplane distal femur deformity after failed lateral opening wedge DFO. Preoperative analysis, recorrective osteotomy with use of temporary external fixation, and postoperative result.

h   Leg-alignment check after straightening the external fixator.
i   Temporary crossed K-wire fixation after osteotomy, straightening and locking of the external fixator.
j   After fixation with plate fixator.
k   TomoFix lateral distal femur plate fixator in situ.
l–m   Postoperative clinical and radiological weight-bearing leg alignment.
n–o   AP and lateral view of the knee show the corrected distal femur.

7   Results

As already stated in the introduction, only a few reports can be found on the treatment of failed osteotomies with recorrective osteotomies around the knee [1–3]. These publications are descriptions of a single case or small case series and reflect the authors' personal experience with specific techniques. Additional case examples can be found in the literature on complications after osteotomies. The authors' experience working in referral centers where large numbers of osteotomies are performed are described in this chapter. Even in our centers the number of recorrective osteotomies performed is relatively small and no other guidelines than formulated in this chapter can be given. In general, it is strongly advised to refer patients with malunited osteotomies to specialist centers.

8   Conclusion

Osteotomies for failed osteotomies around the knee can be performed successfully if taken into account the cause of failure of the osteotomy, symptoms and clinical findings of the patient, and deformities found at the radiological work-up. Preoperative planning, awareness of possible intraoperative technical errors, and specific pitfalls of the osteotomy techniques help the surgeon to find the best surgical solution to recorrect a malunited osteotomy.

9   Bibliography

[1]   **Tsuda E, Ishibashi Y, Sasaki K, et al** (2004) Opening-wedge osteotomy for revision of failed closing-wedge high tibial osteotomy. A case report. *J Bone Joint Surg Am;* 86(9):2045–2049.

[2]   **Schaller TM, Roehr B** (2007) Salvage of failed opening wedge tibial osteotomy using a locking plate. *Orthopedics;* 30(2):161–162.

[3]   **Watanabe K, Tsuchiya H, Matsubara H, et al** (2008) Revision high tibial osteotomy with Taylor spatial frame for failed opening-wedge high tibial osteotomy. *J Orthop Sci;* 13(2):145–149.

[4]   **Teitge RA** (1996) Complications of high tibial osteotomy: a personal experience. Seminars in arthroplasty; 7(2):167–178.

[5]   **Handal EG, Morawski DR, Santore RF** (1994) Complications of high tibial osteotomy. *Fu FH, Harner CD, Vince KG (eds), Knee Surgery.* Baltimore: Lippincott Williams & Wilkins, 1153–1171.

[6]   **Spahn G** (2004) Complications in high tibial (medial opening wedge) osteotomy. Arch Orthop Trauma Surg; 124(10):649–653.

[7]   **Rose T, Imhoff AB** (2007) Complications after transgenicular osteotomies. *Op Tech Orthop;* 17(1):80–86.

[8]   **Van de Bekerom MP, Patt TW, Kleinhout MY, et al** (2008) Early complications after high tibial osteotomy: a comparison of two techniques. *J Knee Surg;* 21(1):68–74.

[9]   **Van Heerwaarden RJ, Mast JW, Paccola CA** (2008) Diagnostics and planning of deformity correction: formation of a surgical plan. *Marti RK, van Heerwaarden RJ, Osteotomies for posttraumatic deformities.* AO Publishing, Stuttgart New York: Thieme Verlag, 33–55.

[10]   **Hofmann S, van Heerwaarden RJ** (2007) [General patient selection criteria and indication for double osteotomies around the knee.] *Orthopädische Praxis;* 43(3):142–146. German.

[11]   **Teitge RA** (1996) Supracondylar osteotomy for lateral compartment osteoarthritis. *Seminars in arthroplasty* 7(2):192–211.

[12]   **Müller ME** (1967) *[Posttraumatic angular deformity of the lower extremities.]* 1st ed. Bern Stuttgart: Verlag Hans Huber. German.

[13]   **Van Heerwaarden RJ, Marti RK** (2008) Posttraumatic deformities and osteotomies. *Marti RK, van Heerwaarden RJ, Osteotomies for posttraumatic deformities.* AO Publishing, Stuttgart New York: Thieme Verlag, 3–15.

[14]   **Gugenheim JJ, Brinker MR** (2003) Bone realignment with use of temporary external fixation for distal femoral valgus and varus deformities. *J Bone Joint Surg;* 85(7):1229–1237.

Future developments

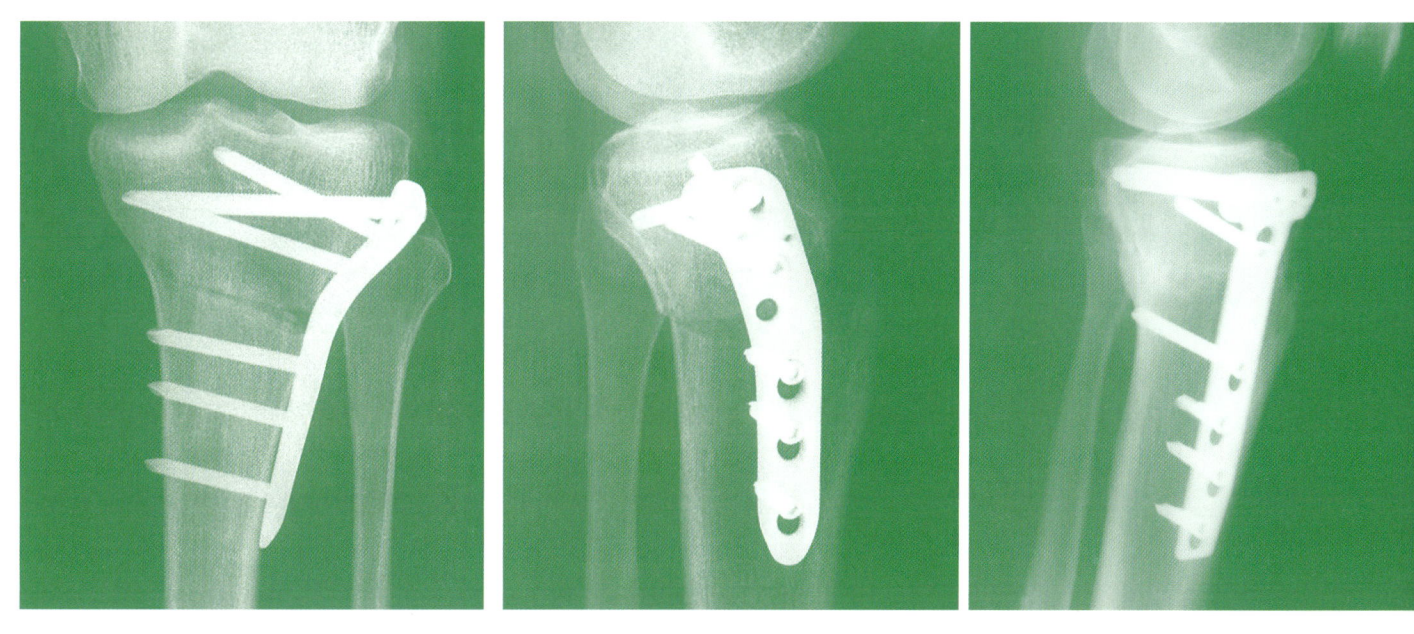

Authors   Urs W Müller, Gongli Wang, Guoyan Zheng, Alex E Staubli, Lutz-Peter Nolte

19   Computer-assisted navigation in proximal tibial osteotomy

1   Introduction

Osteotomies around the knee are well-established methods for treatment of deformities of the lower extremity and monocompartmental osteoarthritis due to congenital or posttraumatic etiology. Numerous osteotomy procedures exist, including open-wedge technique with or without interposition of bone grafts [1], closed-wedge technique [2], and dome-shaped osteotomies. The choice of treatment method is based on clinical findings, taking into account the severity of the deformity, its location, the knee base line, the range of motion, possible rotational malalignment, patellofemoral tracking, leg-length differences, and soft-tissue condition [3].

Osteotomies around the knee, in particular osteotomies at the proximal tibia, are regarded as technically demanding surgical methods with a steep learning curve. Retrospective clinical studies demonstrate that the most frequent complication after osteotomy is insufficient postoperative alignment [4, 5]. An evaluation of recently published clinical findings reveals that only 60–80% of postoperative outcomes reach satisfactory alignment [1, 6–10]. This can often be attributed to inadequate preoperative planning or failure to examine the mechanical axis of the extremity intraoperatively. Another cause may be unstable fixation of the osteotomy during the bone healing process, resulting in secondary correction loss with revarization or valgus overcorrection. Improperly performed osteotomies or incorrect orientation of the chisel or saw blade can cause intraoperative tibial plateau fractures and injury to the neurovascular structures.

The occurrence of complications related to preoperative planning and intraoperative mistakes can be decreased by computer-assisted, navigated procedures. The exact result achieved in this way must nevertheless be securely stabilized by internal fixation so that the surgical outcome is maintained. Ideal fixation can be achieved with angular stable internal plate fixators.

Computer-assisted surgical techniques (CAS) with CT-based intraoperative guidance systems [11] and robot-assisted systems [12] have been developed for closed-wedge correction osteotomies. These systems have proven effective in aiding the surgeon to excise a precise bone wedge. Despite this advantage, these systems also include certain disadvantages, eg, high radiation dose and increased risk of infection after preoperative implantation of the marker pins. For these reasons, a new intraoperative planning and navigation system has been developed that is applied with a fluoroscopic C-arm instead of preoperative CT scans.

In addition to conventional closed-wedge osteotomy, the presented system also allows for open-wedge and dome-shaped osteotomies. It permits the user to measure the deformity precisely, to plan the osteotomy intraoperatively, and to perform the planned operation accurately under navigated guidance.

2 System components

The development of this system was based on the SurgiGATE system (PRAXIM/Medivision, La Tronche, France). An infrared camera fixed to an adjustable stand (Opto Track 3020, Northern Digital Inc, Ontario, Canada) is used for permanent tracking of optical targets that are equipped with infrared light-transmitting diodes. These diodes are attached as dynamic reference bases to relevant anatomical structures (distal tibial shaft, tibial head segment, distal femur), to the image intensifier of the C-arm, and to all relevant surgical instruments, thus permitting real time navigation. A Sun-ULTRA-10 workstation (Sun Microsystems Inc., Mountain View, Canada) is used for image processing and visualization on the monitor. This workstation is connected to the video output of the C-arm in order to receive the radiographic images. The workstation communicates with the infrared system via specially designed software.

The navigated system can be categorized into three groups according to their function:
1. Image acquisition and recording: Intraoperative movements and changes are tracked with the calibrated fluoroscopic C-arm, a reference measuring instrument, a control system, and a percutaneous pointer.
2. Navigated instruments: drill, saw, and chisel.
3. Dynamic reference bases (DRB): The three reference bases are attached at the distal tibial shaft, the tibial head segment, and the distal femur and record all steric changes at these anatomical structures during the operation.

3 Surgical procedure

Preoperative planning is not necessary for application of the described navigation system. The patient is placed in supine position on a radiolucent table. Two dynamic reference bases (DRB) are fixed with 3 mm K-wires to the distal femur and the distal tibia. It is important to ensure rigid fixation of these reference bases. After radiographic imaging and registration of the anatomical landmarks, the deformity is calculated intra-operatively and interactive planning of the osteotomy can be performed. A third DRB is attached to the proximal segment of the tibia before performing the osteotomy in order to monitor relative movements between the proximal and distal osteotomy segments of the tibia. The planned osteotomy and correction of the deformity are then conducted under navigated control.

3.1 Recording of image data and landmarks

At the beginning of surgery a total of six x-rays—AP and lateral view of the hip joint, the knee joint, and the upper ankle joint— are obtained (Fig 19-1). Based on these images the anatomical landmarks are digitally captured with a 3-D reconstruction concept [13, 14]. First, the center of the hip joint is defined as the center of the femoral head using a virtual Mose circle. Second, the center of the talus is defined as the center of the ankle joint. Third, the tangent to the posterior femoral condyles is determined. In the next step, the contours of the tibial plateau are defined by the most lateral, most medial, most anterior, and most posterior point of the tibial plateau. The center of the knee joint is then calculated as the geometric center of the recorded contours of the tibial plateau. This procedure permits all anatomical bone structures that cannot be reached directly with the pointer to be registered. Alternatively, the pointer can be inserted percutaneously to digitally record the midpoint on the transmalleolar axis (distance from the lateral to medial malleolus) as the center of the upper ankle joint.

3.2   Measurement of the deformity

After registration of the landmarks, a patient-specific coordinate system is established. For geometric description of bone and joint geometry, each reference point requires its own coordinate system. The frontal plane of the femur passes through the hip and knee joint centers and lies parallel to the posterior tangent of the femoral condyles. The sagittal plane passes through the hip and knee centers and lies perpendicular to the frontal plane. The transverse plane lies in a 90° angle to the other two mentioned planes.

The functional biomechanical parameters of the extremities are measured intraoperatively. Considering the digital hip joint (H), knee joint (K), and ankle joint (A) centers, the femoral mechanical axis, the tibial mechanical axis, and the mechanical weight bearing axis can be defined as the line HK, KA, and HA. The varus/valgus angle and the flexion/extension angle are defined as the intersection angles of the projected lines of the tibial and femoral mechanical axes in both the frontal and sagittal planes [3]. The inclination angle of the tibial plateau in the sagittal plane (tibial slope) corresponds to the intersection angle between the tangent to the tibial plateau and the mechanical tibial axis. Deviation from the mechanical axis is measured as the distance of the mechanical axis to the knee center (mechanical axis deviation = MAD) in the frontal plane and is given in mm [3]. Accurate definition of the above mentioned parameters is mandatory to correctly identify and adequately correct a deformity.

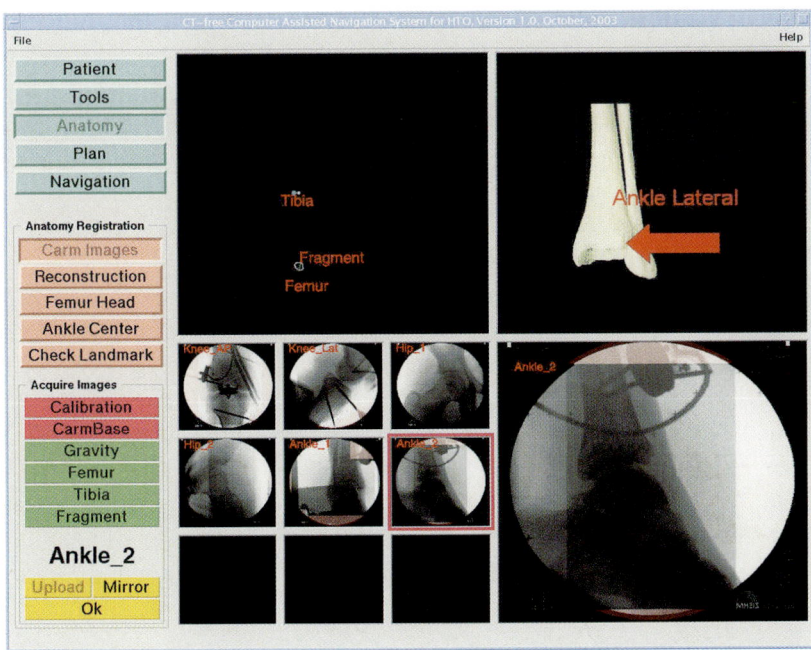

Fig 19-1   Recording the anatomical landmarks. X-rays of the hip joint, the knee joint, and the upper ankle joint are obtained in both planes with the fluoroscopic C-arm (bottom left). The dynamic reference bases (DRBs) can be seen attached to the distal femur and the proximal and distal tibia. Based on these x-rays, the centers of the femoral head and the upper ankle joint as well as other important anatomical landmarks will be defined on the monitor with a cursor. Alternatively, the center of the ankle joint can be recorded percutaneously with a digital pointer (top right).

Another important aspect is ligament and soft-tissue laxity. In addition to skeletal varus or valgus deformity, asymmetric joint-gap width may be caused by separation of the lateral or medial compartments due to ligament laxity [15]. This must be taken into account when planning the correction angle (see chapter 4 "Basic principles of osteotomies around the knee"). The skeletal and ligamentous causes must be differentiated. A mathematical formula is given in chapter 5 "Detailed planning algorithm for high-tibial osteotomies". Alternatively, skeletal deformities can be differentiated from ligament laxities by exerting varus and valgus stress [16]. The convergent angle of the joint surface (see chapter 1 "Physiological axes of the lower limb", Fig 1-6), which is defined as the intersection angle between the tibial and femoral knee base line, can be calculated with the system software.

3.3   Planning and navigation of the osteotomy

The system offers the possibility of interactive planning and navigation of both open-wedge and closed-wedge procedure. Fig 19-2, Fig 19-3, Fig 19-4, and Fig 19-5 show the sequence of navigated surgical technique on the monitor.

Open-wedge osteotomy

Open-wedge osteotomy is a widespread surgical technique for the treatment of monocompartmental osteoarthritis [1]. The osteotomy starts at the medial cortex at the upper margin of pes anserinus and ends 10 mm from the lateral cortex (Fig 19-2a). Complete transection of the lateral cortex leads to instability that makes fixation of the osteotomy more difficult. In addition, osteotomies that are performed improperly, eg, oblique saw cut, may lead to fractures of the tibial plateau or damage to the neurovascular structures [4]. These technical problems indicate the importance of a tool for intraoperative planning and monitoring of the osteotomy.

The system used by the authors offers visualization of every intraoperative step. The consequences of changing parameters, eg, the orientation of the osteotomy plane, the angle of the osteotomy in the frontal plane and the distance of the osteotomy plane to the tibial plateau can be accurately assessed. The planned osteotomy is then performed under navigated guidance. The surgical instruments are also projected on the monitor during operation (Fig 19-4). This means that the surgeon maintains constant control over instrument application. In addition, deviations of the instruments from the planned osteotomy are calculated in real time (Fig 19-4). Thus, instrument handling can be accurately evaluated and modified in accordance with preoperative planning to achieve precise implementation of the calculated correction. The difficulty of dissociation of the monitor and the surgical site that is familiar from arthroscopic and endoscopic surgical procedures should not be underestimated.

Closed-wedge osteotomy

Closed-wedge osteotomy as described by Coventry [2] is still a popular procedure today. Planning and navigated guidance are similar to those for open-wedge osteotomy, except that two osteotomy planes need to be defined in this case. After planning both osteotomies, the wedge angle between the two saw cuts is automatically determined.

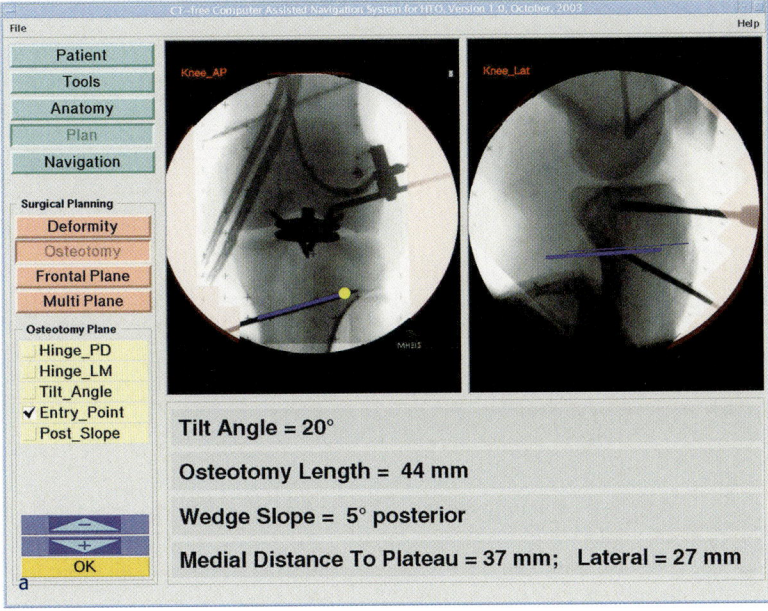

Tilt Angle = 20°

Osteotomy Length = 44 mm

Wedge Slope = 5° posterior

Medial Distance To Plateau = 37 mm; Lateral = 27 mm

a

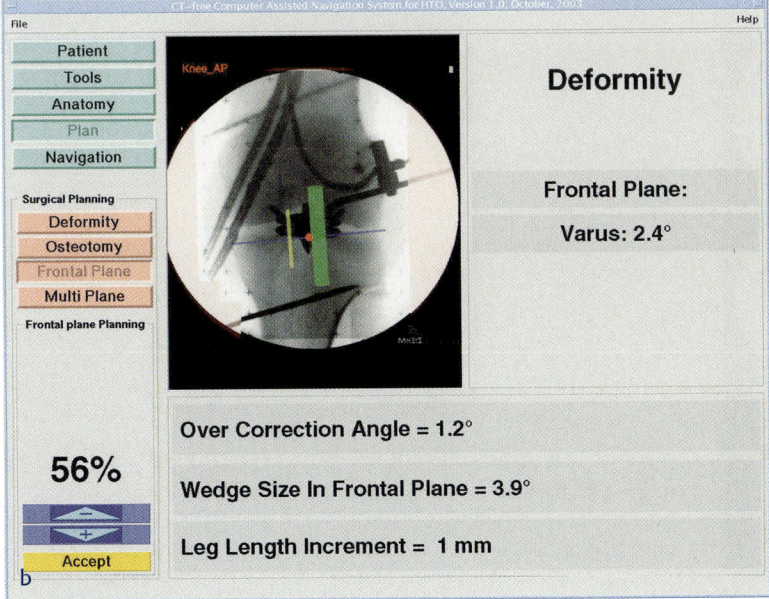

Deformity

Frontal Plane:

Varus: 2.4°

Over Correction Angle = 1.2°

Wedge Size In Frontal Plane = 3.9°

Leg Length Increment = 1 mm

b

Fig 19-2a–b   Planning an open-wedge osteotomy of the proximal tibia on the monitor.

a   Planning of the osteotomy plane (blue) based on the image data in the frontal and sagittal plane. The osteotomy aims at the upper third of the proximal tibiofibular joint and ends 10 mm from the lateral cortex (yellow mark).

b   Definition of the weight-bearing axis. The preoperative mechanical axis passes through the medial compartment (yellow) medial to the knee center (red) due to varus deformity. The postoperative alignment of the weight-bearing axis is defined (green). Ideally, the corrected weight-bearing axis should intersect with the knee base line (blue) at the 62% point of the width of the tibial plateau as defined by Fujisawa [17].

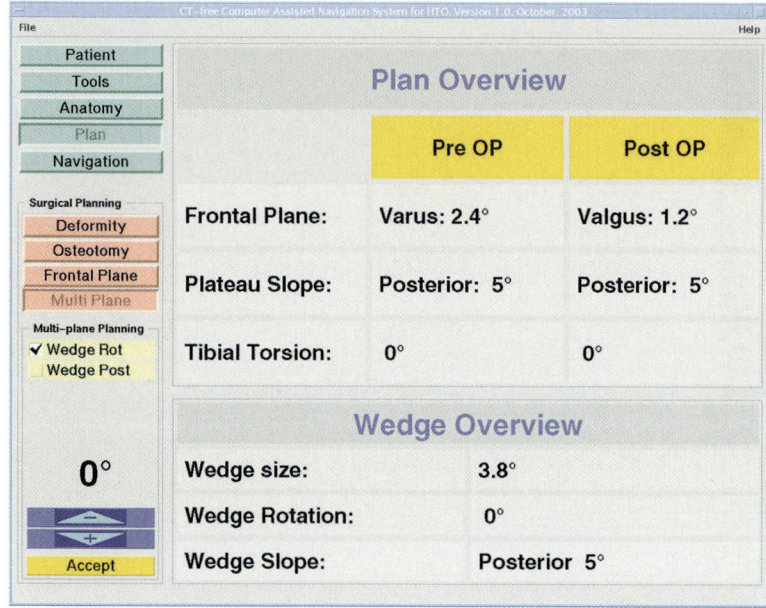

Fig 19-3   Planning overview. The required amount of correction is calculated from the preoperatively measured angles and values and the desired postoperative angles respectively values in all three planes.

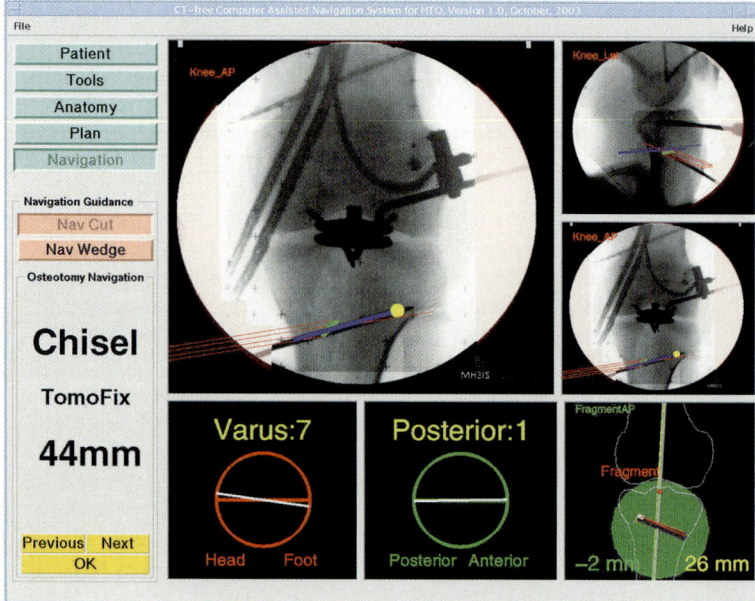

Fig 19-4   Navigated instruments. The position of the chisel (red) in relation to the osteotomy plane can be visually assessed in the frontal plane and in the sagittal plane. If the chisel diverges out of the calculated plane, the deviation will be recorded immediately (bottom row).

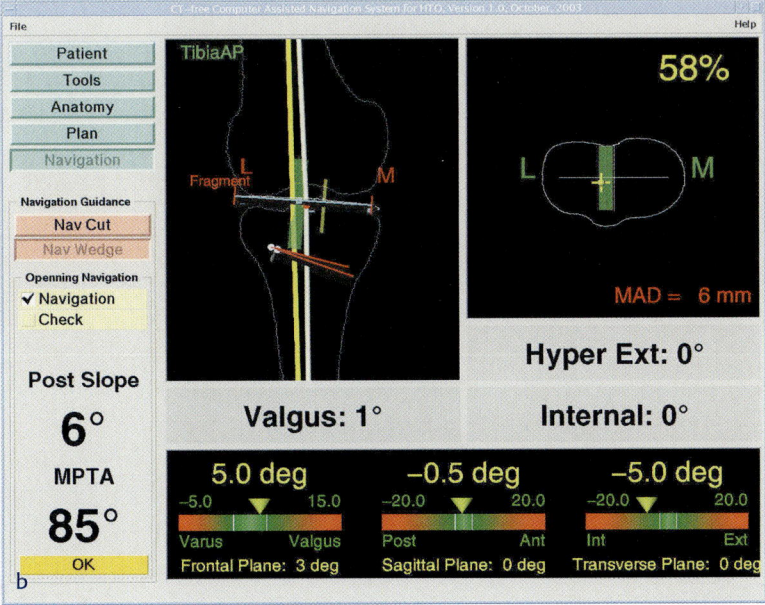

Fig 19-5a–b   Spreading of the osteotomy is monitored on the screen. When the osteotomy gap is opened the mechanical weight bearing axis (yellow) shifts from medial to lateral within the planned correction range (green). View in the frontal plane (top left) and view in the transverse plane (top right). Mechanical axial deviation (MAD) from the knee center is given in mm. Conformity with the planned correction outcome can be monitored in all three planes (bottom).

3.4   Navigated guidance of deformity correction

The aim of all osteotomy techniques is correction of the deformity and realignment of the mechanical axis. Particularly in open-wedge osteotomy, an asymmetrical gap in the sagittal plane due to excessive anterior or posterior opening of the osteotomy gap, can lead to undesirable secondary deformities arising from changes of the tibial slope in the sagittal plane. In addition, internal and external rotational malalignment may occur. Navigation recognizes these errors intraoperatively prior to fixation since the following parameters are calculated in real time:

- The correction angle between the proximal and distal fragments in the frontal, sagittal, and transverse plane
- Mechanical medial proximal tibial angle (mMPTA)
- Mechanical lateral distal femoral angle (mLDFA)
- Tibial slope
- Shift of the mechanical axis at the tibial plateau

4   Discussion

Realignment of the mechanical axis of the lower extremity is a complex and technically demanding operation [8, 18]. The success of this surgical technique depends on accurate recognition of the deformity, the correct indication for osteotomy and its precise implementation. The planned correction angle does not only depend on the extent of the deformity, but also on the height of the osteotomy. Conventional preoperative planning may be inadequate. In less experienced hands, manual planning based on conventional x-ray images may be associated with the risk of over- or undercorrection. Likewise, conventional intraoperative measuring techniques may be inaccurate. Given a lack of objective intraoperative evaluation options, it may be difficult to achieve the desired correction of the essential parameters. The advantages of the presented system are the multidimensional monitoring option and the visualization of intraoperative changes.

Numerous studies show that exact postoperative alignment is essential for good long-term outcomes following osteotomy of the proximal tibia [5, 17–19]. More recently published studies report over- or undercorrection in 20–40% [1, 6, 8–10, 20]. However, in the authors' patient sample, the desired correction with subsequent physiological weight-bearing axis was achieved in all cases. We attribute this significant improvement to the advantages of intraoperative control of all parameters and navigated guidance of the osteotomy. The navigation system conducts "plastic bone evaluation" of the anatomical structures and is therefore more accurate than measurements made on radiological full-length weight-bearing images.

Operation time was extended by 10–30 minutes according to our observations. This time was required primarily for set up of the system and for attachment of the dynamic reference bases. An increased intra- or postoperative complication rate compared with other patient samples was not observed.

■ Computer-assisted, navigated implementation of high-tibial osteotomy permits accurate intraoperative measurement of the deformity, exact interactive planning, and precise conduction of the osteotomy. Since all surgical procedures and changes in relevant parameters are visualized, deviation from the planned correction is recognized immediately. The navigation system described here can be used to avoid preoperative planning and intraoperative surgical errors prior to fixation of the osteotomy. Thus, correct postoperative alignment of the mechanical weight-bearing axis is achieved, which is indispensable for a good outcome of osteotomy procedures.

5   Bibliography

[1]   **Staubli AE, De Simoni C, Babst R, et al** (2003) TomoFix: a new LCP-concept for open wedge osteotomy of the medial proximal tibia—early results in 92 cases. *Injury;* 34 Suppl 2:B55–B62.

[2]   **Coventry MB** (1973) Osteotomy about the knee for degenerative and rheumatoid arthritis. *J Bone Joint Surg Am;* 55(1):23–48.

[3]   **Paley D** (2002) *Principles of deformity correction.* Berlin Heidelberg New York: Springer-Verlag, 451–464.

[4]   **Fu FH, Harner CD, Vince KG** (1996) *Knee surgery.* 2nd ed. Baltimore: Lippincott Williams and Wilkins, 1153–1171.

[5]   **Phillips MJ, Krackow KA** (1998) High tibial osteotomy and distal femoral osteotomy for valgus or varus deformity around the knee. *Instr Course Lect;* 47:429–436.

[6]   **Magyar G, Ahl TL, Vibe P, et al** (1999) Open-wedge osteotomy by hemicallotasis or the closed-wedge technique for osteoarthritis of the knee, a randomized study of 50 operations. *J Bone Joint Surg Br;* 81(3):444–448.

[7]   **Mathews J, Cobb AG, Richardson S, et al** (1998) Distal femoral osteotomy for lateral compartment osteoarthritis of the knee. Orthopedics; 21(4):437–440.

[8]   **Murphy SB** (1994) Tibial osteotomy for genu varus. Indications, preoperative planning, and technique. *Orthop Clin North Am;* 25(3):477–482.

[9]   **Sprenger TR, Doerzbacher JF** (2003) Tibia osteotomy for the treatment of varus gonarthrosis. Survival and failure analysis to twenty-two years. *J Bone Joint Surg Am;* 85-A(3):469–474. (2003) Erratum in: *J Bone Joint Surg Am;* 85-A(5):912.

[10] **Takahashi T, Wada Y, Tanaka M, et al** (2000) Dome-shaped proximal tibial osteotomy using percutaneous drilling for osteoarthritis of the knee. *Arch Orthop Trauma Surg;* 120(1–2):32–37.

[11] **Ellis RE, Tso CY, Rudan JF, et al** (1999) A surgical planning and guidance system for high tibial osteotomy. *Comput Aided Surg;* 4(5):264–274.

[12] **Phillips R, Hafez MA, Mohsen AM, et al** (2000) Computer and robotic assisted osteotomy around the knee. *mmVR 2000 – 8th Annual Medicine Meets Virtual Reality Conference*. Newport Beach, 265–271.

[13] **Hofstetter R, Slomczykowski M, Sati M, et al** (1999) Fluoroscopy as an imaging means for computer-assisted surgical navigation. *Comput Aided Surg;* 4(2):65–76.

[14] **Zheng G, Marx A, Langlotz U, et al** (2002) A hybrid CT-free navigation system for total hip arthroplasty. *Comput Aided Surg;* 7(3):129–145.

[15] **Noyes FR, Barber-Westin SD, Hewett TE** (2000) High tibial osteotomy and ligament reconstruction for varus angulated anterior cruciate ligament-deficient knees. *Am J Sports Med;* 28(3):282–296.

[16] **Paley D, Bhatnagar J, Herzenberg JE, et al** (1994) New procedures for tightening knee collateral ligaments in conjunction with knee realignment osteotomy. *Orthop Clin North Am;* 25(3):533–555.

[17] **Fujisawa Y, Masuhara K, Shiomi S** (1979) The effect of high tibial osteotomy on osteoarthritis of the knee. An arthroscopic study of 54 knee joints. Orthop Clin North Am; 10(3):585–608.

[18] **Hernigou P** (2002) Open wedge tibial osteotomy: combined coronal and sagittal correction. *Knee;* 9(1):15–20.

[19] **Iorio R, Healy WL** (2003) Current concept review, unicompartimental arthritis of the knee. *J Bone Joint Surg;* 85A: 1351–1364.

[20] **Müller W** (2001) High tibial osteotomy, conditions, indications, techniques, problems. *European Federation of National Associations of Orthopaedic and Trauma;* 28:194–204.

Authors Philipp Lobenhoffer, Denise Freiling

20 Development of plate fixators: current status and perspectives

1 Introduction

Plate fixators have already replaced conventional plating systems in fracture treatment to a large extent. Internal fixators with angular stable locking screws provide for stable fixation, especially in osteoporosis or in highly instable fractures. "Biological" internal fixation can be achieved by application of a suitable implant: reduction should be performed as far as possible indirectly without exposure or direct manipulation of the fragments followed by bridging fixation without contouring the implant to the shape of the bones at the fracture site. The fixation distant from the fracture with angular stable bolts combined with the elasticity of the implant across the fracture zone stimulates osteogenesis. In angular stable systems fracture healing generally progresses via callus formation so that primary and secondary cancellous bone grafting is now seldom needed (Fig 20-1). The most widely used system, and the one applied by the authors, is that, which currently only permits unidirectional locking of the screws in the plate. Therefore, the anatomical alignment of the screws, especially in areas adjacent to the joints, is of great importance. For this reason, special precontoured plates for different regions of the skeleton have already been developed. Their design is anatomically adapted and allows for optimal insertion of the fixation screws in the joint segment.

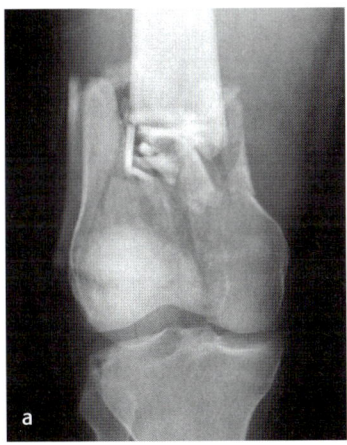
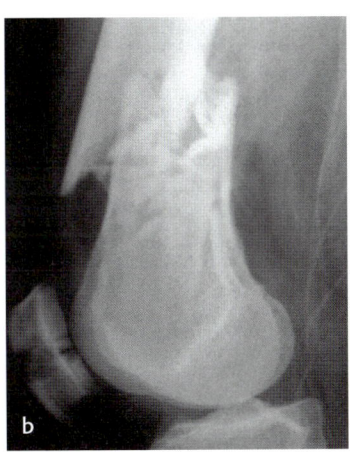
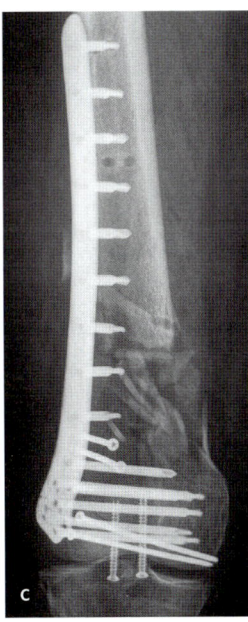
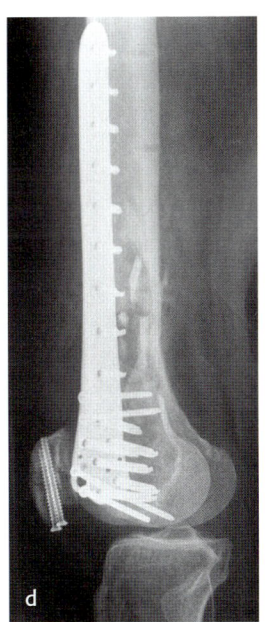

Fig 20-1a–h Osteogenesis as a result of elastic stable fixation with a plate fixator.
a–b Closed distal femur fracture with extensive metaphyseal comminuted zone (Müller AO 33-C2) and transverse patellar fracture.
c–d Bridging fixation with LISS plate for the distal femur.

Due to the long lever arms and the heavy loading stress on the implant, osteotomies around the knee have always been problematic regarding stability and bone healing. Therefore, it seemed reasonable to transfer the approved principles of fracture stabilization with plate fixators to osteotomy procedures around the knee joint. The first operative technique to be developed was open-wedge valgization osteotomy of the proximal tibia. TomoFix MPT (medial proximal tibia) developed by Alex E Staubli and co-workers, Luzern, is finding ever increasing acceptance worldwide due to its outstanding biomechanical properties [1, 2]. The work of the AO Knee Expert Group has helped to design special plate fixators which meet the anatomic requirements of the specific skeletal region and the type of osteotomy.

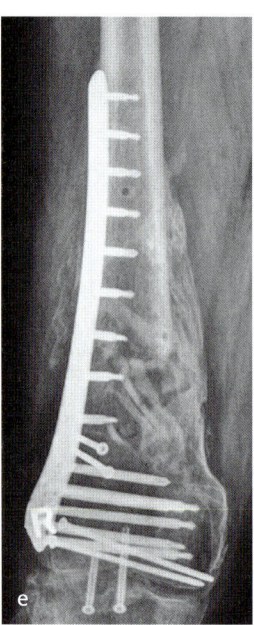 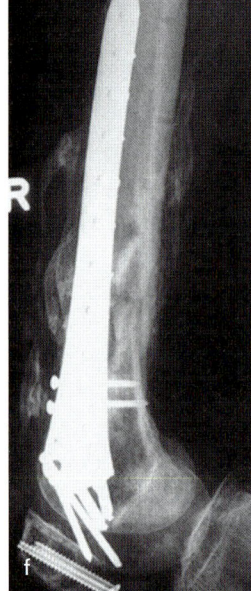 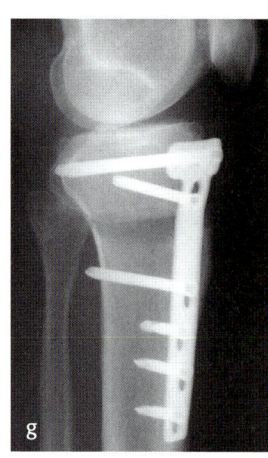 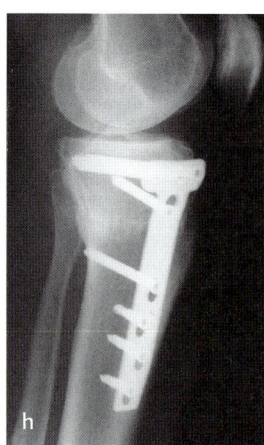

Fig 20-1a–h (cont)   Osteogenesis as a result of elastic stable fixation with a plate fixator.
e–f Six months postoperatively, callus formation without cancellous bone graft.
g Open-wedge valgization osteotomy of the proximal tibia (9 mm) stabilized with a plate fixator. The osteotomy gap was not filled with bone graft.
h Six months postoperatively, extensive callus formation is seen, especially at the posterior aspect.

2   Proximal lateral tibia

2.1   Closed-wedge valgization osteotomy

Closed-wedge valgization osteotomy of the proximal tibia has been a standard technique for many years. Various implants have been developed for this procedure, but the incidence of instability and loss of correction with nonangular stable implants is significant. Mechanical problems can be expected especially if a fracture of the medial cortex occurs intraoperatively which subsequently leads to loss of support on the medial side. Pape carried out an RSA analysis and noticed up to 3 mm interfragmental instability in the first three postoperative weeks for corrections of more than 8 mm that were stabilized with nonangular stable plates [3, 4]. However, the mechanical stability of this type of osteotomy can be markedly improved by application of a plate fixator. Van Heerwaarden, using the TomoFix LPT (lateral proximal tibia), found interfragmental movement of less than 0.3 mm in his RSA analysis, ie, ten times less. This indicates that the application of a special plate fixator can clearly increase the stability of closed-wedge tibial valgization osteotomy. The authors recommend that a biplanar cutting technique should be used for this procedure in the manner that it is advised for medial open-wedge osteotomy of the tibia. The authors only perform closed-wedge osteotomy in exceptional cases because of the risk of damage to the extensor muscles and the peroneal nerve, which make the medial technique preferable in most cases.

2.2   Open-wedge varization osteotomy

Posttraumatic valgus deformities, eg, after fracture of the lateral tibial head, sometimes require open-wedge varization osteotomy of the lateral tibia. This can be achieved by application of the TomoFix LPT. The technique is similar to that for the medial tibia. In general, fibula osteotomy is required and can be performed either in the diaphyseal mid-third or in the region of the fibula neck (with exposure of the peroneal nerve). In our cases, we always inserted autogenous cancellous bone graft into the osteotomy gap (Fig 20-2).

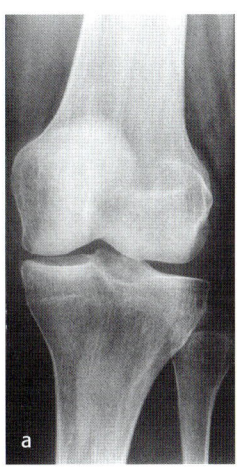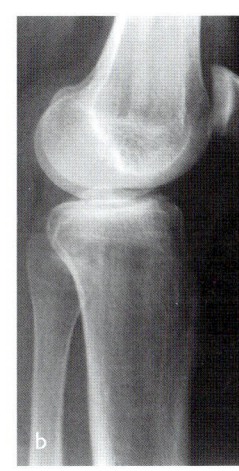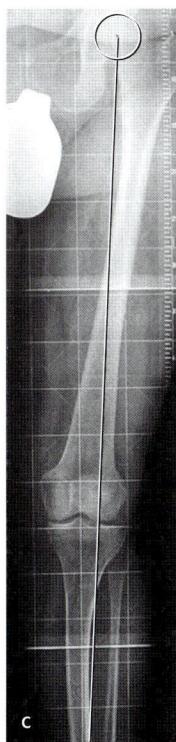

Fig 20-2a–e
a–c Lateral open-wedge varization osteotomy of the proximal tibia. Symptomatic valgus deformity of the tibia with hyperextension and posterior knee instability. Indication for open-wedge varization and flexion osteotomy of the tibia.

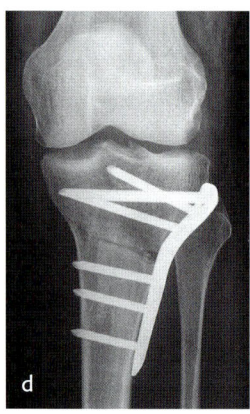
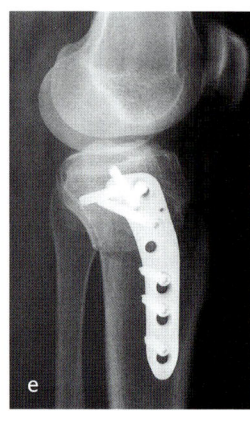

Fig 20-2a–e (cont)
d–e Biplanar open-wedge osteotomy of the proximal tibia (valgization, flexion), fibula osteotomy, autogenous cancellous bone graft, fixation with TomoFix LPT.

3 Proximal medial tibia

3.1 Open-wedge valgization osteotomy

The technique of open-wedge osteotomy of the proximal tibia is becoming increasingly established. Advantages of this technique are simple approach, preservation of lateral muscle insertions and the peroneal nerve, and minor morbidity of this procedure. TomoFix medial proximal tibia (MPT) provides optimal biomechanical properties for this procedure and the complication rate is correspondingly very low [1, 2, 5, 6]. The implant is relatively bulky, but this is of limited importance in percutaneous implantation technique. The plate shaft, however, may cause symptoms at the tibia in small patients. The current design is probably too large for Asian patients, in particular. This is why two modifications have been developed. The new standard plate has conventional locking head holes and not combination holes in the distal part of the plate so that the shaft is designed narrower in this area. In addition, the edges of the entire implant are rounded in an effort to reduce local soft-tissue irritation. Furthermore, a plate with overall smaller dimensions was developed for small people and especially for the Asian population. It is possible to apply this small implant in patients with up to 75 kg body weight. With these new designs, suitable implants should be available for all anatomical conditions.

3.2 Closed-wedge varization osteotomy

The closed-wedge varization osteotomy presents an attractive technique for valgus deformity localized in the proximal tibia. A similar biplanar cutting technique as in open-wedge osteotomy is used, but in this method a wedge of appropriate size ending 5 mm before the lateral cortex is removed (see chapter 17 "Management of complications after high-tibial open-wedge osteotomy", Fig 17-2d–e). The authors use the osteotomy guiding device (OGD) as cutting jig (see chapter 13 "Supracondylar varization osteotomy of the femur with plate fixation"), but the wedge can also be marked with wires placed under fluoroscopic control. Clinical and experimental work by van Heerwarden has demonstrated that no loosening of the medial collateral ligament occurs. The TomoFix MPT can be applied in these cases. If necessary, the tensioning device can be connected to the most distal plate hole in order to close the osteotomy gap.

4   Distal lateral femur

4.1   Open-wedge varization osteotomy

Correction of valgus deviation of the leg is preferably performed at the distal femur. The lateral open technique seems to be the first choice because the lateral approach is simple and correction can still be modified intraoperatively. A special plate fixator is available for this procedure: the TomoFix LDF. This plate has been derived from the LISS system providing screw position adapted to the anatomy of the lateral distal femur. In contrast to LISS, the TomoFix plate holes have been designed for locking head screws. The proximal combination holes permit additional application of a lag screw to compress the osteotomy. However, practice has shown that open-wedge varization osteotomy may cause problems due to overtensioning of the iliotibial tract. Furthermore, bone healing was not as reliable and reproducible

as at the proximal tibia. The authors are now only applying the open-wedge technique in special cases in which there is shortening of the lateral distal femur (eg, as a result of a malaligned distal femur fracture). In lateral opening osteotomy of the distal femur autogenous cancellous bone graft should be added (see chapter 14 "Double osteotomies of the femur and the tibia", Fig 14-5).

4.2   Closed-wedge valgization osteotomy

TomoFix LDF can be used this method as well, whereby application of dynamic compression by means of the combination holes and the tensioning device is also possible (see chapter 18 "Osteotomies for failed osteotomies around the knee", Fig 18-14).

5   Distal medial femur

5.1   Closed-wedge varization osteotomy

Because of the difficulties seen with femoral lateral open-wedge osteotomy the authors have been working to improve the technique of closed-wedge varization osteotomy from the medial approach. The anatomy of the medial distal femur differs greatly from that of the lateral distal femur, which necessitated the development of a special implant. In particular, at the medial condyle the distal T-arm of the plate lies at an angle of 25° to the frontal plane resulting in a considerable posterior direction of the distal locking screws in the condyle. TomoFix MDF

(medial distal femur) has distal screws that are angled 20° anteriorly and is therefore available in two different versions for the left and the right leg. Four locking screws can be inserted into the distal section and four combination holes are available proximally in the plate shaft. Biomechanical tests have proven that the stability of this internal fixation is very similar compared to the conventional condylar plate [7]. Since the success of this osteotomy type depends very much on the exact congruence of the bone surfaces, a special osteotomy guiding device (OGD) was developed to ensure precise sawing and wedge extraction.

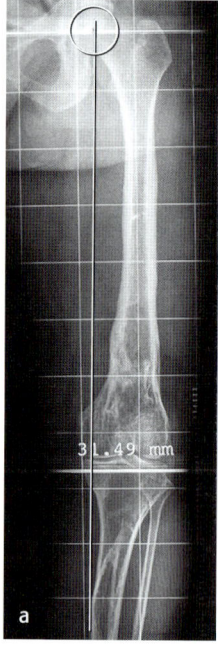
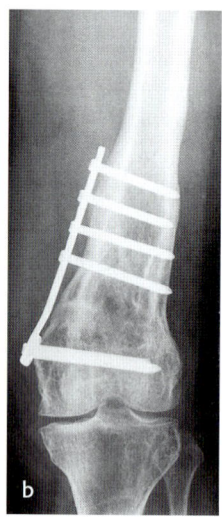
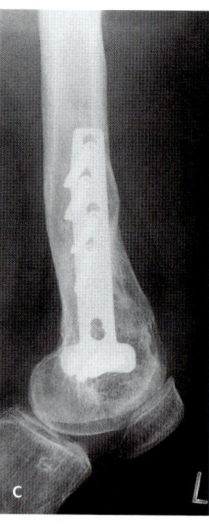

a

b

c

5.2   Open-wedge valgization osteotomy

This method also presents an exceptional indication and is only performed in patients with shortening of the medial distal femur, eg, after malunited distal femur fracture. The authors´ technique of biplanar open-wedge osteotomy with incomplete transection of the metaphyseal femur and medial distraction of the osteotomy can be applied in these cases. Stabilization can be achieved with TomoFix MPT (medial proximal tibia) or TomoFix MDF (Fig 20-3).

Fig 20-3a–c   Open-wedge osteotomy of the medial distal femur.
a–b   Patient with posttraumatic varus deformity located at the distal femur.
c   Open-wedge osteotomy of the medial distal femur, autogenous cancellous bone graft, stabilization with TomoFix MPT. The implant can be modeled to fit the anatomy of the distal femur.

6   Developments

A number of angular stable implants specially designed for osteotomies around the knee are available facilitating stable correction of deformities at the distal femur and proximal tibia. The authors' own results show that the range of indications for one-stage correction with internal fixation can be extended including complex deformities around the knee joint reducing the need for external ring fixators for gradual correction. Based on our experience, further improvements can be expected less in terms of implant development, but more concerning planning and intraoperative control of osteotomies.

6.1   Computer-assisted planning

A system with easy handling for the analysis of leg geometry and planning of correction osteotomies is especially required for complex corrections. Ideally, the system addresses both the frontal and sagittal plane and the rotation of the region of interest. Appropriate programs are already available, but have not yet gained wide acceptance and could certainly be improved in terms of user-friendliness.

6.2   Navigation

The importance of navigation systems for osteotomy procedures is still unclear. Currently, it seems to be too time-consuming since the only information provided by available navigation systems is axial alignment in the frontal and sagittal plane. In this situation, conventional intraoperative fluoroscopy can provide equal information. However, intraoperative navigation could be useful in regard of evaluation of mechanical loading on the cartilage. At present, our recommendations for the amount of correction by osteotomies are only based on clinical data. In particular, it is largely unknown which correction angle actually results in unloading of the damaged cartilage. Possibly, redistribution of the peak load areas (maximum loading) within the damaged joint compartment is of greater importance than the quantitative unloading of the entire compartment. Initial tests with pressure-sensitive sensors have provided some unexpected results (see chapter 10 "Effect of osteotomies on cartilage pressure in the knee" and chapter 11 "Osteotomy and ligament instability: tibial slope corrections and combined procedures around the knee joint"). When more knowledge of the biomechanical effects of osteotomies is available, computer-assisted planning and navigation in osteotomies may gain more importance.

6.3   Osteoinductive substances

In most cases, open-wedge osteotomies with plate fixation consolidate without interposition of cancellous bone, especially at the tibia. The healing process, however, requires 6–12 months. The osteotomy is protected during this period by the plate fixator. Acceleration of bone regeneration is desirable. Osteoconductive substances like hydroxyapatite and tricalcium phosphate in solid form or as granulate have been found to heal in equal bone healing time [8] and not faster than in nongrafted HTO's. In some cases, the application of these substances resulted in delayed consolidation of the osteotomy and increased the complication rate. In a biologically favorable host bed and a stable osteosynthesis, only osteoinductive substances can accelerate osteogenesis. Osteoinductive substances of this kind are already used in maxillofacial surgery for repair of mandibular tumor defects. Clinical studies investigating these substances in tibial open-wedge osteotomy have been initiated.

6.4   Osteotomy and knee instability

Tibial osteotomies can be also applied in treatment of ligament instabilities of the knee (see chapter 11 "Osteotomy and ligament instability: tibial slope corrections and combined procedures around the knee joint"). The authors have proved that alteration of the tibial slope influences the sagittal stability of the knee joint effectively and improves function of the joint, especially in patients with posterior knee instability [9]. The technique of open-wedge osteotomy with plate fixator is particularly suitable for three-dimensional correction, where stable fixation is indispensable.

- Plate fixators substantially increase biomechanical stability of osteotomies around the knee.
  Stable fixation and soft-tissue preserving insertion of the implant promote bone healing.
  Special implants are available for the different types of osteotomy.
  Further developments are to be expected in planning and intraoperative monitoring of osteotomies.

7 Perspectives

In summary, the development of plate fixators has stimulated interest in osteotomies for axis correction around the knee. Plate fixators provide safe, soft-tissue preserving internal stabilization and substantially reduce the risk of secondary loss of correction. However, it remains the surgeon's responsibility to review the indications for osteotomies around the knee critically, to evaluate the consequences carefully, and to improve the techniques to perfection. The supreme responsibility of our medical actions, never to harm the patient, is particularly valid in this difficult and complex area. The present book aims to summarize current knowledge. The authors and publishers hope to have made a contribution to the further development of osteotomies around the knee.

8 Bibliography

[1] **Agneskirchner JD, Freiling D, Hurschler C, et al** (2006) Primary stability of four different implants for opening wedge high tibial osteotomy. *Knee Surg Sports Traumatol Arthrosc;* 14(3):291–300.

[2] **Staubli AE, De Simoni C, Babst R, et al** (2003) TomoFix: a new LCP-concept for open wedge osteotomy of the medial proximal tibia—early results in 92 cases. *Injury;* 34 Suppl 2:B55–B62.

[3] **Pape D, Adam F, Rupp S, et al** (2004) [Stability, bone healing and loss of correction after valgus realignment of the tibial head. A roentgen stereometry analysis.] *Orthopäde;* 33(2):208–217. German.

[4] **Pape D, Adam F, Scil R, ct al** (2005) Fixation stability following high tibial osteotomy: a radiostereometric analysis. *J Knee Surg;* 18(2):108–115.

[5] **Lobenhoffer P, Agneskirchner JD** (2003) Improvements in surgical technique of valgus high tibial osteotomy. *Knee Surg Sports Traumatol Arthrosc;* 11(3):132–138.

[6] **Lobenhoffer P, Agneskirchner JD, Zoch W** (2004) [Open valgus alignment osteotomy of the proximal tibia with fixation by medial plate fixator.] *Orthopäde;* 33(2):153–160. German.

[7] **Brinkman JM, Hurschler C, Agneskirchner JD, et al** (2008) Axial and torsional stability of supracondylar femur osteotomies: a biomechanical investigation of five different plate osteotomy configurations. *Clin Orthop Relat Res;* submitted.

[8] **Van Hemert WL, Willems K, Anderson PG, et al** (2004) Tricalcium phosphate granules or rigid wedge performs in open wedge high tibial osteotomy: a radiological study with a new evaluation system. *Knee;* 11(6):451–456.

[9] **Agneskirchner JD, Hurschler C, Stukenborg-Colsman C, et al** (2004) Effect of high tibial flexion osteotomy on cartilage pressure and joint kinematics: a biomechanical study in human cadaveric knees. *Arch Orthop Trauma Surg;* 124(9):575–584.

Appendix

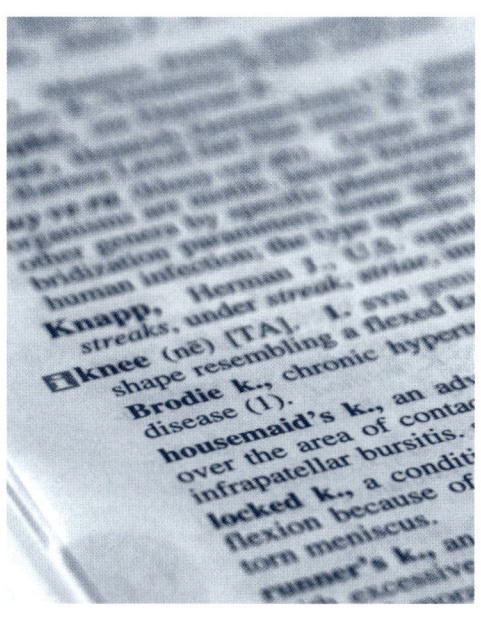
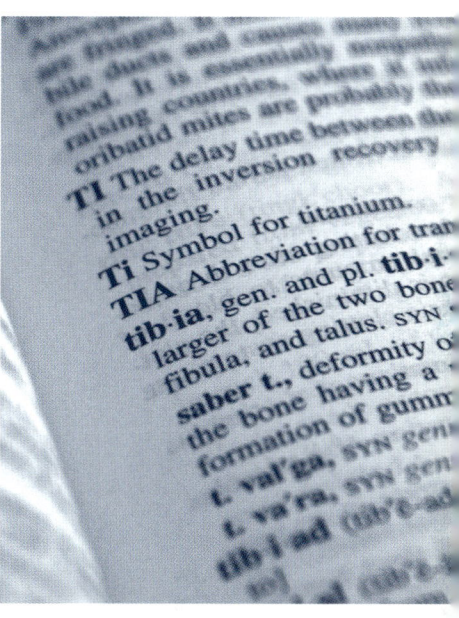

Glossary

This glossary provides the working definitions for terms that have been used by authors within this book.

(Parts of this glossary are taken from **Rüedi TP, Buckley RE, Moran CG** (2007) *AO Principles of Fracture Management.* Second expanded edition. Stuttgart New York: Georg Thieme Verlag, A2–A14.)

additive technique   Osteotomy technique aimed at adding of bone after correction and bone healing.

biological internal fixation   Internal fixation preserving bone and soft-tissue biology.

biplanar deformity   Bone deformity in two planes of one bone segment, eg, frontal and sagittal plane—see uniplanar deformity, multiplanar deformity.

biplane osteotomy   Osteotomy technique combining bone cuts in two planes at one osteotomy level.

C-arm   Image intensifier.

callus   A tissue of immature bone and cartilage that is formed at the site of bony repair to bridge a fracture—see healing, indirect.

callus distraction   See distraction osteogenesis.

combination hole   The plate hole of the locking compression plate (LCP) that consists of two parts: the nonthreaded dynamic compression unit (DCU); shaped like the holes of a dynamic compression plate (DCP), and the threaded part which has a reciprocal thread for the insertion of a locking head screw (LHS).

compartment syndrome   Raised pressure in a closed fascial compartment that results in painful local tissue ischemia.

complete osteotomy   Osteotomy technique including cutting of the contralateral cortex.

contact bone healing   See primary bone healing.

conventional screw   Any screw with a smooth outer surface of the head (ie, without threads) that is used for osteotomy, fracture, or plate fixation.

custom-made total knee replacement   Total knee replacement (TKR) made specifically to accommodate alignment of the TKR in a severely deformed proximal tibia and/or distal femur, ie, after failed osteotomy.

cupula   Dish-formed defect of the proximal tibia found in lateral view x-rays of the knee, indicating fixed anterolateral subluxation of the tibia.

deformity   Any abnormality of the form of a body part or bone.

delayed union   Bone healing is not taking place in what is accepted as the expected time for a particular fracture or osteotomy (and the patient's age)—see nonunion.

distraction osteogenesis   The induction of bone formation by the application of tension to soft tissue that has the potential to form bone, eg, the organized hematoma, periosteum, and endosteum at the site of an osteotomy or osteoclasis. This phenomenon was first described by Bier (1927) and scientifically investigated by the Russian surgeon Ilizarov.

double osteotomy   Combination of two osteotomies in one bone segment or around a joint.

double varus deformity   Combination of varus bone deformity, medial joint space narrowing, and increased lateral distraction—see primary varus deformity, triple varus deformity.

dynamic compression plate (DCP)   A plate with chamfered oval holes through which eccentrically placed screws can be inserted to provide compression across a fracture site.

dynamic compression unit (DCU)   The nonthreaded part of a combination hole of a locking compression plate (LCP), which is shaped like the hole of a dynamic compression plate (DCP).

dynamic locking   When an interlocking screw is placed into the oval hole of an intramedullary nail, controlling rotation and alignment, but allowing some (controlled) impaction of the osteotomy during weight bearing—see dynamization.

dynamization   Diverting the mechanical load from a fixation device to load the osteotomy site in order to enhance bone formation.

external fixation   Skeletal stabilization using pins, wires, or screws that protrude through the skin and are linked externally by bars or other devices.

fasciotomy   The surgical division of the wall of a muscle compartment, usually to release high intracompartmental pressure—see compartment syndrome.

fixed-angle device   An implant with two or more parts that are solidly connected at an angle so that it will resist forces tending to angulate one part with respect to the other. Such devices are used to prevent angular displacement of fractures or osteotomies. Fixed-angle devices may be manufactured as a single, solid device, eg, 95° angled blade plate, or produced by mechanically coupling two implants, eg, a locking compression plate (LCP) with a locking head screw (LHS).

Fujisawa point   Intersection point of weight-bearing axis at 62% of the tibial plateau entire width measured from its medial cortex. Named after Dr Fujisawa in regards to recommended position of weight-bearing axis after high-tibial osteotomy (HTO).

gap bone healing   See secondary bone healing.

healing, indirect   Bone healing by callus formation in osteotomies or fractures treated either with relative stability or left untreated.

hemicallotasis   See distraction osteogenesis.

incomplete osteotomy   Osteotomy technique leaving a bone bridge intact not violating the contralateral cortex.

interlocking screw   Also called (inter)locking bolt. It couples an intramedullary nail to the bone to maintain length, alignment, and rotation.

internal fixator   A mechanical device underneath the skin that bridges an osteotomy site or a fracture zone—similar to external fixation—providing an angularly locked, extramedullary splint resulting in relative stability (eg, LCP, LISS, TomoFix).

intrinsic stability   Stability provided by a corrected bone with or without bone grafting before bone fixation is applied.

limited-contact plate   A plate designed to limit contact with the underlying bone which preserves the most possible periosteal blood supply. The most common variety is the limited-contact dynamic compression plate (LC-DCP).

locking compression plate (LCP)   See locking plate and internal fixator.

locking head screw (LHS)   A screw with a thread cut into its head which provides a mechanical couple, or linkage to a threaded screw hole in a plate, thereby creating a fixed-angle device.

locking plate   A plate with threaded screw holes that allow mechanical coupling to a locking head screw (LHS). The less invasive stabilization system (LISS) will accept only this type of screw, while locking compression plates (LCPs) have a combination hole that will accept conventional screw heads or threaded screw heads.

malunion   A fracture which has healed in a position of deformity.

Mikulicz line   Mechanical leg axis from the center of the femoral head to the center of the ankle joint.

midjoint line   Line centered between the knee base line of the femur and the baseline of the tibial plateau.

multiplanar deformity   Bone deformity that coexists in more than two planes in one bone segment—see uniplanar deformity, biplanar deformity.

navigated instruments   Surgical instruments used in computer-assisted surgery, equipped with infrared light transmitting diodes which enables real time navigation in combination with an infrared camera used in computer-assisted surgery.

nonunion   A bone fracture caused by the osteotomy is still present and healing has stopped. The bone will not unite without surgical intervention. A nonunion is usually due to inadequate mechanical or biological conditions–see union, pseudarthrosis, and delayed union.

offset stem   Stem connected to the tibial or femoral component of a total knee replacement offset in a position that corresponds to stem position in line of the bone diaphysis.

orthosis   An external device that is applied to the body in order to protect and/or stabilize a body part, to prevent or correct scarring and deformities, or to aid movement.

osteotomy   Controlled surgical division of a bone which may be aimed at restoration of normal bone anatomy, joint anatomy, and limb function. Further aims to unload joints, or parts of joints, or straighten a limb to prevent progression of cartilage damage or osteoarthritis of the neighboring joints.

plate fixator   See internal fixator.

primary bone healing   Bone healing process in a stable environment with osteons regenerating in three phases; activation, resorption, and formation—see secondary bone healing.

primary varus deformity   Axial deviation exclusively caused by bony deformity of the tibiofemoral anatomy—see double varus deformity, triple varus deformity.

pseudarthrosis   Literally meaning "false joint". When a nonunion is mobile and allowed to persist for a long period, the bone ends become sclerotic and the intervening soft tissues differentiate to form a type of synovial articulation—see delayed union, union.

push view   Planning drawing of simulated push of the tibia on the femur to avoid overcorrection in osteotomies of knee joints with increased collateral ligament laxity.

Rosenberg view   Weight-bearing view of the knee in 45° flexion.

scouring effect = cold welding   Deformation of the head of a screw during insertion as a result of inadequate, overthightened screw fixation.

secondary bone healing   Bone healing process in a (controlled) unstable environment with bone formation in two phases; fibrous bone and lamellar bone formation—see primary bone healing.

sintering   Collapse of immature bone after too early plate removal in open-wedge osteotomies.

stability, relative   A fixation or support construction that allows small amounts of motion in proportion to the load applied. This results in indirect healing by callus formation.

tension band   The principle by which an implant, attached to the tension side of a fracture, converts the tensile force into a compressive force at the cortex opposite the implant. While wires, cables, and sutures are often used for tension band fixation, plates, and external fixators, when appropriately placed, can also function as tension bands.

tibial bone varus angle (TBVA)   Angle between the proximal tibial epiphyseal axis and the mechanical tibial axis used to differentiate a constitutional tibial varus from an acquires tibial varus deformity.

torsion angle   The angle of alignment of the distal joint axis in relation to the alignment of the proximal joint in the transverse plane

torsion malalignment syndrome   Combination of pathological femoral internal torsion and compensatory pathological external torsion in one leg.

triple varus deformity   Combination of varus bone deformity, medial joint-space narrowing and increased lateral distraction, and increased external rotation of the tibia due to posterolateral instability—see primary varus deformity, double varus deformity.

TT-TG scan   CT scan measurement method to assess patellofemoral tracking by projecting two transverse plane scans showing highest point of the tibial tuberosity (TT) and the deepest point of the trochlear groove (TG) onto each other.

union   The bone has healed and regained its normal stiffness and strength. In clinical terms this means there is no movement or tenderness at the fracture site and no pain on stressing the fracture site. Radiologically, there should be evidence of bone trabeculae bridging the fracture site.

uniplanar deformity   Bone deformity that exists in only one plane and bone segment—see biplanar deformity, multiplanar deformity.

varus thrust   Lateral joint subluxation due to lateral and/or posterolateral ligament insufficiency combined with varus leg deformity causing instability during weight bearing.

Abbreviations

aFTA	anatomical femorotibial angle
aLDFA	anatomical lateral distal femoral angle
aLDTA	anatomical lateral distal tibial angle
aMFA	anatomical mechanical femoral angle
aMPTA	anatomical medial proximal tibial angle
CORA	center of rotation of angulation
JLCA	joint line convergence angle
MAD	mechanical axis deviation
MJL	midjoint line
mLDFA	mechanical lateral distal femoral angle
mLDTA	mechanical lateral distal tibial angle
mMPTA	mechanical medial proximal tibial angle

For further explanations see chapter 1 "Physiological axes of the lower limbs".